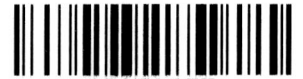

Dictionary⁺
of
Eldercare Terminology

Walter Feldesman

ISBN 978-0-615-28136-0

Publisher
Walter Feldesman
300 East 56th Street, 16-C
New York, NY 10022

NOTE:

The content of this book is designed to provide information on the subjects it covers. It is published and/or otherwise disseminated with the understanding that neither the author, nor any person or entity associated with him, is engaged in rendering legal, accounting, or other professional services with respect to any of the subjects of the book. If legal or other expert assistance is required, the services of a competent professional should be sought. Although the author has endeavored to ensure the accuracy and completeness of information contained in the book, he assumes no responsibility for errors, inaccuracies, omissions, or inconsistencies.

To the memory of my dear wife, Lucille

✦

CONTENTS

TABLE OF OVERVIEWS

APPEALS

ELIGIBILITY AND ENROLLMENT

MEDICAID

MEDICARE

MEDICARE ADVANTAGE

INTRODUCTION

Eldercare is very much on the minds of America's policymakers and families. This is as true today as it was when the first (1997) and second (2000) editions of my *Dictionary of Eldercare Terminology* were published. And this will remain true for the foreseeable future, as the number of older Americans grows and as they live longer.

When it first appeared in 1997, the *Dictionary* was the first and only comprehensive guide to the language of eldercare. It remains so today. The vocabulary of the subject of eldercare can be bewildering and seem like a foreign tongue that needs both interpretation and translation. This third edition updates and expands the dictionary so that it better serves this purpose. The inclusion of the symbol "+" in this book's title – *Dictionary⁺ of Eldercare Terminology* – is intended to highlight its expanded scope.

Eldercare terminology cannot be adequately understood simply from a compendium of words and phrases or unrelated entry definitions. To assist readers seeking an in-depth understanding of the defined terms, the entries are cross-referenced to other related entries.

Further and most importantly, the *Dictionary⁺* includes Overviews of major eldercare fields (including Home Care, Long-term Care Insurance, Medicaid, Medicare, Medicare Supplemental Insurance and the Social Security Program). The overviews contain the key words and phrases (repetitions of the entries) and their relationships in each major field of eldercare.

Unlike any other reference tool on the subject of eldercare, the *Dictionary+* offers readers narrow explanations of specific terms and words, while at the same time giving them a broad operational context with the related Overviews. The *Dictionary+* thus uniquely combines the functions of an encyclopedia and a dictionary.

In both its print and electronic versions, the *Dictionary⁺* strives to be user-friendly. This goal is accomplished in several ways. First, the outline style allows readers to peruse entries and Overviews quickly. Second, the extensive cross-referencing helps readers find relevant information. And finally, the availability of the *Dictionary⁺* as an e-Book and online conveniently enables readers to search it at a very detailed level. This makes the process of consulting the *Dictionary+* quite dynamic. (The section "Navigating the *Dictionary⁺* Online" explains how to conduct searches.)

An effective way for readers to use the *Dictionary+* is first to turn to the Contents pages and scan the Table of Overviews and the subheadings listed under each Overview. Find the subtopic relevant to the specific term the reader wishes to learn about. Since the subheadings are hyperlinked, a simple click will take readers to the desired section. After learning the broad background about the term found in the Overviews, then the reader can turn to the specific entry for the term.

To demonstrate the unparalleled utility of the *Dictionary⁺*, an example of the way one term – "assignment" – is treated will explain the advantages of the *Dictionary⁺*. "Assignment" is a term of art that pertains specifically to Medicare. The *Dictionary⁺* defines it in a separate entry and also provides cross-references to other relevant terms. And then in the Overview on Medicare, readers are given an operational context to the way the term is functionally used in the system of Medicare.

The goals of this *Dictionary⁺* are to be comprehensive, clear, current and correct. The entries are meant to include almost every non-medical term used today in eldercare. Readers will find a wide mix of gerontological terms (e.g., activities of daily living, cluster care) as well as financial, estate planning and legal terms related to eldercare (e.g., generation skipping tax, grantor retained income trust). However, scientific terms, the names of organizations relevant to the field of aging, and terminology pertinent to veteran's affairs and Federal civil service retirement have not been incorporated.

In the preparation of the *Dictionary's* first edition (published in 1997), a panel of highly qualified editors and experts (their names and occupational associations in that year are stated below) reviewed drafts and contributed to its overall quality. While they were not consulted for the second or current edition, the results of their previous collaboration nevertheless are still evident. I owe a continuing debt of thanks to them – Robert B. Friedland, National Academy on an Aging Society; Priscilla Itzcoitz, AARP; William Lessard, Virginia Department of Medical Assistance Services; Patricia B. Nemore, Esq., Center for Medicare Advocacy; Mark D. Olshan, B'nai B'rith International; Anne Werner, United Seniors Health Cooperative; and Ira S. Wiesner, Esq., Wiesner Associates, Chartered, Sarasota, Florida.

Another group of individuals (their names and associations held in 1997 are stated below) graciously shared advice, encouragement, and information valuable to development of the first edition. Thanks goes to Diane Archer, Medicare Rights

Center; Robert Blancato, Matz, Blancato & Associates; Bonnie Burns, a California-based consultant on Medicare, health policy and insurance for older Americans; John Cutler, Esq., U.S. Department of Health and Human Services; Stephanie Exarhakis, Visiting Nurses Service of New York; Carol Fraser Fisk, American Academy of Audiology; Carla Herman, Catholic Health Care Network, New York; Edward Howard, Alliance for Health Reform; Mary Gardiner Jones, Consumer Interest Research Institute; Janet Sainer, consultant to the Brookdale Foundation Group; Annabel Seidman, National Council of Senior Citizens; Jane Stenson, Catholic Charities USA; and Janis Gray Thompson, Texoma Area Agency on Aging, Texas.

The second edition of the *Dictionary*, published in 2000, was reviewed by highly qualified experts (names and associations in that year are set forth below); their generous comments are set forth on the back cover of that book. Amongst them were the following – James P. Firman, President and CEO, The National Council on the Aging, Inc.; Sia Arnason, CSW, Co-Director, Samuel Sadin Institute on Law, Brookdale Center on Aging of Hunter College, CUNY; Rona S. Bartelstone, LCSW, BCD, CMC, Vice President, National Academy of Certified Care Managers, Past President, National Association of Geriatric Care Managers; and Gene Cohen, M.D., Ph.D., former Acting Director, National Institute on Aging, Past President, Gerontological Society of America, Professor, George Washington University Medical Center.

This third edition is the work-product solely of the author. It is available in three formats. Hard copies can be purchased through the Barnes & Noble and Lulu.com websites. Digital versions are compatible for both Amazon's Kindle and Barnes & Noble Nook devices. Finally, *Dictionary*⁺ can be accessed online without charge at the website www.biblioline.com/eldercare/dictionaryplus.

I invite the readers of this third edition of the *Dictionary*⁺ to submit their comments to the book's website with a view of improving the public's understanding and helping keep current the vocabulary of the ever-growing subject of eldercare.

Walter Feldesman, J.D.
Harvard

GUIDE TO THE *DICTIONARY*⁺

Entries vary in style – classic definitional compositions; entries which are overviews of major eldercare subjects; and entries which are culled from the Medicare handbook, *Medicare & You 2011*.

The key defined terms constitute the infrastructure of the Overviews. Reference is made in the Table of Overviews by page number to eldercare topics within a major eldercare subject, providing the reader with an Introduction to these major subjects and to the relationship and nexus of key words and phrases entered and defined in the *Dictionary*⁺.

The Medicare handbook entries (preceded by an asterisk and printed in italics) are instructional in style, repetitive of the Medicare definition entries, and show the use and function of the terminology employed.

When the definition of a term relates to a particular topic within a broad major subject of eldercare, the focus of the definition is identified by the subject following a slash (/) after the term. For example, the entry *Disability/Social Security* indicates that the term "disability" is defined in the context of the subject, "Social Security." The major eldercare subject used after the slash – such as, Medicare, Medicare Advantage, Medicaid, Social Security, Home Care, Long-term Care Insurance (LTCI) and Medicare Supplemental Insurance (Medigap) – thus identifies a definition's focus.

Abundant cross-references, appearing in italics, are added to many definitions to further amplify the meaning and context of a particular term.

All dollar figures cited in the *Dictionary*⁺ for deductibles, copayments, income limitations, premiums, and other similar matters are for the year 2012, unless otherwise noted.

NAVIGATING THE *DICTIONARY*⁺ ONLINE

The *Dictionary*⁺ can be downloaded and searched without charge. Visit www.biblioline.com/eldercare/dictionaryplus. According to the copyright restrictions set by the author, only limited portions of the book may be printed by users.

The *Dictionary*⁺ can be searched using BiblioLineᴿᴹ or Adobe Acrobat Reader. Instructions for searching the text with BiblioLineᴿᴹ can be found on the website.

A search the *Dictionary*⁺ by using Adobe Acrobat Reader requires users of the *Dictionary*⁺ to employ version 9.0 or higher of Acrobat Reader. It can be downloaded at no cost at www.adobe.com/products/acrobat/readstep2.html or by clicking this icon 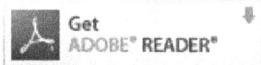 To activate an Acrobat search, click on the binocular icon on the extreme right-hand side of the opening screen.

ABBREVIATIONS & ACRONYMS

AAA	Area agency on aging
AAPPC	Adjusted average per capita cost
ADL	Activity of daily living
AIME	Average indexed monthly earnings
ALJ	Administrative law judge
AoA	Administration on Aging
BBA	Balanced Budget Act of 1997
BIPH	Benefit Improvement and Protection Act (2000)
CCHA	Certified Home Health Agency
CCP	Coordinated care plan
CCRC	Continuing Care Retirement Community
CMS	Centers for Medicare and Medicaid Services
CNO	Community Nursing Organization
CNS	Clinical Nurse Specialist
COBRA	Consolidated Omnibus Budget Reconciliation Act
COLA	Cost-of-Living Adjustment
CORF	Comprehensive Outpatient Rehabilitation Facility
CPI	Consumer price index
CSRA	Community Spouse's Resource Allowance
DAB	Departmental Appeals Board

DHHS	Department of Health and Human Services
DME	Durable Medical Equipment
DNR	Do Not Resuscitate
DRA	Deficit Reduction Act (2005)
DRG	Diagnosis-Related Group
ECHO	Elder Cottage Housing Opportunity
EMSN	Electronic Medicare Summary Notice
EOMB	Explanation of Medicare Benefits
EPO	Exclusive Provider Organization
ERISA	Employee Retirement Income Security Act
ESRD	End-stage Renal Disease
FFS	Fee for Service
FPL	Federal Poverty Level
GRAT	Grantor Retained Annuity Trust
GRIT	Grantor Retained Income Trust
GRUT	Grantor Retained Unitrust
HCFA	Health Care Financing Administration
HDHP	High deductible health policy
HEDIS	Health Plan Employer Data and Information Set
HHA	Home health agency
HHS	Health and Human Services, Department of
HICAP	Health Insurance Counseling and Assistance Program

HIO	Health Insuring Organization
HIPAA	Health Insurance Portability and Accountability Act
HMO	Health Maintenance Organization
HOME	Home Investment Partnerships Program
HUD	Housing and Urban Development, Department of
IADL	Instrumental Activities of Daily Living
ICF	Intermediate Care Facility
IPA	Independent Practice Association
IRA	Individual retirement Account
IRE	Independent review entity
LTCI	Long-term Care Insurance
LPN	Licensed Practical Nurse
LSDP	Lump-sum death benefit
M+C	Medicare+Choice
MA	Medicare Advantage (formerly Medicare+Choice)
MAC	Medicare Appeals Council
MA-PDP	Medicare Advantage prescription drug plan
MAGI	Modified Adjusted Gross Income
MAP	Medicare Advantage plan
MMA	Medicare Prescription Drug Improvement and Modernization Act (2003)
MNIL	Medically needy income level
MSA	Medical Savings Account

MSO	Management Services Organization
MSN	Medicare Summary Notice
NORC	Naturally Occurring Retirement Community
NP	Nurse Practitioner
OAA	Older Americans Act
OASDI	Old-age, Survivors and Disability Insurance
OASIS	Outcome and Assessment Information Set
OBRA	Omnibus Budget Reconciliation Act
PA	Physician assistant
PACE	Program for All-inclusive Care of Elderly
PBGC	Pension Benefit Guaranty Corporation
PCCM	Primary care case management
PCP	Primary care physician
PDP	Prescription drug plan
PEBE	Personal Earnings and Benefits Estimate
PERS	Personal Emergency Response System
PFFS	Private fee-for-service
PHA	Public housing agency
PHO	Physician Hospital Organization
PHP	Prepaid Health Plan
PIA	Primary Insurance Amount
PNA	Personal Needs Allowance

POS	Point of Service
PPO	Preferred Provider Organization
PRO	Peer Review Organization
PSO	Provider-sponsored Organization
QDWI	Qualified disabled and working individual
QI	Qualifying individual
QIC	Qualified Independent Contractor
QIO	Quality improvement organization
QMB	Qualified Medicare Beneficiary
QPRT	Qualified Personal Residence Trust
QTIP	Qualified Terminable Interest Property
RFBP	Religious Fraternal Benefits Plan
RBRVS	Resource-based Relative Value Scale
RRB	Railroad retirement beneficiary
RUG	Resource Utilization Group
SEP	Special Enrollment Period
SHMO	Social Health Maintenance Organization
SLMB	Specified Low-income Medicare Beneficiary
SNF	Skilled Nursing Facility
SNP	Medicare Advantage Specialized Plans for Special Needs Beneficiaries
SSA	Social Security Administration
SSI	Supplemental Security Income

TEFRA   Tax Equity and Fiscal Responsibility Act

URC   Utilization Review Committee

A

Accessory Apartments

Living quarters created within a single family residence constituting complete living units with separate kitchen and bath.

Accessory Units

Private housing arrangements in existing family homes, small cottages, or apartments that are in, attached to, or adjacent to living facilities. Examples of such units are ECHO units which are situated on the exterior of a single family residence, and accessory apartments which are created within the single family home.

Accounting, judicial

A judicial proceeding that reviews an executor's or trustee's transactions.

Accreditation Organization/Medicare Advantage

A private, independent national organization approved by CMS to evaluate and accredit a Medicare Advantage organization and its plan. Accredited organizations are deemed to be in compliance with the Balanced Budget Act of 1997 and to have quality assessment and performance improvement programs.

Activities of Daily Living (ADL)
See also *Instrumental activities of daily living (IADL)*.

Activities usually performed for oneself in the course of a normal day. Although definitions differ, ADLs are usually considered to be mobility (e.g., transfer from bed to chair), dressing, bathing, self-feeding and toileting.

People may need assistance with ADLs regardless of their living arrangements. Assistance to a person limited in his/her ADLs is customarily performed by a

---

All entries preceded by an asterisk (*) are culled or copied from the official U.S. government **Medicare** handbook (*Medicare & You 2011*).

1

family member, a home health aide or attendant, or a nurse's aide in a nursing facility. The assistance is of a non-medical nature, commonly characterized as personal care, custodial care or physical care. Assistance provided in a home setting may extend beyond ADLs and include such non-medical activities as housekeeping (e.g., cleaning, cooking), laundry and shopping.

Medicare cannot be looked to, except to a limited extent, for coverage of assistance with ADLs. (See also *Home health aide services/Medicare*). Medicare pays for acute care services and does not provide coverage for chronic, personal or custodial care.

Medicaid, unlike Medicare, will cover Medicaid-eligible persons for many home care services including personal care, and in certain cases ancillary services such as housekeeping. (See also *Home health care services/Medicaid*.)

Activities of Daily Living (ADL) Trigger/LTCI

A long-term care insurance policy that has an ADL trigger releases benefits after the covered person suffers limitations in a certain number of activities of daily living (ADLs), usually two or three. Not all policies use the same ADLs or the same definition of the ADLs. Restrictive definitions may be used in a way that makes it unlikely that benefits will be collected.

The Health Insurance Portability and Accountability Act of 1996 established certain standards regarding the ADL trigger in order for policies issued after January 1, 1997 to be considered tax-qualified; that is, for a portion of their premiums to be eligible for treatment as a medical deduction on income tax returns. For details see *Long-term care insurance, tax status*.

Actual Charge/Medicare
See also *Balance billing/Medicare; Approved charge/Medicare.*

The amount a health care provider charges for a service, which is frequently larger than the amount approved by Medicare.

Actuarial Equivalence/Medicare Part D Drug Coverage
See also *"As good as"/Medicare Part D Drug Coverage.*

This term refers to drug coverage in a Medicare prescription drug plan which is considered to be at least as good as another plan. Drug coverage, computed in dollar amounts, must be at least actuarially equivalent to the standard Part D plan.

Actuarial Tables

Tables that calculate present value of a future interest in money or other property. They are commonly used by the Internal Revenue Service.

Acute Care

Short-term, as compared to chronic, health care required by a patient, usually in a hospital, following the onset of an acute illness, which begins over a brief time span.

Adaptive Devices

Specialized products, hardware and clothing that help people compensate for their disabilities and function with some independence.

Additional Benefits/Medicare Advantage Plans (MAP)

As distinguished from basic and supplemental benefits, additional benefits in the context of Medicare Advantage include health care services not covered by Medicare (e.g., outpatient prescription drugs) as well as premium reductions or cost-sharing for Medicare-covered services.

Adjusted Average Per Capita Cost (AAPCC)
See also *Adjusted community rates (ACR); Competitive bidding process/Medicare Advantage Plans.*

Prior to the Balanced Budget Act of 1997, Medicare paid risk contractors according to the adjusted average per capita cost payment methodology to provide health care to Medicare beneficiaries. The AAPCC – an estimate of the average payment made per beneficiary to a Medicare-approved, fee-for-service risk contractor – was based on Medicare fee-for-service expenditures by county. These fee-for-service expenditures were adjusted for the demographic factors of age, sex, institutional welfare and employment status. The AAPCC methodology was criticized for the disparity of payment rates among geographic regions, sometimes as much as a twenty- (20%) percent difference between adjacent countries.

The Balanced Budget Act of 1997 introduced a different payment methodology – adjusted community rate process (ACR) – that addressed these concerns. Medicare capitation rates paid to risk contractors for each county are the greater of a blended capitation rate, a minimum amount rate, or a minimum percentage increase. According to the adjusted community rating process, the blended capitation rate is the average of the historic per capita cost in a particular county and the national annual per capita cost adjusted for local differences in the price of care. The blended capitation rate is then adjusted by a budget-neutral factor.

Adjusted Community Rate (ACR)
See also *Competitive bidding process/Medicare Advantage Plans.*

This is a process, prescribed in the Balanced Budget Act of 1997, to determine, according to the same formula for all Medicare Advantage plans, the amount of the annual capitation payment to each plan. The adjusted community rate blends local, historical per capita cost in each county and the national annual per capita cost, adjusted for local differences in the price of care.

The ACR process, a form of administered pricing process has been replaced by a competitive bidding process prescribed by the Medicare Prescription Drug Improvement and Modernization Act (2003), which amended the Balanced Budget Act of 1997.

Adjusted Gross Income
See also *Gross income; Modified adjusted gross income/Social Security.*

A taxpayer's taxable income is his/her adjusted gross income less prescribed statutory deductions (exclusions). These deductions from gross income result in a figure known as adjusted gross income.

Administration of Medicaid Program
See *Medicaid Introduction*

Administration of Medicare Program/Medicare

Overall responsibility for the administration of the Original Medicare program rests with the Secretary of the Department of Health and Human Services (DHHS).

The Centers for Medicare and Medicaid Services (CMS), previously known as Health Care Financing Administration (HCFA), a division of DHHS, directly manages and administers the Original Medicare program. Its day-to-day administration of payment of Part A and B bills is operated through private companies under contract with the Secretary of DHHS. In the case of Part A services, they are called "fiscal intermediaries," and in the case of Part B services except for homebound beneficiaries whose claim administration is through fiscal intermediaries), they are called "carriers." The Medicare Prescription Drug and Improvement Modernization Act of 2003 (MMA) mandates that the Secretary of DHHS replace the fiscal intermediaries and the carriers with Medical administrative contractors. The implementation of this replacement was phased in during 2005-2011.

Medicare independent review entities, consisting of groups of practicing physicians and other health care experts, participate (as private contractors for DHHS) in the administration of the Medicare program. These entities are called Quality Improvement Organizations (QIO) (formerly known as Peer Review Organizations (PRO)). The QIO's functions consist of the following: (i) responsibility for making determinations regarding the necessity and reasonableness of health care provided by Medicare; (ii) reviewing of non-coverage notices issued by hospitals to Medicare beneficiaries changing coverage of their continued stay; (iii) evaluating the efficiency and economy of the health care services provided; (iv) ensuring that such services meet professional and accepted medical quality of care standards; and (v) reviewing the professional activities of prescription drug sponsors pursuant to contracts under Medicare Part D. In addition, the QIOs review complaints by beneficiaries relating to the quality of care in settings such as inpatient hospitals, hospital outpatient departments, hospital emergency rooms, skilled nursing facilities, home health agencies, private fee-for-service plans, and ambulatory sites. QIOs make initial determinations in hospital cases, but do not issue payments; they authorize the appropriate contractor to issue payment.

CMS has established new entities called Qualified Independent Contractors (QICs) to conduct a second level of administrative reviews (called reconsideration(s)) of Part A claim denials made by fiscal intermediaries, carriers and QIOs.

The MMA created the role of Ombudsman as the principal point of contact with CMS for Medicare beneficiaries. The Ombudsman's responsibilities include: 1) responding to complaints, grievances and inquiries concerning any aspect of the Medicare program; 2) assisting beneficiaries in collecting information needed to file appeals; 3) helping beneficiaries with enrollment and disenrollment problems; 4) assisting beneficiaries with issues related to premiums; and 5) working with the aging and disability communities to improve beneficiaries' understanding of their rights and protections within the program.

Administration of Social Security Program/Social Security

Social Security is the popular name for the Old Age, Survivors and Disability Insurance program (OASDI) authorized under Title II of the Social Security Act. It is a social insurance program funded through employee and employer payroll taxes under the Federal Insurance Contributions Act (FICA) and the Self-Employment Contributions Act. The Social Security Independence and Program Improvements Act of 1994 (SSIPIA) removed the Social Security Administration (SSA) from the aegis of the Department of Health and Human Services and made the SSA an independent agency in the executive branch of the Federal government. The agency is responsible for administering the Old-Age, Survivors, and Disability Insurance (OASDI) and Supplemental Security Income (SSI) programs, and programs providing health benefits (including black lung benefits) to coal industry workers. The SSIPIA provides for the establishment of a seven- (7) member Social Security Advisory Board selected partially by the executive branch and partially by the legislative branch. The Board's function is to advise the commissioner on policies related to the OASDI and SSI programs. The board meets at least quarterly and serves without pay.

The Social Security Administration (SSA) is headed by a Commissioner of Social Security appointed by the President, with the advice and consent of the Senate, to serve a six-(6) year term. The Commissioner is responsible for the exercise of all powers and the discharge of all duties of the Administration, and has authority and control over all personnel and activities thereof. The Commissioner may prescribe rules and regulations (subject to established rule making procedures) to carry out the functions of the agency.

Administration on Aging (AoA)/Older Americans Act
See *Older Americans Act (Area Agency on Aging)*

Administrative Law Judge (ALJ)
See also *Appeals/Social Security; Appeals/Medicare; Appeals/Medicare Advantage.*

The appeals structure of the Social Security Administration involves appeals relating to Social Security, Supplemental Security Insurance claims and Medicare claims from decisions at the initial determination and reconsideration levels.

Appeals from these decisions are brought before an ALJ at a hearing. ALJs have special training to review the lower level determinations and have the authority to accept or review decisions.

Administratively Necessary Days of Care/Medicare

In large towns or large hospitals, Medicare may pay for administratively necessary days of care – that is, days when a patient should be at a nursing home – but no bed is available. The attending physician must certify the need for care before Medicare will pay.

Adult Community
See *Independent living retirement community.*

Adult Congregate Living Facility (ACLF)
See *Assisted living facility.*

(continued on next page)

ADULT DAY CARE CENTERS

INTRODUCTION

An adult day care center for elderly people living in the community provides on a daily basis, recreation and social services, hot meals, and, in many adult day centers, medical, nursing and rehabilitation services. Programs which include medical services are commonly referred to as adult day health centers. They are state-licensed and may be covered by Medicaid or partially covered by Medicare Part B. When programs provide no medical services, licensure depends on the particular state requirements. Adult day care is designed to provide not only the foregoing services to the elderly but also relief to family caregivers during ordinary office hours when they are at work. As part of a company's cafeteria plan of benefits, some corporations provide care for an employee's parent(s) in an adult care center. The employee's share of the cost, if any, is usually funded by a salary reduction which makes the benefit non-taxable.

Regular attendance at an adult day care center may cause a participant to lose coverage of the Medicare home health benefit since it may affect his/her required homebound status. However, attendance at an adult day care center for the sole purpose of receiving medical care probably will not affect the participant's homebound status.

I.   GENERAL.

Adult day care centers provide frail elderly people living in the community a variety of services on a yearly basis (usually four (4) or five (5) days a week, approximately six (6) to eight (8) hours per day): recreation, social services, hot meals, and often medical, nursing and rehabilitative services. Programs which include medical services are state licensed. If programs provide no medical services, licensure depends on the particular state. Adult day care centers sometimes provide transportation to their location.

There are basically two (2) types of programs depending upon services rendered:

> Programs that emphasize social services, recreation, meals, and transportation. They offer few, if any, medical services.

> Programs, many affiliated with a health care institution, that provide medical care and rehabilitation treatment, in addition to meals, transportation, social and recreational activities.

The National Adult Day Services Association has established three (3) levels of care, or service, provided by adult day care programs: core, enhanced, and intensive. Participants in need of core services are those whose physical condition is stable, but who require some supervision, supportive services, minimal assistance with activities of daily living (ADLs), and socialization. Individuals needing enhanced services require moderate assistance with one to three (3) ADLs, and possibly therapy services at a maintenance level. Intensive services provide maximum assistance, regular monitoring, or intervention by a nurse, and possibly therapy services at a rehabilitative or restorative level.

The New York State Office for the Aging defines adult day care as a community-based, non-residential program providing four (4) core services for frail individuals: socialization, supervision, monitoring or personal care, and nutrition.

II.   PAYMENTS FOR SERVICE.

The fee of adult day care centers varies from a flat fee to no fee, or a sliding fee depending upon the participant's income. (In some adult day centers, charges may be covered by Medicaid and in part by Medicare.) Many long-term care insurance policies, where a fixed amount is paid for nursing home and home care, may include care in adult day centers as an additional benefit.

Some corporations provide dependent care at an adult day care center covering parents of employees. This benefit is included as part of an employee's cafeteria plan and is funded by salary reductions, thereby constituting a non-taxable benefit.

III. ADULT DAY CARE CENTER ATTENDANCE'S EFFECT ON HOMEBOUND STATUS.

Regular absences to participate in therapeutic, psychosocial or medical treatment at a licensed or accredited adult day care program will not disqualify a beneficiary from being considered homebound.

Home health agencies enrolling patients eligible for Medicare home health benefits are responsible for demonstrating that the adult day center is licensed or certified/accredited as part of determining whether a patient is homebound for purposes of Medicare eligibility.

(continued on next page)

Adult Day Health Care

A medically oriented long-term medical service provided in a congregate setting such as a hospital or a clinic. An example of such care is a mobile patient going to a clinic to have daily medication administered there.

Adult Foster Home

Like board-and-care homes, an adult foster home, usually a single family residence, is a care home in a non-medical setting. Elderly persons live with a foster family which provides meals, housekeeping and personal care.

Unlike board-and-care homes, the maximum number of residents permitted in foster care homes is limited. Thus, Iowa, Massachusetts and Pennsylvania permit only two (2) residents, Texas permits eight (8), and sixteen (16) are allowed in Colorado. Other states permit three (3), four (4) or five (5) residents per home. In about half of the twenty-six (26) states with foster care home programs, the homes are required to be licensed by a state health agency. Other states use a voluntary certification standard by which the homes can optionally apply for certification by a social service or aging agency. Foster homes are funded in large part through SSI and Medicaid home and community-based waivers.

Adult Guardian

The person appointed by a court, usually a probate court under a modern protective services statute, to perform the court-ordered tasks of caring for an incapacitated adult's financial affairs and/or personal needs.

Three (3) different types of guardians have varying degrees of authority:

> **Plenary guardian** with total authority over personal and property matters;
>
> **Guardian of the person** with authority only over personal matters such as medical decisions and residential questions; and
>
> **Guardian of the estate** with authority over property only.

Adult Home
See *Alternative Housing Facilities.*

Adult Retirement Community
See *Alternative Housing Facilities*.

*Advance Beneficiary Notice/Medicare

If you have Original Medicare, your health care provider or supplier may give you a notice called an "Advance Beneficiary Notice of Noncoverage" (ABN). This notice says Medicare probably (or certainly) won't pay for some services in certain situations. You will be asked to choose whether to get the items or services listed on the ABN. If you choose to get the items or services listed on the ABN, you will have to pay if Medicare doesn't. You will be asked to sign the ABN to say that you have read and understood it. An ABN isn't an official denial of coverage by Medicare. You could choose to get the items listed on the ABN and still ask your health care provider or supplier to submit the bill to Medicare or another insurer. If Medicare denies payment, you can still file an appeal. However, you will have to pay for the items or services if Medicare determines that the items or services aren't covered (and no other insurer is responsible for payment).

Advance Beneficiary Notice to Beneficiaries (ABN)/Medicare
See *Home health agency advance beneficiary notice /Medicare; Medicare/Denial Notices, sections I and IV.*

*Advance Directives/Medicare

Advance directives, are legal documents that allow you to put in writing what kind of health care you would want or name someone who can speak for you if you were too ill to speak for yourself. Advance directives most often include the following:

> *A health care proxy*
> *A living will*

A health care proxy (sometimes called a "durable power of attorney for health care") is used to name the person you wish to make health care decisions for you if you aren't able to make them yourself.

A living will is another way to make sure your voice is heard. It states which medical treatment you would accept or refuse if your life is threatened. Dialysis for kidney failure, a breathing machine if you can't breathe on your own, CPR (cardiopulmonary resuscitation) if your heart and breathing stop, or tube feeding if you can no longer eat are examples of medical treatment you can choose to accept or refuse.

Advance Directive

See also *Durable power of attorney for health care; Living will.*

A declaration expressing an individual's health care preferences, including both the routine treatment preferences as well as direction on withholding or withdrawal of life-prolonging procedures. An advance directive may include designation of an agent or surrogate, sometimes called a health care proxy, to make medical decisions if an individual is unable to do so.

Affordable Care Act

The Patient Protection and Affordable Care Act of 2010 (PPACA) was amended by the Health Care and Education Reconciliation Act of 2010 and, as amended, was signed into law by President Obama on March 23, 2010. PPACA is colloquially referred to as the Affordable Care Act. It reforms certain aspects of the private health industry and public insurance programs, including increasing coverage of pre-existing health conditions and expanding access to insurance for over thirty (30) million Americans. Under PPACA individuals affected by the Medicare Part D coverage gap are entitled to receive from Medicare a $250 rebate; fifty (50%) percent of the gap will be eliminated in 2011, and all of the gap will be eliminated by 2020.

Many states, numerous organizations, and many persons have filed actions in Federal court challenging the constitutionality of PPACA. The Supreme Court has upheld the constitutionality of the ACT.

Age-restricted Housing

Age-restricted housing refers to a facility that restricts residence to households containing at least one older person. The eligible age of that older person will vary according to the type of housing facility. For example, most adult retirement communities set the minimum age limit at 55 years of age, while most government-subsidized apartments for the elderly require that at least one person be 62 years of age or older.

It is against the Federal Fair Housing Amendments Act of 1988 to establish the age limit lower than 55 years of age. However, a housing sponsor can limit its development to individuals of a higher age, or state that everyone in a household must be of minimum age. For example, it is legal for a sponsor of a continuing care retirement community to require that all residents be at least 65 years of age.

Aging in Place

A phenomenon when a person becomes elderly, and perhaps frail, while continuing to live his in his/her same place of residence over a number of years, or even decades.

Aid Continuing/Medicaid
See *Appeals/Medicaid, section I.*

Aide
See also *Home health aide; Home attendant.*

A general term relating to an individual such as a home health aide who under the supervision of skilled medical personnel (e.g., registered nurse) performs medically oriented as well as non-medically oriented services, and/or an unsupervised individual (personal care aide or attendant) who performs non-medical custodial tasks relating to a patient's activities of daily living. Unlike a home health aide, an attendant or personal care aide performs duties that do not require any particular education or training.

Aliens, Eligibility/Medicare
See also *Eligibility and enrollment/Medicare, section A.1.*

The following individuals may purchase Medicare coverage by payment of a monthly premium: voluntary enrollees who (a) attained age 65, (b) are not eligible for either Social Security or Railroad Retirement benefits, and (c) are aliens lawfully admitted for permanent residence (i.e., they have continuously resided in the United States for not less than five (5) years immediately before the month in which application for enrollment is made). In order to receive coverage in Medicare Part A, a lawful alien must enroll in Medicare Part B.

As in the case of Medicare Part A benefits, an alien age 65 or over who is a permanent resident alien residing in the United State for at least five (5) years immediately prior to application, can purchase Medicare Part B benefits by filing an application and paying monthly premiums which CMS fixes annually.

All-payer System

A uniform system in which the prices charged for health services are the same to the health provider without regard to who is paying for medical services. In an all-payer system, the government, an insurer, a large corporation or any other payer will pay a uniform fee for health services at the same institution.

Allied Health Professional

A person, like a laboratory technician, with specialized training in a field related to medicine who works in collaboration with physicians or other health professionals.

Allowed Charge/Medicare

See *Approved Charges/Medicare.*

Alternative Delivery Systems/Managed Care

Forms of structured managed care health delivery systems, other than traditional fee-for-service indemnity health care, such as the classic HMO or preferred provider organizations.

Alternative Prescription Drug Coverage Plan/Medicare Part D

Part D drug plans are not required to offer the standard benefit coverage, but can offer alternative prescription drug coverage. Alternative coverage must be actuarially equivalent to the standard benefit (i.e., the value of the benefit package must be equal to or greater than the value of the standard benefit package). In an actuarially equivalent plan, cost sharing may vary by the use of such tiered copayments. However, a plan that offers an alternative benefit package cannot impose a higher annual deductible ($320 in 2012) or require a higher out-of-pocket threshold ($4,700 in 2012) than required by the standard benefit. Plans can offer enhanced alternative coverage that may include changes to the deductible and the initial coverage limit, though the deductible cannot be higher than the $320 (2012). Enhanced alternative coverage under Part D might include coverage of some drugs that are excluded under Part D, or that are in the coverage gap ("doughnut hole"). A prescription drug plan (PDP) that wants to offer a drug plan with enhanced alternative coverage in a service area must also offer a PDP with the basic benefit prescription package in that area.

ALTERNATIVE HOUSING FACILITIES

INTRODUCTION

When persons reach a particular age or level of frailty, they often decide to move from their home to an alternative living situation, other than a nursing home, for which they must pay and which may better meet their changing physical and/or psychosocial needs. Alternative living facilities reflect the range of options that most often exist in the community short of a skilled medical institution. Generally, they are residential in nature and incorporate a variety of psychosocial support and personal care services that may be required to permit an individual to remain living in that community, independent of a nursing home.

The facilities are best described by categorizing them into the levels of care provided by the facility where the resident lives. Most of the facilities named below have independent entries that describe them more fully.

I.   INSTITUTIONAL, NON-MEDICAL FACILITIES FOR DEPENDENT RESIDENTS.

These facilities are care homes in a non-medical, institutional setting. Residents are supervised to varying degrees and are dependent to varying extents. These facilities range in size from a private home housing two or three seniors, to small facilities with approximately a dozen beds, to multi-unit complexes accommodating dozens of individuals. Licensure for these facilities varies by state.

The facilities are known as:

Adult congregate living facility   Domiciliary care home
Adult foster home   Group home

Adult home

Assisted living facility

Board-and-care home

Home for the aging

Personal care home

Residential care home

These facilities have no uniform definition around the country. Terms for them are fuzzy and lack a common meaning. They may be called something different in a given state and also have a popular name that differs from a regulatory name. Thus, for example, a board-and-care facility is a lot like an assisted living facility, but the term sounds more déclassé and now seems to be used only in connection with a facility for low-income people. Similarly, an assisted living facility commonly is less institution*al (or non-institutional) than a board-and-care home.

II. NON-INSTITUTIONAL, NON-MEDICAL FACILITIES FOR SEMI-DEPENDENT RESIDENTS.

These shared housing facilities and arrangements are for elderly persons who do not wish an institutional or medical setting but require some minimal supportive services. Examples of this type of living arrangement are:

Elderly owners of homes with housemate(s);

Elderly persons who move in with relatives;

Elderly persons who are matched up with younger persons and live in their homes;

Foster homes for elderly semi-independent residents who move in with another non-related family that provides meals and other supportive services; and

Accessory units.

III. NON-INSTITUTIONAL, NON-MEDICAL FACILITIES FOR INDEPENDENT RESIDENTS.

These facilities for elderly persons are neither medical facilities nor care homes. Supportive services and amenities such as meals, health, transportation, and some social activities are provided. The residents are basically well and capable of living independently, although they may have functional limitations. The facilities commonly consist of town houses, garden apartments or condominiums in which the resident generally has an equity interest, although sometimes these accommodations are on a rental basis. The cost of living in these facilities ranges from moderate to very expensive. These facilities are sometimes referred to as:

Continuing care retirement community;

Independent living retirement community;

Life care community;

Residential apartment; and

Residential village.

_____

(continued on next page)

Alternative Medicine

A system of therapeutics, such as acupuncture, holistic medicine, or osteopathic medicine, that is different from traditional medical care.

Alzheimer's Disease

A form of progressive dementia, resulting from degeneration of brain cells, that causes severe intellectual deterioration. It is currently considered irreversible.

*Ambulance Services/Medicare

Ground ambulance transportation when you need to be transported to a hospital or skilled nursing facility for medically necessary services, and transportation in any other vehicle could endanger your health. Medicare may pay for ambulance transportation in an airplane or helicopter to a hospital if you need immediate and rapid ambulance transportation that ground transportation can't provide.

In some cases, Medicare may pay for limited non-emergency ambulance transportation if you have orders from your doctor saying that ambulance transportation is medically necessary. Medicare will only cover services to the nearest appropriate medical facility that is able to give you the care you need. You pay 20% of the Medicare-approved amount, and the Part B deductible applies.

Ambulance Transportation/Medicare

Transportation by ambulance of a Medicare beneficiary who is receiving Part A benefits while a patient at a hospital, critical access hospital (CAH) or skilled nursing facility (SNF) is covered by Part A.

Medicare Part B helps pay for medically necessary ambulance transportation of a beneficiary who is not a patient of a hospital, CAH or SNF but only if the ambulance, equipment and personnel meet Medicare requirements, including origin and destination requirements described below, and if transportation in any other vehicle would endanger a patient's health. Ambulance use from one's home to a doctor's office is not covered.

For ambulance transportation to be covered by Part B, there must be a medical necessity for such transportation, and other requirements need be met also. The medical necessity requirement is met when a beneficiary is unable to get up from bed without assistance, ambulate or sit in a chair or wheelchair and when another means of transportation would be contra-indicated. A physician's certificate of medical necessity is required unless the beneficiary resides at home or is a patient of a facility and not under the direct care of a physician.

If the criteria for coverage are met, ambulance service is covered from any point of origin to the nearest hospital, CAH or SNF capable of furnishing the required level and type of care, from a hospital, CAH or SNF to the beneficiary's home, or from a SNF to the nearest supplier of medically necessary services not available at the SNF where the beneficiary resides. Transportation from the home of a beneficiary receiving renal-dialysis for treatment of end-stage renal disease to the nearest facility providing renal-dialysis is covered under Part B.

Ambulance services, unlike most other Part B services which are paid on a prospective payment basis, are paid under a negotiated fee schedule established by the Secretary of HHS.

Ambulatory Care

Health services that do not require an overnight hospital stay which are rendered to an outpatient.

Ambulatory Setting

A site at which health services are provided to an outpatient such as a clinic or surgery center.

*Ambulatory Surgical Center/Medicare

Facility fees for approved surgical procedures provided in an ambulatory surgical center (facility where surgical procedures are performed, and the patient is released within 24 hours). Except for certain preventive services (for which you pay nothing), you pay 20% of the Medicare-approved amount to both the ambulatory surgical center and the doctor who treats you, and the Part B deductible applies. You pay all facility fees for procedures Medicare doesn't allow in ambulatory surgical centers.

Ambulatory Surgical Center

This freestanding facility, which may be a separate part of a hospital, performs outpatient surgery.

*Amyotrophic Lateral Sclerosis (ALS)/Medicare

Amyotrophic Lateral Sclerosis (also called Lou Gehrig's disease), is a disease of the nerve cells in the brain and spinal cord that control voluntary muscle movement. If you have ALS you automatically get Part A and Part B the month your disability benefits begin.

Annual Aggregate Bidding/Medicare Advantage Plan

See also *Capitation/Medicare Advantage plans; Competitive bidding process/Medicare Advantage.*

Payments by Medicare to Medicare Advantage plan organizations (MA) are based on competitive bids. MA organizations submit to CMS an annual aggregate bid amount for each MA plan. An aggregate plan bid is based upon its determination of expected costs in the plan's service area for the national average beneficiary for providing (i) non-drug benefits, (ii) Part D basic prescription drugs, and (iii) supplemental benefits if any. To determine the amount of payments to a plan, by Medicare, CMS will compare the non-drug portion of the aggregate bid to the local or regional plan benchmark (an amount which is an average of county rates). Annual Deductible/Medicare, Medicare Part B beneficiaries must pay a $155 (2012) deductible each calendar year. This deductible is offset against the first incurred covered expenses (determined on the basis of Medicare's approved charges) for the calendar year. In addition, Medicare Parts A and B also require an annual deductible of the first three pints of blood used.

Annual Deductible, Medical Savings Account

See *Medical savings account; Medical savings account/Medicare Advantage.*

Annual Earnings Exemption/Social Security

This is the amount of annual earnings (earned income) of a retired individual, up to age 70, without reducing his/her Social Security benefits.

Annual Gift Tax Exclusion

See also *Unified tax credit.*

A gift by a donor of $13,000 (2012) per donee in any one calendar year, if one's spouse consents, is free of any gift tax liability.

ANNUITIES

INTRODUCTION

The funds obtained by an individual from an insurance company of an annuity are one of the sources that can be utilized to fund eldercare.

I.   DEFINED.

A financial arrangement, such as a pension plan payout, an intrafamily transaction or an investment sold by an insurance company, under which, for a consideration, a continuing stream of payments is promised for a person's life, or for the joint lives of two people or for a term of years to the purchaser or his/her assignee(s). The more common types of annuities are:

Deferred annuity. A contract is entered into with the insurer whereby the insurer will commence payments at a specified date in the future, called the annuity start date. The purchaser of the annuity may either pay a single premium or an initial premium plus periodic later premium payments.

Fixed annuity. A contract is entered into with the insurer who agrees to pay a specified rate of return for a period of years.

Immediate annuity. A contract is entered into with an insurer whereby funds are transferred to the insurer. A single premium is paid, and an immediate stream of payments will begin.

Joint survivor annuity. A contract is entered into with the insurer who makes payments until the second of two annuitants, such as a husband and wife or parent and child, has died.

Single life annuity. A contract is entered into with the insurer who makes payments during the annuitant's life.

Variable annuity. A contract is entered into with the insurer with arrangements similar to those of a mutual fund. The annuitant is given a number of investment choices, and the annuitant's return will depend upon performance of the investments chosen.

Annuity payments can be made in several ways including, term certain (a specified number of years), single life (straight life) or other variations of the foregoing.

II.   TAXABILITY.

The annuity recipient is not taxed on the portion of the annuity payout that represents his/her original investment. Taxes must be paid, however, upon any increased value of the annuity's accumulated balance resulting from interest, dividends or capital gains.

Usually until the original investment has been fully recovered, each annuity payment will be multiplied by an exclusion ratio to determine the taxable amount. The exclusion ratio is calculated by dividing the annuitant's investment in his/her contract by the expected return. The expected return in a life annuity is determined by multiplying the person's life expectancy figure, based upon Internal Revenue Code tables, by one-year's annuity payment. In the case of a variable annuity, determination of the taxable amount of payouts is calculated in a somewhat different, more complicated manner.

III.   MEDICAID TRANSFER PENALTY RULE.

In the context of the Medicaid transfer of assets penalty rule, an annuity is included as a transfer of assets unless it:

Falls under IRC § 408(b) or (q); or

Is purchased with the proceeds from a trust or account under IRC § 408(a)(c) or a simplified employee pension, or a Roth IRA; or

Is irrevocable and non-assignable, "actuarially sound" (using actuarial publications of the office of the SSA Chief Actuary), and provides payments in equal amounts during the annuity term. There can be no deferred annuity or annuity with balloon payments which pay interest, plus a relatively small amount of principal monies rather than being actuarially sound, with equal monthly payments.

The purchase of an annuity will be treated as the "transfer of an asset" for less than fair market value unless the annuity meets specific requirements:

The state is either the remainder beneficiary in the first position for at least the full amount of medical assistance received by the Medicaid recipient; or

The state is listed as the beneficiary in the second position after the community spouse or disabled or minor child; and the state is named in the first position if either the spouse or the child's representative disposes of the remainder for less than fair market value.

IV. RECOVERY BY MEDICAID.

Annuities will be subject to estate recovery upon the death of the Medicaid recipient unless there is a surviving spouse or disabled or minor child or unless the Medicaid recipient purchased a qualified long-term insurance contract, which sheltered the annuity (see *Robert Wood Johnson Program/LTCI*).

V. APPLICATIONS FOR MEDICAID.

State Medicaid applications, including recertification applications, must include a description of any interest the applicant or community spouse has in an annuity or a similar financial instrument, even though the annuity is considered as actuarially sound. The recertification application must include a statement that the state, by providing Medicaid, becomes the remainder beneficiary under the annuity or instrument.

(continued on next page)

Annuity Trust

See *Charitable remainder trust.*

Any Willing Provider Bill

This legislation proposed in many states and enacted in some protects physicians who find themselves left out of the health care networks. It requires a managed care organization to include in the network any health care provider willing to abide by the plan's contractual requirements. In some instances, this legislation contains freedom of choice provisions that would restrict a health plan's ability to induce subscribers with financial incentives to choose network providers (instead of providers who are outside the network), such as requiring a higher copayment for choosing an out-of-network provider.

*Appeal/Medicare (Part A/Part B/Part D)

An appeal is the action you can take if you disagree with a **coverage or payment** *decision made by Medicare.*

Do the following to file an appeal:

- *Get the Medicare Summary Notice (MSN) that shows the item or service you're appealing. Your MSN is the statement you get every 3 months that lists all the services billed to Medicare and tells you if Medicare paid for the services.*
- *Circle the item(s) you disagree with on the MSN, and write an explanation on the MSN of why you disagree.*
- *Sign, write your telephone number, and provide your Medicare number on the MSN.*
- *Send the MSN, or a copy, to the Medicare contractor's address listed on the MSN.*

If you're getting Medicare services from a hospital, skilled nursing facility, home health agency, comprehensive outpatient rehabilitation facility, or hospice, and you think your Medicare-covered services are ending too soon, **you have the right to a fast appeal**. *Your provider will give you a notice before your services end that will tell you how to ask for a fast appeal. With a fast appeal, an independent reviewer, called a Quality Improvement Organization (QIO), will decide if your services should continue. You must call your local QIO to request a fast appeal no later than the time shown on the notice you get from your provider.*

You have the right to appeal a Medicare Drug [Part D] Plan's decision in all of the following ways:

*Get a written explanation (called a **"coverage determination"**) from your Medicare drug plan. A coverage determination is the first decision made by your Medicare drug plan (not the pharmacy) about your benefits, including whether a certain drug is covered, whether you've met the requirements to get a requested drug, how much you pay for a drug, and whether to make an **Exception** to a plan rule when you request it.*

*Ask for an **Exception** if you or your prescriber (your doctor or other health care provider who is legally allowed to write prescriptions), believes you need a drug that isn't on your plan's formulary.*

*Ask for an **Exception** if you or your prescriber believes that a coverage rule (such as prior authorization) should be waived.*

*Ask for an **Exception** if you think you should pay less for a higher tier (more expensive) drug because you or your prescriber believes you can't take any of the lower tier (less expensive) drugs for the same condition.*

You or your prescriber may make a standard request by phone or in writing, if you're asking for prescription drug benefits you haven't received yet. If you're asking to get paid back for prescription drugs you already bought, you or your prescriber must make the standard request in writing.

*You or your prescriber can call or write your plan for **an expedited (fast) request**. Your request will be expedited if you haven't received the prescription and your plan determines, or your prescriber tells your plan, that your life or health may be at risk by waiting.*

*If you're requesting an **Exception**, your prescriber must provide a statement explaining the medical reason why the exception should be approved.*

*If you disagree with your Medicare drug plan's **Coverage Determination** or **Exception** decision, you can appeal. <u>There are five levels of appeal</u>. The first level is appealing to your plan. Once your Medicare drug plan gets your appeal, it has 7 days (for a standard appeal) or 72 hours (for an expedited appeal) to notify you of its decision. If you disagree with the plan's decision, you can ask for an independent review of your case. The notice you get with the plan's decision will explain the next level of appeal.*

APPEAL (STANDARD)/MEDICARE

INTRODUCTION

There is a uniform standard process for handling Medicare Part A and Part B claims. All first level appeals are subject to a qualified independent contractor's (QIC) reconsideration. The appeal process consists of the steps set forth below.

(See also *Appeal (Expedited), Non-hospital provider's service termination/Medicare; Appeal (Expedited), Discharge of hospital patient/Medicare; Medicare/Denial Notices*)

I.   STANDARD APPEAL PROCESS.

Initial Determinations by the Fiscal Intermediary (FI). When the FI makes a determination (called "initial determination") with respect to a claim, the beneficiary may appeal the determination and seek re-determination from the FI.

Re-determination by the FI. This is the <u>first</u> level of appeal. The FI will make a re-determination of its initial determination.

Reconsideration by the QIC. If the FI upholds its re-determination, this is the <u>second</u> level of appeal by the beneficiary. The QIC, a new review entity, will reconsider the re-determination of the FI.

Hearing before the Administrative Law Judge (ALJ). If the QIC upholds the re-determination decision of the FI, this is the <u>third</u> level of appeal by the beneficiary. The ALJ will review the reconsideration decision of the QIC.

Review by Departmental Appeals Board (DAB). If the ALJ upholds the reconsideration decision by the QIC, this is the <u>fourth</u>

level of appeal by the beneficiary. The DAB will review the ALJ decision.

Federal District Court. If the DAB upholds the ALJ decision, this is the <u>fifth</u> and final level of appeal.

(See Illustrative Chart in section II, a restatement of the foregoing description of the Medicare appeal process.)

II.   ILLUSTRATIVE CHART.

The chart below illustrates the levels in the standard appeal process, the amount in controversy (AIC) to qualify for an appeal, the number of days to file an appeal, and the time limit for a decision.

<u>Levels of the Standard Appeal Process</u>

<u>Initial Determination by FI</u>	<u>Second Level of Appeal – Reconsideration by the QIC</u>
• The required **amount** in **controversy** (AIC) – $0 • The number of days to file an appeal for re-determination by the FI of the initial determination – 120 days	• The required AIC – $0 • The time limit for a **reconsideration** by the AIC – 60 days • The number of days to file appeal for a hearing to ALJ – 60 days
<u>First Level of Appeal – Re-determination by FI</u>	<u>Third Level of Appeal – ALJ Hearing</u>
• The required AIC – $0 • Time limit for a **re-determination** – 60 days • The number of days to file for a **reconsideration** by the QIC – 120 days	• The required AIC - $120 • The time limit for ALJ decision – 90 days • The number of days to file for review by DAB – 60 days

Levels of the Standard Appeal Process	
Fourth Level of Appeal – DAB Review	**Final Appeal – Federal District Court**
• The required AIC – $0 • The time limit for DAB decision – None • The number of days to file appeal to the Federal District Court – 60 days	• The required AIC – $1,180 • The time limit for decision – None

(continued on next page)

APPEAL (EXPEDITED), DISCHARGE OF HOSPITAL PATIENT/MEDICARE

INTRODUCTION

Hospital inpatients denied continued stay by the hospital may resort to an expedited appeal process to appeal the denial. The appeal process is different depending on whether the patient's physician agrees with the hospital's decision to discharge the patient or not, as discussed below.

I. WHEN THE PATIENT'S PHYSICIAN CONCURS WITH THE DISCHARGE DECISION OF THE HOSPITAL.

Notice of Non-Coverage

When a patient disagrees with the hospital's discharge decision, before any discharge from the hospital, the hospital must deliver to a patient a notice of non-coverage. The notice is generic and simple and must be given by the hospital on the day before the patient is to be discharged.

A beneficiary who has received a notice of non-coverage has the right to, and may request, an expedited determination by the quality improvement organization (QIO).

Expedited Determinations by QIO

Should the patient seek an expedited determination by the QIO, he/she must submit a request for the expedited determination to the QIO. The request may be in writing or by telephone. The patient's request must be submitted by noon of the first working day after he/she has received the hospital's notice of non-coverage.

On the day the QIO receives the patient's request, the QIO must notify the hospital that the beneficiary has filed a request for immediate review of the hospital's discharge decision. The hospital in turn must deliver a detailed notice to the patient, explaining why services are no longer reasonable or necessary, or are otherwise no longer covered by Medicare. The notice must be given by the close of business on the date of the QIO's notification to the hospital of the patient's request for an expedited determination.

The QIO's review must take place, and the QIO's determination must be made within three (3) working days from the request by the patient for such determination. When the QIO issues its expedited determination, the QIO must notify the patient, the physician of the patient and the hospital of its decision by telephone and subsequently in writing. If the QIO affirms the hospital discharge, the patient may request expedited reconsideration by the qualified independent contractor (QIC).

Expedited Reconsideration By QIC

If the individual is still a patient in the hospital, and is dissatisfied with the QIO's initial determination, he or she may request an expedited reconsideration by the QIC. The QIC must make its decision within seventy-two (72) hours of the patient's request for an expedited reconsideration.

If the patient is dissatisfied with the decision of the QIC following the reconsideration (or following the QIO's initial determination), the patient may pursue the regular appeals process. However, appellate review is available only when the amount in controversy exceeds $200 to obtain an administrative hearing and $2,000 to receive judicial review.

II.   WHEN THE PHYSICIAN DISAGREES WITH THE HOSPITAL'S DISCHARGE DETERMINATION.

If the hospital, directly or through its utilization review committee, believes that the beneficiary does not require further inpatient hospital care but is unable to obtain the agreement of the physician, it may request an expedited determination by the QIO. The hospital must notify the beneficiary of its request.

Expedited Determination by QIO

On the date the QIO receives the hospital's request for a review, it must notify the patient and the patient's physician of the hospital's request. The QIO must make a determination and notify the hospital, the patient and the patient's physician within two (2) working days, of its determination. The QIO's notification must be done telephonically and subsequently with a written notice.

The notice must contain a basis for determination, a rationale for determination, and, if the determination affirms the hospital's discharge decision, a statement informing the beneficiary of his/her appeal rights.

Expedited Reconsideration by QIC

If the patient is dissatisfied with the QIO's determination, he/she may request an expedited reconsideration by the appropriate QIC in writing or by telephone, by no later than, noon of the calendar day following initial notification of the QIO's determination.

On the day the QIC receives the patient's request for an expedited reconsideration, the QIC must notify the QIO of the request. No later than seventy-two (72) hours after receipt of the patient's request for an expedited reconsideration, the QIC must notify the QIO, the patient and the patient's physician of its determination. The notice may be done by telephone, followed by a written notice and will set forth the patient's right to appeal the QIC's reconsideration decision.

(continued on next page)

APPEAL (EXPEDITED), NON-HOSPITAL PROVIDER'S SERVICE TERMINATION/MEDICARE

INTRODUCTION

Set forth below is the expedited appeal process when a non-hospital provider (as defined below) terminates services to a beneficiary.

The term "provider" (as used in a non-hospital process of termination of services) includes a skilled nursing facility (SNF), a home health agency (HHA), a comprehensive outpatient rehabilitation facility (CORF), and a hospice. A termination of Medicare coverage service is (i) discharge of the beneficiary by the provider of services or, (ii) a complete cessation at the end of a course of treatment. Termination does not include a reduction of services.

Before any termination of services, the provider must deliver a written general standard notice (provider's standard notice) to the beneficiary of the provider's decision to terminate services. The provider must give such notice to the beneficiary no later than two (2) days before the proposed end of the services and must provide a description of the beneficiary's right to obtain an expedited determination by the quality improvement organization (QIO) of whether the provider's decision was correct, and how to request an expedited determination by the QIO and expedited reconsideration by a qualified independent contractor (QIC). Beneficiaries may seek expedited review of the service termination.

The expedited appeal process is described below.

I. EXPEDITED DETERMINATION BY QIO.

A Request by Beneficiary. A beneficiary, who wishes to exercise the right to an expedited determination, must submit a request for such determination to the QIO by no later than noon of the calendar day following receipt of the provider's standard notice.

Continuing Coverage. The coverage of the provider's services will continue until the date and time designated in the notice.

Notice by QIO. On the day that the QIO receives a request for expedited determination, it must notify the provider that a request for an expedited determination has been made.

Notice by Provider to Beneficiary. The provider must send a detailed notice (detailed explanation of non-coverage) to the beneficiary by the close of business of the QIO's notification, setting forth why the services are either no longer necessary or no longer covered.

QIO's Determination. Not later than seventy-two (72) hours after receipt of the beneficiary's request for an expedited determination, the QIO must notify the beneficiary, the beneficiary's physician and the provider of the QIO's determination as to whether the termination by the provider was a correct decision. The QIO's notification may be by telephone followed by a written notice.

The QIO's notice of its determination should set forth the rationale for the determination, and the beneficiary's rights to an expedited reconsideration by the QIC, of the QIO's determination including information about how to request such expedited reconsideration.

II.   EXPEDITED RECONSIDERATION BY QIC.

The beneficiary has the right to expedited reconsideration by an appropriate QIC of the QIO's expedited determination. A beneficiary who wishes to obtain expedited reconsideration must submit a request for the reconsideration to the appropriate QIC, in writing or by telephone, no later than noon of the calendar day following the receipt of the QIO's notice of termination.

On the day the QIC receives a request for an expedited reconsideration, it must immediately notify the QIO and the provider of the request by the beneficiary for an expedited reconsideration.

No later than seventy-two (72) hours after receipt of the request for expedited reconsideration, the QIC must notify the QIO, the beneficiary, the beneficiary's physician, and the provider of its decision. The QIC's initial notification may be done by telephone, followed by written notice (QIC notice). The QIC notice will set forth the rationale for the QIC's decision, and information about the beneficiary's right to appeal the QIO's reconsideration to an Administrative Law Judge, including how to request an appeal and the time period for doing so. When a beneficiary requests an expedited reconsideration by the QIC, the provider may not bill the beneficiary for any services until the QIC makes its decision.

(continued on next page)

APPEAL (STANDARD)/MEDICARE ADVANTAGE ORGANIZATIONS (MA)

INTRODUCTION

The appeals procedure in Medicare Part C (Medicare Advantage (MA)) plans is different from that applicable to Original Medicare. The MA standard appeals process entitles enrollees of these plans to the right to:

1. An **organization determination**

   - Standard (service related, payment related)
   - Expedited (only if service related);

2. A **reconsideration by the MA organization** of an adverse organization determination

   - Standard (service related)
   - Standard (payment related)
   - Expedited (service related);

3. A **review by the independent review entity**;

4. An **Administrative Law Judge (ALJ) hearing**;

5. Request a **Departmental Appeals Board** (DAB) review of the ALJ hearing decision; and

6. A **judicial review** (see section V below) of the hearing decision.

(continued on next page)

41

The foregoing process is described below.

I.   ORGANIZATION DETERMINATIONS BY MA ORGANIZATION.

An organization determination is any determination made by a MA organization regarding:

Payment for temporary out-of-area renal dialysis services, emergency services, post-stabilization care, or urgently needed services;

Payment for any other health services furnished by a provider other than the MA organization that the enrollee believes is covered under Medicare;

The MA organization's refusal to provide or pay for services, including the type or level or services, that the enrollee believes should have been furnished, arranged for, or reimbursed by the MA organization;

Denial, reduction or termination of a service if the enrollee believes that continuation of the services is medically necessary; or

Failure of the MA organization to timely furnish or pay for health care services.

The time frames within which an organization must make its organization determinations depends upon whether they are related to services or to payment, and are divided into two categories – standard (service related, payment related) and expedited (only service related) as set forth below:

Standard MA Organization Determinations (service related)

When an enrollee or representative requests a service, the organization must notify the enrollee in writing of its determination as expeditiously as the enrollee's health condition requires, but no later than (that is, not to exceed (NTE)) fourteen (14) days after the date on which the organization received the enrollee's request for a determination. This time frame is subject to a possible extension requested by the enrollee, or by the organization if there is a justified need for additional information on the part of the organization and the extension is in the interest of the enrollee.

Standard MA Organization Determinations (payment related).

A difference is made in the time frames within which determinations must be made where a claim for payment is (i) a "clean claim", and (ii) other claims for payment. When there is a request for payment (other than a clean claim), the organization must make a determination NTE sixty (60) days from the date of receipt of the payment request. However, clean claims must be paid NTE thirty (30) days of receiving the payment request. Clean claims are claims that have no defect or impropriety, do not lack any required substantiating documentation, and do not require special treatment that prevents timely payments.

Expedited MA Organization Determinations (only service related).

An enrollee or physician (whether affiliated with the organization or not) can orally or in writing request an expedited organization determination with respect to the organization's refusal to provide service (when the enrollee has not received the service outside the plan) or its discontinuance of the service. Requests for determination as to payments are not subject to expedited organization determinations.

If the organization approves the request for an expedited organization determination or if a physician (whether affiliated with the organization or not) requests an expedited time frame, indicating that to apply the standard time frame (i.e., fourteen (14) days) for making the determination could serious jeopardize the life or health of the enrollee, or the enrollee's ability to regain maximum function, then the organization must:

> make its determination, NTE seventy-two (72) hours after receiving the request, (subject to possible extension of time, if the enrollee requests the extension or the organization justifies a need for additional information and that the delay is for the benefit of the enrollee); and

> first notify the enrollee of the determination orally, and then send written notification within two (2) days of the oral notification.

If the organization denies a request for expedited action, it must give the enrollee oral notice of the denial, and within three (3) days, send a letter explaining that a determination will be made NTE fourteen (14) days of receiving the request, and that the enrollee can file a grievance with the organization, if he/she so desires. If the organization denies a service request, it must so notify the enrollee, and inform the enrollee of his/her right to a reconsideration determination and to the rest of the appeal process.

II. RECONSIDERATION DETERMINATION BY MA ORGANIZATION.

This is the first step in the review of an adverse organization determination. A reconsideration request may be made by the enrollee or his/her representative, an enrollee's assignee, or a legal representative of a deceased enrollee's estate.

The request for reconsideration must be in writing and filed with the organization that made the organization determination or a Social Security office or, in the case of a qualified railroad retirement beneficiary, a Railroad Retirement Benefit office. The request must be made NTE sixty (60) days of the date of the notice of the organization determination. The request may be for a standard reconsideration determination (service related or payment related) or an expedited reconsideration determination (only service related):

Standard Reconsideration Determination by MA Organization (service related).

Should the organization make a reconsideration determination that is completely favorable to the enrollee, then the organization must issue the determination as expeditiously as the enrollee's health condition requires, and must authorize or provide the service, NTE thirty (30) days from receipt of the request for reconsideration.

Should the organization affirm in whole or in part its adverse organization determination (by making a determination that is wholly or partially unfavorable to the enrollee), the case file and the issues that remain in dispute must be sent to, and reviewed and resolved by an independent review entity (IRE) selected by the CMS. This submission must be made as expeditiously as the enrollee's condition requires, but not after more than thirty (30) days (subject to extension) from the date of the request for review by the IRE. When the IRE makes its determination, it must mail notice of this determination to the parties and to the CMS not later than thirty (30) days from the date of the request for IRE review. If the IRE determination is adverse, the enrollee must be informed of his/her right to an ALJ hearing, if the amount in controversy is $100 or more. However, if the entity should rule in favor of the enrollee, the organization must authorize or provide the service as expeditiously as the enrollee's health requires, but not later (NTE) than sixty (60) days from the date the organization receives notice reversing its organization determination.

Standard Reconsideration Determination by MA Organization (payment related)

Should the organization make a reconsideration determination that is completely favorable to the enrollee, the organization must issue its determination and pay the requested payment NTE sixty (60) days from the date it receives the request for reconsideration.

Should the organization make a reconsideration determination that is partially or completely unfavorable to the enrollee, it must send the case file to an IRE, selected by the CMS, for review and resolution NTE sixty (60) days from the date it receives the reconsideration request for review and resolution. The entity must render its decision as expeditiously as an enrollee's health condition requires, but not more than (NTE) thirty (30) days (subject to extension in certain cases) from the date it received the request for IRE review.

The IRE must send the enrollee and the CMS written notice of its determination, stating the reasons for its determination. Should the entity's decision be adverse to the enrollee, the notice must inform the enrollee of his/her right to an ALJ hearing, if the amount in controversy is $100 or more.

Should the entity decide in favor of the enrollee, the organization must pay for the service as expeditiously as the enrollee's health condition requires, but not more than (NTE) sixty (60) calendar days from the date the organization receives notice reversing the organization determination.

Expedited Reconsideration Determination by MA Organization (services related)

Enrollees, their representatives, or physicians may request an expedited reconsideration of an organization determination involving a request relating to a service, or discontinuance of a service. Expedited reconsiderations may not involve a payment-related case. The organization can first notify the enrollee orally, but must send a written notice within NTE two (2) days.

If the organization makes an expedited reconsideration, which is completely favorable to the enrollee, it must issue such determination as expeditiously as the enrollee's health condition requires, but not more than seventy-two (72) hours after receiving the request. If the organization does issue such an expedited reconsideration (i.e., one which is completely favorable to the enrollee), the organization must authorize or provide the service as expeditiously as the enrollee's health condition requires, but not later than thirty (30) days from the date the organization received the reconsideration request.

The organization may deny an enrollee's request for expedited reconsideration but must grant the request of any physician for an expedited reconsideration.

If an organization denies the request for an expedited reconsideration, it must give the enrollee prompt oral notice and follow up, NTE three (3) days with a written notice that (i) the request was denied and (ii) the reconsideration determination will be made by the organization in the standard time frame for reconsiderations NTE thirty (30) days of receiving the request.

If the organization makes an expedited reconsideration that is partially or wholly unfavorable to the enrollee, it must deliver the case file to the IRE as expeditiously as the enrollee's health condition requires, but not later than (NTE) twenty-four (24) hours of its determination. The IRE must make its decision as expeditiously as the enrollee's condition requires, but not later (NTE) than seventy-two (72) hours (subject to a possible extension in certain cases). The entity must mail a written notice of its determination to the enrollee, and to the CMS, stating the reasons for its decision. If the decision is adverse to the enrollee, the notice must notify the enrollee of his/her right to a hearing before the ALJ, if the amount in controversy is $100 or more. If the IRE should decide in favor of the enrollee, the organization must authorize or provide the requested service as expeditiously as the enrollee's health requires, but not later than seventy-two (72) hours from the date the organization receives notice reversing its organization determination.

III.   HEARING BEFORE ALJ.

If the amount in controversy is $100 or more, the enrollee (or other proper party acting on his/her behalf), if dissatisfied with the IRE determination, has a right to a hearing before an Administrative Law Judge (ALJ). The written request for a hearing is made before either the organization that issued the organization determination, a Social Security office or, in the case of a qualified railroad retirement beneficiary, a Railroad Retirement Benefit office, whereupon the aforesaid organization must forward the request to the IRE that made the IRE determination, and the entity must transfer the case to the appropriate ALJ hearing office. The enrollee must file his/her request for a hearing NTE sixty (60) days of the date of the determination by the IRE.

IV.   DEPARTMENTAL APPEALS BOARD REVIEW.

If the enrollee is dissatisfied with the ALJ hearing decision, he/she may request the Departmental Appeals Board to review the decision.

V.   JUDICIAL REVIEW.

Any party, including the organization, may request judicial review of an ALJ final decision, if the amount in controversy is $1,000 or more.

(continued on next page)

APPEAL (EXPEDITED), DISCHARGE OF HOSPITAL PATIENT/MEDICARE ADVANTAGE ORGANIZATION

INTRODUCTION

There is an alternative means for a hospital inpatient, who is an enrollee of a MA organization, to appeal to the quality improvement organization (QIO) for its immediate review of a determination made by the organization or the hospital that the enrollee/patient is no longer entitled to hospital care. This alternative process of appeal is described below.

I. ISSUANCE OF NOTICE OF NON-COVERAGE.

Where an MA organization has authorized coverage of the inpatient admission of an enrollee, either directly or by delegation (or the admission constitutes emergency or urgently needed care), the MA organization (or hospital that has been delegated by the organization to make the discharge decision) must provide a written notice of non-coverage to the patient when:

>The beneficiary disagrees with a discharge decision; **or**

>The MA organization (or hospital delegated the authority to make the discharge decision) is not discharging the individual but no longer intends to continue coverage of the inpatient stay.

The written notice of non-coverage must be issued no later than the day before hospital coverage ends. The written notice must include the following:

>The reason why inpatient hospital care is no longer needed.

>The effective date and time of the enrollee's liability for continued inpatient care.

The enrollee's appeal rights.

An enrollee is entitled to coverage until at least noon of the day after such notice is provided.

II.   PHYSICIAN CONCURRENCE REQUIRED.

Before notice of non-coverage is provided, the entity that makes the non-coverage/discharge determination (the MA organization or the hospital by delegation of the MA organization) must obtain the concurrence of the physician who is responsible for the enrollee's inpatient care.

III.   EXPEDITED REVIEW OR RECONSIDERATION.

An enrollee who wishes to appeal a determination by an MA organization or hospital that inpatient care is no longer necessary may request immediate QIO review of the determination. An enrollee who requests immediate QIO review may remain in the hospital with no additional financial liability. Persons who fail to ask for an immediate review may request expedited reconsideration, but will be subject to financial liability for costs of the hospital stay and care.

An enrollee who fails to request immediate QIO review may request expedited reconsideration by the MA organization, but the financial liability rules (see section IV below) do not apply.

For the immediate QIO review process, the following rules apply:

The enrollee must submit the request for immediate review to the QIO that has an agreement with the hospital, in writing or by telephone, by noon of the first working day after he or she receives written notice that the MA organization or hospital has determined that the hospital stay is no longer necessary.

On the date it receives the enrollee's request, the QIO must notify the MA organization that the enrollee has requested immediate review.

The QIO must make a determination and notify the enrollee, the hospital, and the MA organization by close of business of the first working day after it receives all necessary information from the hospital, or the organization, or both.

IV.   LIABILITY FOR COSTS OF CONTINUED STAY.

If the MA organization authorized coverage of the inpatient admission directly or by delegation, the organization continues to be financially responsible for the costs of the hospital stay, from the time an appeal is filed until noon of the calendar day following the day the QIO notifies the enrollee of its review determination.

If coverage of the hospital admission was never approved by the MA organization (or the admission does not constitute emergency or urgently needed care), the MA organization is liable for the hospital costs only if it is determined on appeal that the hospital stay should have been covered under the MA plan.

The hospital may not charge the MA organization if:

> It was the hospital (acting on behalf of the enrollee) that filed the request for immediate QIO review; and

> The QIO upholds the non-coverage determination made by the MA organization.

If the hospital determines that inpatient hospital services are no longer necessary, and the enrollee could not reasonably be expected to know that the services would not be covered, the hospital may not charge the enrollee for inpatient services received before noon of the calendar day following the day that the QIO notifies the enrollee of its review determination.

(continued on next page)

APPEAL (FAST TRACK), TERMINATION OF NON-HOSPITAL SERVICES/MEDICARE ADVANTAGE ORGANIZATIONS

INTRODUCTION

Before an MA organization may terminate services, an advance written notice must be provided to an enrollee by providers of the services (i.e., home health agencies (HHAs), skilled nursing facilities (SNFs) and comprehensive outpatient rehabilitation facilities (CORFs)). Hence, prior to any termination of service, the provider must deliver advance written notice to an enrollee of the MA organization's decision to terminate service. The advance notice is to be provided no later than two (2) days before the proposed end of services.

The advance notice must include: date that coverage ends; date of enrollee's liability; a description of the enrollee's right to a fast-track appeal to an independent review entity (IRE); an enrollee's right to submit evidence that services should continue; availability of other MA appeal procedures; the right to receive detailed information about the IRE process (see below); and other information required by the Secretary of HHS.

Delivery of notice is not valid unless: (i) the enrollee (or authorized representative) has signed and dated the notice to indicate receipt and comprehension of content; and (ii) notice is delivered. An MA organization is financially liable for continued services until two (2) days after the enrollee receives valid notice.

The fast track appeal process is set forth below.

I. APPEAL TO IRE – IRE DETERMINATIONS.

An enrollee of an MA organization has a right to a fast-track appeal of an MA organization decision to terminate provider services, which can be requested of an IRE (a QIO selected by CMS) in writing or by telephone by noon of the first day after the day of delivery of the termination notice. If the enrollee fails to make a timely request to the IRE, he or she may resort to the standard appeal process and request expedited reconsideration by the MA organization (see *Appeals (Standard)/Medicare Advantage Organizations*).

Coverage of provider services continues until the date and time designated on the termination notice, unless the enrollee appeals and the IRE reverses the MA organization decision.

On the date or receipt of enrollee's request for an appeal, the IRE must immediately notify the MA organization and the provider of the appeal request, and its responsibility to submit documentation as requested by the IRE. The IRE must make a determination and notify the enrollee, the MA organization, and the provider, by close of business of the day after it receives the necessary information for decision. It can defer the determination until it receives necessary information from the MA, and coverage continues until the IRE makes its determination.

II. IRE – RECONSIDERATION.

An enrollee may request an IRE reconsideration of its decision no later than sixty (60) days after notification that the IRE has upheld the decision. The reconsideration must be rendered expeditiously, but no later than within fourteen (14) days of receipt of the enrollee's request. If affirmed in whole or part, the enrollee may appeal the IRE reconsideration decision in turn to the ALJ, the DAB or a Federal court.

(continued on next page)

APPEALS/MEDICAID

INTRODUCTION

Medicaid applicants and recipients are entitled to a notice and a full evidentiary hearing to challenge any agency action to terminate, suspend or reduce Medicaid eligibility or services. If an individual is already eligible, he/she is entitled to continued assistance until the hearing Medicaid claimants have the right to appeal adverse decisions made by the Medicaid program. These decisions involve, among other matters, eligibility requirements; the denial, suspension or reduction of benefits; and the number of hours of homecare services. Claimants have a right to written notice about their claims and the reason for a decision. Generally, the state or local Medicaid agency must mail the notice at least ten (10) days before benefits are reduced or discontinued. This period may be shortened to five (5) days in a fraud matter.

To appeal a decision, a claimant should follow the process and procedures outlined below.

I.   REQUEST FOR A FAIR HEARING.

To request a fair hearing review of a claim, a Medicaid applicant or recipient is entitled to a reasonable time, not to exceed ninety (90) days, from the mailing of the notice of an adverse decision. If a Medicaid recipient (not a new applicant) requests a fair hearing within ten (10) days of the mailing of the notice of the adverse decision, he/she has a right to receive continuing Medicaid benefits, known as aid continuing, until a decision has been reached after a fair hearing.

The right to aid continuing applies to those already receiving Medicaid benefits, not to new applicants.

II.   FAIR HEARING.

A hearing officer who has not participated in the local Medicaid agency's initial adverse decision conducts a fair hearing. The hearing officer's decision is mailed to the Medicaid claimant four (4) to six (6) weeks following the hearing.

III.   *DE NOVO* HEARING.

Within fifteen (15) days of the mailing of the fair hearing decision, a claimant may appeal to the state Medicaid agency for a new hearing, commonly called a *de novo* hearing. If a claimant does not specifically request a *de novo* hearing but merely a general request for a new hearing, the state agency will review only the record of the local hearing, as contrasted to a hearing that includes new and independent evidence. Following the hearing, the claimant will receive a written notice of the decision within ninety (90) days from the date of the request for a hearing.

IV.   JUDICIAL REVIEW BY A STATE COURT.

A claimant may appeal an adverse fair hearing decision to a state court.

Note: In addition to the above formal procedures, a claimant may seek an informal review by calling or meeting with a caseworker at the Medicaid agency. The request for this type of conference review is not a fair hearing request and does not replace such a request nor extend the time limitation for seeking a hearing or a continuation of benefits. A request for an informal review customarily is and should be made together with a request of a fair hearing.

(continued on next page)

APPEALS/SOCIAL SECURITY

INTRODUCTION

All claims and all questions relating to benefits are initially acted upon by the Social Security Administration, which makes an initial determination. (In the case of a disability claim, the initial determination is made after a determination as to disability by the state disability determinations service agency in accordance with rules and regulations of the SSA). In each case the persons concerned are notified in writing of the decision. If they are dissatisfied with the SSA's findings, they may pursue the Social Security appeals process.

The Social Security appeals process consists of the five (5) steps set forth below (I – V). Two further steps are available to a claimant in special cases (see note after section V below).

(See also Social Security Program, section II.)

I. INITIAL DETERMINATION.

A SSA decision relating to an individual's application for claims and matters generally affecting entitlement or payment. Issues involving determinations other than disabilities are for the most part made by staff in the SSA district office without a prior hearing. Determinations about disability and blindness are made by state agencies under contract by SSA and not by SSA itself.

II. RECONSIDERATION.

A claimant who is dissatisfied with an initial determination can request reconsideration within sixty (60) days after date of receipt of notice of an initial determination. The reconsideration review is conducted in the same SSA office that made the initial determination, but generally by staff members who had no part in the initial determination. Generally no adversarial proceeding is involved.

However, where an individual has been the recipient of disability benefits and has been determined not to be disabled or blind, he/she is entitled to a hearing if requested.

III. HEARING.

After receiving an adverse reconsideration determination, a claimant can request a hearing within sixty (60) days from the date of the notice of determination. The hearing is heard by an ALJ whose writing decision contains findings of fact for the basis of the decision. The role of the ALJ at a hearing is to act as a fact-finder and a decision-maker, not an advocate for the government. In disability cases the ALJ may accept post-hearing reports from doctors or other experts. In cases involving termination of disability benefits, the ALJ will consider the claimant's ability to perform substantial gainful activity at the time of the hearing, not at the time of the original termination.

The ALJ, instead of making the initial decision, also may send the case to the appeals council with a recommended decision.

IV. APPEALS COUNCIL REVIEW.

The appeals council is the basic body within the SSA that hears appeals from an ALJ's decision. A claimant, following an adverse decision, may seek review by the council within sixty (60) days after receipt of the ALJ's adverse decision. An appeal to the appeals council is the final stage of administrative review of a person's claim in the Social Security and Medicare appeal process. It is an administrative appeal of a claim by an unsuccessful claimant following a hearing before an ALJ.

V. JUDICIAL REVIEW.

Following an adverse decision by the appeals council, a claimant may appeal that decision by filing a complaint in Federal district court within sixty (60) days after SSA mails the decision.

Note: Expedited appeals to the Federal district court are available to a claimant:

Where request is for SSA to reopen and reverse a determination or decision filed within twelve (12) months of initial determination, or within four (4) years with good cause, or at any time if fraud or similar fault is present in action.

Where request is made after a reconsideration determination or ALJ decision, appeals council review without final decision, or agreement of claimant and SSA, when the only factor preventing favorable decision for claimant is a provision of law which claimant believes is unconstitutional.

(continued on next page)

Appliances/Medicare
See *Durable medical equipment/Medicare.*

Application for Disability Benefits/Social Security

Disability applications are made to the SSA at one of their local offices. The application is more complicated than an application for retirement benefits. The applicant is required to submit substantially the same documents which Social Security requires in support of applications for retirement benefits, plus medical and employment related information. Eligibility will depend on medical conditions and the inability of the worker to work.

Application for Enrollment/Medicare Part A
See *Enrollment/Medicare (Part A, Part B); Eligibility and enrollment/Medicare, sections A.3 and 4.*

Application for Enrollment/Medicare Part B
See *Enrollment/Medicare (Part A, Part B, Part D); Eligibility and enrollment/ Medicare, sections B.2 and 3; Application for enrollment/Medicare Advantage Plan (Part C); Enrollment/Medicare Advantage Plan (Part D).*

Application for Enrollment/Medicare Part D Drug Coverage
See *Enrollment/Medicare Advantage Plan (Part D); Medicare Advantage (MA)/Outpatient Prescription Drugs, section G.*

Application for Medical Assistance/Medicaid

An individual eligible for Medicaid may apply for assistance by following the application process described below:

> A written application on a state-prescribed Medicaid application form is submitted by the applicant to the state agency designated to handle Medicaid applications. A personal interview is necessary. The state agency will accommodate a disabled individual by sending a worker to his/her home. The state agency will require extensive documentation to establish eligibility, (e.g., age 65 or over, citizenship, and income and resources at or below the levels established by the state);

The state agency will make a determination on the applicant's Medicaid eligibility and provide the applicant with a written notice of acceptance or denial. Medicaid reimbursement is generally retroactive to the third month preceding the month of application, if the applicant met eligibility requirements during that period;

Medicaid is usually for an authorized period such as one year. At the end of the authorized period, the Medicaid recipient is required to submit a state Medicaid form seeking recertification for continued eligibility; and

Applications for home care, private duty nursing and personal care require completing further information and nursing assessments and other assessments prescribed by the state agency. (See *Application for personal care/Medicaid*).

Application for Personal Care/Medicaid
See also *Application for medical assistance/Medicaid.*

An application for personal care generally follows the procedures set forth below:

The applications based upon a physician's order will be processed by Medicaid offices, designated by the state, to review such applications;

A physician's order form will customarily provide required information including the client's medical condition and his/her need for assistance with personal care services tasks. The physician or the patient must forward the completed signed form to the appropriate state office together with a Medicaid application if the patient is not yet receiving Medicaid;

Upon receipt of the physician's order, the state Medicaid agency will require a nursing assessment by a registered nurse. The nursing assessment must contain an evaluation of the functions and tasks required by the patient, the degree of assistance required for each function, and, together with the patient, the development of a plan of care. The nurse's assessment will recommend services for a designated number of days per week, and hours per day of personal care services;

Upon receipt of a personal care application, the state Medicaid agency will make a social assessment of the need for personal care services. An assigned case manager will visit the patient and then complete a social assessment form; and

When personal care services will be required for more than sixty (60) continuous days, then additional assessments will be made: an assessment of other services and efficiencies to ensure that the most cost-effective services are being used in every plan of care; and a fiscal assessment. The home health agency which is to deliver the services customarily will perform these assessments, subject to approval by a state Medicaid agency.

Application for Retirement Benefits/Social Security
See also *Social Security Program, section VIII.*

An application is filed at the claimant's local Social Security office and processed by that office. The application can be requested by phone, but is not considered filed until the SSA receives a completed and signed form.

An application may be filed before the claimant is actually eligible for payment of the benefit. Many claimants will file several months before they reach the age of 62 (early retirement) or 67 (normal retirement) so that by the time they reach the respective retirement age, the application will have been approved.

Application for SSI Benefits/Supplemental Security Income
See *Supplemental Security Income, section I.*

Approved Charge (Approved Amount)/Medicare
See also *Fee schedule charge/Medicare; Balance billing/Medicare.*

When a doctor or other provider contracts with Medicare to provide Medicare-covered services under the assignment method, the doctor or other provider accepts the fee schedule amount approved by Medicare as total payment for covered services. Such amount is known as the Medicare-approved charge or Medicare-approved amount. The doctor or other provider will send the patient's claim to Medicare and will be paid directly eighty (80%) percent of the approved charge less any portion of the annual $140 (2012) deductible which the patient may not have paid. The doctor will bill the patient the difference between the approved charge and the amount received from the Medicare carrier.

When the provider does not accept assignment (see *Assignment/Medicare*), the beneficiary must pay for the service and wait until the claim is processed by Medicare for reimbursement. The carrier will pay eighty (80%) of the approved fee directly to the beneficiary, less any amount of the $140 (2012) annual deductible that has not been met. The beneficiary is responsible for paying the full amount of the bill for services which in the case of a doctor or the provider who does not accept assignment may not exceed one-hundred fifteen (115%) percent of the approved charge. This excess charge is banned in several states which have taken the position that by forbidding billing beyond one-hundred fifteen (115%) percent of the Medicare-approved rate, Congress has not created an affirmative entitlement for physicians to balance bill up to that amount.

If an individual receives outpatient therapy services at a hospital, he/she must pay an amount equal to that established by CMS by the Balanced Budget Act of 1997. (See *Outpatient occupational therapy, physical therapy and speech-language pathology/Medicare*)

If an individual receives outpatient services at a hospital, he/she is responsible for paying twenty (20%) percent of the Medicare-approved amount. If an individual receives outpatient mental health services, his/her coinsurance share is fifty (50%) percent of the approved amount.

Area Agency on Aging

See *Older Americans Act (Area Agency on Aging)*.

Artificial Nutrition and Hydration/Medicare

Nutrients and liquids may be provided to a patient through a tube that is inserted into the stomach via the nose or through one that is placed directly into the stomach through which liquid nourishment is delivered. Medicare covers this.

"As good as"/Medicare Part D Drug Coverage

This term is used to compare the cost of a drug insurance plan to the Medicare prescription drug coverage insurance. If the other drug insurance is as good as the Medicare prescription drug coverage insurance, and a plan enrollee chooses to stay with that insurance, there will be no penalty if he/she decides at some time in the future to enroll in the Medicare prescription drug plan.

Assessment (Home Care)/Medicare

See also *Medicare qualifying criteria.*

Before a Medicare beneficiary who meets Medicare qualifying criteria can obtain covered services from a Medicare-certified home health agency, the agency is required to make an initial visit assessment and a comprehensive assessment of a patient's need for Medicare home health care services.

In an initial assessment visit, a registered nurse determines the immediate care and support needs of the patient and the eligibility for the Medicare home health benefits, including homebound status. When rehabilitation therapy (speech-language pathology, physical therapy or occupational therapy) is the only service ordered by the physician and if the need for that service establishes program eligibility, the initial assessment visit may be made by the appropriate skilled professional.

A patient-specific comprehensive assessment must also be conducted by a registered nurse to identify a patient's need for home care, and his/her medical, nursing, rehabilitative, social and discharge planning needs. This assessment must include a review of all medications that the patient is currently using and the outcome and assessment information items prescribed by CMS. When physical therapy, speech-language pathology or occupational therapy is the only serviced ordered by the physician, a physical therapist, speech-language pathologist or occupational therapist may complete the comprehensive assessment and determine the beneficiary's eligibility for the Medicare home health benefit, including homebound status.

Assessment/Medicaid

See *Application for personal care/Medicaid; Snapshot rule/Medicaid; Fiscal assessment/Medicare.*

Assets/Medicaid

See also *Robert Wood Johnson programs/LTCI; Countable resources/Medicaid.*

The term "assets," as used in the context of Medicaid transfer penalty rules, refers to the income and resources of an individual or the individual's spouse which either have been placed in a trust or have been transferred to someone else for less than fair market value. Included are income or resources which such individual is entitled to but does not receive because of his/her own actions, such as a disclaimer, waiver of pension income, waiver of an inheritance, or because of the action of an entity or another person with legal authority to act in place of the individual, such as a court guardian or attorney-in-fact. In contrast, Medicaid eligibility rules treat income and resources separately from each other.

The term also includes an annuity, unless it:

> falls under IRC § 408(b) or (q); <u>or</u>

> is purchased with the proceeds from a trust or account under IRC §408(a)(c) or (p), a simplified employee pension, or a Roth IRA; <u>or</u> is irrevocable and non-assignable, "actuarially sound" (using actuarial publications of the office of the SSA chief actuary), and provides payments in equal amounts during the annuity term. There can be no deferred annuity or annuity with balloon payments which pay interest, plus a relatively small amount of principal monies rather than being actuarially sound, with equal monthly payments.

The Deficit Reduction Act of 2005 (DRA) treats the purchase of an annuity as the transfer of an asset for less than fair market value unless the annuity meets specific requirements including: (i) the state is either the remainder beneficiary in the first position for at least the full amount of medical assistance received by the Medicaid recipient; or (ii) the state is listed as the beneficiary in the second position after the community spouse or disabled or minor child; and the state is named in the first position if either the spouse or the child's representative disposes of the remainder for less than fair market value.

The term "assets" also includes funds used to purchase a mortgage, or for a loan or promissory note unless the repayment term is actuarially sound, provides for payments in equal amounts during the term of the loan without deferrals or balloon payments, and prohibits the cancellation of the balance on the lender's death. For those mortgages, loans or notes that do not satisfy these requirements, the value of the mortgage, loan or a note is the outstanding balance on the date of the individual's Medicaid application.

The term "assets" also includes funds used to purchase a life estate in another's home unless the individual buyer resides in the home for at least one (1) year after the purchase.

Assets/Medicare Part D Drug Coverage

Assets and income are used to determine if a person is eligible for a low-income drug subsidy. Assets include bank accounts, stock accounts, real estate, homes and cars. A primary residence and one car are not included. Assets of both spouses, if married and living in the same household, will be added together to determine eligibility for extra help. (See *Extra help subsidy/Medicare Part D Drug Coverage*).

Assets/Supplemental Security Income (SSI)
See *Countable resources/SSI.*

*Assignment/Medicare

Assignment means that your doctor, provider, or supplier has signed an agreement with Medicare (or is required by law) to accept the Medicare-approved amount as full payment for covered services. Some providers who are enrolled in Medicare don't accept assignment.

Most doctors, providers, and suppliers accept assignment. In some cases, doctors, providers, and suppliers must accept assignment, like when they have a participation agreement with Medicare and give you Medicare-covered services.

If your doctor, provider, or supplier accepts assignment:

Your out-of-pocket costs may be less.

They agree to only charge you the Medicare deductible and coinsurance amount and usually wait for Medicare to pay its share.

They have to submit your claim to Medicare directly. They can't charge you for submitting the claim.

If your doctor, provider, or supplier doesn't accept assignment, they're supposed to submit a claim to Medicare when they give you Medicare-covered services. They can't charge you for submitting a claim. You might have to pay the entire charge at the time of service, and then submit your claim to Medicare to get paid back.

They may charge you more than the Medicare-approved amount, but there is a limit called **"the limiting charge."** They can only charge you up to 15% over the

Medicare-approved amount. The limiting *charge* applies only to certain services and doesn't apply to some supplies and durable medical equipment.

Assignment/Medicare

See also *Approved charge/Medicare; Billing and payment of bills by non-hospital providers for Part B services and supplies/Medicare.*

The understanding by which physicians agree to limit their charges to the amounts approved by Medicare and accept Medicare payment as full payment for services rendered. Doctors who accept this agreement are said to "accept or take assignment." Medicare is directly billed for a doctor's services. Medicare will pay the doctor eighty (80%) percent of the approved charge, less any part of the $140 (2012) Part B annual deductible that the beneficiary has not already met. The

patient is responsible for paying the doctor twenty (20%) percent of the approved charge plus any portion of the $140 (2012) Part B annual deductible not already paid.

(continued on next page)

ASSIGNMENT OF DEATH BENEFITS OF A LIFE INSURANCE POLICY (ACCELERATED BENEFITS)

INTRODUCTION

An individual who is insured under a life insurance contract and who is terminally ill or chronically ill may access during his/her life the death benefits covered by the contract tax-free. These benefits are called accelerated benefits, or sometimes, living benefits.

There are two methods by which the insured may accelerate death benefits of a life insurance contract. The first method is called a viatical settlement. Upon the sale by the insured to a viatical provider of a life insurance contract on the insured's life, or upon the assignment to the provider of the death benefits under the contract, the provider pays the insured all or a portion of the insured's death benefits (see *section I* below). Under the second method, an insurance company directly pays to the insured during his/her life a percentage of the death benefits pursuant to the provision of the life insurance contract (see *section II* below).

Medicaid treats accelerated benefits when collected as resources in determining Medicaid eligibility. It is unclear whether the existence of a living benefits option makes an insurance policy an available resource for Medicaid eligibility purposes.

I. VIATICAL SETTLEMENT.

A. Definition of a Viatical Settlement.

Viatical settlement denotes a transaction whereby an individual who is terminally or chronically ill (as defined in section II below) and is insured under a life insurance contract on his/her life sells the contract, or assigns the death benefits under such contract, to a viatical settlement provider.

B.   Tax Status of a Viatical Settlement.

A viatical settlement provider is any person regularly engaged in the trade or business of purchasing or taking assignment of the death benefit of a life insurance contract of an insured who is terminally ill or chronically ill. Such person must be licensed for such purposes in the state in which the insured resides. Or in the case of an insured who resides in a state that does not require the licensing of such person, he/she must meet the requirements of the Viatical Settlement Model Act and Long-term Care Insurance Model Act of the National Association of Insurance Commissioners.

The insured, if chronically or terminally ill, may receive the proceeds of such a sale or assignment tax-free. The proceeds received are excluded from gross income as if paid by reason of the death of the insured. This exclusion applies, as in the case of accelerated benefits paid to a chronically ill individual under a life insurance contract, only if:

> payment received by the insured is for costs incurred for qualified long-term services rendered to the insured;

> payment or reimbursement of such costs are not made by Medicare; and

> the life insurance contract complies with the consumer protection provisions of the Health Insurance Portability and Accountability Act (HIPAA) applicable to long-term care insurance contracts.

II.   ACCELERATED LIFE INSURANCE BENEFITS UNDER PROVISION OF A LONG-TERM INSURANCE CONTRACT.

A.   Definition of a Qualified Long-Term Care Insurance Contract.

HIPAA extends certain tax advantages to a qualified long-term care insurance (LTCI) contract, sometimes informally called a tax-qualified policy. The law defines such a contract as a guaranteed-renewable life insurance contract or as a rider to a life insurance contract, under which the only insurance protection provided is coverage of qualified long-term care services. A qualified LTCI contract does not pay or reimburse expenses reimbursable by Medicare, except for coinsurance or deductible amounts. Nor may a qualified LTCI contract provide for a cash surrender value or other money that can be paid, pledged or borrowed. Further, certain consumer protection provisions set forth in the Long-term Care Services Model Regulations and Model Act of the National Association of Insurance Commissioners must be part of the contract.

To be qualified, LTCI contracts sold after January 1, 1997 must meet Federal standards explained above. Policies issued prior to this date that have met existing state standards are considered qualified policies though they may not meet the Federal requirements. According to the HIPAA, qualified long-term care services comprise necessary diagnostic, preventive, therapeutic, curing, treating, mitigating and rehabilitative services and maintenance or personal care services which are required by a chronically ill individual and provided pursuant to a plan of care prescribed by a licensed health care provider. The phrase "maintenance or personal care services" means any care the primary purpose of which is the provision of needed assistance with any of the disabilities as a result of which the individual is chronically ill, including severe cognitive impairment. The cost of qualified long-term services can be counted as a medical expense deduction for income tax purposes.

B.   Tax Status of Qualified Long-Term Insurance Contract.

If an insured who has a qualified long-term care insurance contract is terminally ill or chronically ill, he/she may receive accelerated benefits tax free, subject in the case of a chronically ill person to a cap as set forth below. The amount of money received is excluded from the insured's gross income, as if it were paid by reason of the death of the insured.

A terminally ill person is an individual who has been certified by a physician as having an illness or physical condition which can reasonably be expected to result in death in twenty-four (24) months or less after the date of the certification.

A chronically ill person is an individual who:

> is unable to perform without substantial assistance at least two (2) activities of daily living (eating, toileting, transferring, bathing, dressing and continence) for at least ninety (90) days; or

> has a level of disability as determined by the Secretary of Treasury;

> orrequires substantial supervision to protect himself or herself from threats to health or safety due to severe cognitive impairment. In order for a chronically ill individual to obtain tax advantages for accelerated benefits paid under the insurance policy, they must be for qualified long-term care services not reimbursable by Medicare. However, if the insurance policy provides for payment of the benefits on a per diem basis without regard to actual costs, they are excluded from gross income, subject to a cap of $310 per day (2012) or approximately $113,150 per year, annually indexed for inflation. In

the case of a terminally ill insured, no limit is set on how accelerated insurance benefits may be used.

(continued on next page)

Assisted Living Facility

Provides a combination of housing and personalized health care in a professionally managed group-living environment designed to respond to the individual needs of persons who require assistance with activities of daily living.

This type of facility is specifically designed to promote maximum independence and dignity in the most residential and homelike setting possible. It may be all or part of a building that houses a few or several hundred persons, or a distinct part of a residential campus. It traditionally serves the frail resident who cannot or chooses not to live alone, but who does not require the twenty-four- (24) hour skilled or custodial care of a nursing home.

Generally, residents or this type of housing pay privately in the form of rent, rent plus service charge, and sometimes a deposit or entry fee. In some states, Medicaid will pay for certain ADL services under home and community-based service waivers. Medicaid will not pay for room and board charges. Private long-term care insurance may also be used for some of the provided services.

Licensure of this housing type varies by state, depending upon each state's own regulatory requirements. These facilities sometimes are called residential care homes, domiciliary care homes, personal care homes, adult congregate living facilities, homes for the aged, catered living facilities, or board-and-care homes.

Attained Age/Medigap
See *Premiums/Medicare Supplemental Insurance.*

Attendant Care
See also *Activities of daily living (ADL).*

A general term covering the range of non-medical services that help with activities of daily living. Also referred to as custodial care and personal care.

Audiologist

A specialist with a graduate degree who is certified by the American Speech-Language-Hearing Association. This specialist can identify and evaluate hearing problems and recommend and provide therapy to rehabilitate or enhance a person's hearing. The audiologist also specializes in determining when hearing aids are needed and will fit one for a patient.

Audiology

The evaluation and rehabilitative treatment by an audiologist of patients who have impaired hearing.

Automatic Enrollment/Medicare Part A

Enrollment is automatic for most persons age 65 or older who are entitled to <u>and</u> are receiving Social Security or Railroad Retirement benefits. Application by these persons for these benefits is considered to be an application for Medicare Part A and Part B (unless they indicate they do not want Part B), and automatically triggers the enrollment process without the necessity of a separate application.

Enrollment is also automatic for a person, irrespective of age, who has been a disability patient receiving benefits under the Social Security Act or Railroad Retirement Act for twenty-four (24) months. Such patient will automatically receive his/her Medicare card for Part A and Part B benefits.

Should a person be eligible for Social Security or Railroad Retirement benefits but not be receiving those benefits, then eligibility for Medicare Part A is not automatic, and he/she must file an application.

Automatic Enrollment/Medicare Part B

Persons age 65 or older who are entitled to Social Security or Railroad Retirement benefits <u>and</u> are receiving such benefits are automatically eligible for Medicare Part B. As in the case of Medicare Part A, a separate Medicare enrollment for Part B is unnecessary.

Automatic Enrollment/Medicare Part D Drug Coverage

This is the process in which one is enrolled in a Medicare prescription drug plan without having to file an application for enrollment. The automatic enrollment will apply to those eligible for Medicare and Medicaid (full benefit dual eligibles).

Availability of Income and Resources/Medicaid

This term refers to the concept that income and resources must be actually in the applicant's possession or obtainable by reasonable efforts to be "counted," that is included, in determining the financial eligibility of a Medicaid applicant. Availability is an important idea in Medicaid and other public benefit programs to ensure that individuals are not asked to rely on sources of funds that they do not actually have to pay for care. The concept has been the subject of much Medicaid litigation. Decisions do not always favor the applicant, even in instances where funds appear not to be available.

Average Cost of Nursing Facility Care/Medicaid
See *Period of ineligibility/Medicaid.*

Average Indexed Monthly Earnings (AIME)/Social Security
See also *Primary insurance amount (PIA)/Social Security; Bend point/Social Security.*

The average indexed monthly earnings of a worker adjusted for inflation are used to calculate Social Security benefits. The AIME is determined by dividing total indexed earnings (the years of highest earnings up to the countable years) by the number of countable years, converted to months. Countable years used in determining the AIME of workers born after 1928 are the highest thirty-five (35) years of earnings, whereas the AIME of older or disabled or deceased workers is based on record (i.e., actual) years.

(continued on next page)

B

Balance Billing/Medicare

See also *Approved charge/Medicare; Outpatient department hospital services, coinsurance/Medicare; Outpatient occupational therapy, physical therapy and speech-language pathology/Medicare.*

This term refers to health care providers charging patients for amounts above the Medicare-approved charge. By Federal law antedating the Balanced Budget Act of 1997, the maximum allowable charge ("charge limit") may not exceed one-hundred fifteen (115%) percent of the Medicare-approved charge. A number of states – Connecticut, Massachusetts, Minnesota, New York, Ohio, Pennsylvania, Rhode Island and Vermont – have by state statute banned the practice of balance billing. Although the statues have been challenged in Federal courts on preemption grounds, each has withstood the challenge.

Under the Balanced Budget Act of 1997 which created Medicare+Choice (now known as Medicare Advantage (MA)) plans, health care providers may or may not be permitted to engage in the practice of balance billing – depending upon the type of plan, and whether or not the provider has a contract with the plan.

> Providers under contract – Under all Medicare Advantage plans, except private fee-for-service (PFFS) plans, physicians and other health care providers who contract with a MA plan may not balance bill. A contracting physician or other health care provider under a PFFS contract that establishes a payment rate for services may balance bill (i.e., charge) for their services an amount not to exceed, including deductibles, coinsurance, copayments or other balance billing, one-hundred fifteen (115%) percent of such payment rate.

> Providers not under contract – Under all Medicare Advantage plans, except Medicare Advantage medical savings accounts (MSA) and

---

All entries preceded by an asterisk (*) are culled or copied from the official U.S. government **Medicare** handbook (*Medicare & You 2011*).

PFFS plans, non-contracting physicians or other health care providers may not balance bill, but must accept as payment in full from a Medicare Advantage plan enrollee, the amount that would have been paid under traditional Medicare fee-for-service arrangement. A non-contracting physician or other health provider under an MSA or PFFS plan may balance bill without limitation.

Balanced Budget Act of 1997 (BBA '97)

The Balanced Budget Act of 1997 (BBA '97) created by Medicare Part C, also known as the Medicare+Choice program, now known as Medicare Advantage. Medicare Part C added an array of managed care plans for Medicare-covered services while retaining the original Medicare program. The plans are: (i) coordinated care plans, including health maintenance organizations (HMOs), provider service organizations (PSOs), private religious fraternal order plans and both local and regional preferred provider organizations (PPOs); (ii) medical savings accounts (MSAs); and (iii) private fee-for-service plans (PFFS).

BBA '97 also created an option for private contracts (see *Medicare/Private Contracts*) between physicians and their Medicare patients for the receipt of Medicare-covered services for which no Medicare payment will be made. Physicians entering into such contracts must agree not to accept Medicare reimbursement for any Medicare-covered service for two (2) years.

*Barium Enema/Medicare

Once every 48 months if 50 or older (high risk every 24 months) when used instead of a sigmoidoscopy or colonoscopy. You pay 20% of the Medicare-approved amount for the doctor's services. In a hospital outpatient setting, you also pay the hospital a copayment.

Basic Benefits/Medicare Advantage

These include all Medicare Part A and Part benefits, except hospice services.

Basis of Property

The cost of property used to calculate a taxable gain or loss on the sale of property.

Bed/Medicare

See also *Durable medical equipment/Medicare.*

Hospital beds are covered by Medicare.

Bed Hold/Medicaid, Medicare

Preservation of a nursing home bed when a nursing home resident is temporarily hospitalized or out of the facility on therapeutic leave. State Medicaid programs may pay for bed holds, but are not required to. Nursing facility residents on Medicaid have a right to return to the first available bed in the facility which they temporarily left, even if the state has not paid to hold their original bed.

Medicare does not itself pay to hold a bed; moreover, it prohibits facilities from taking payment from beneficiaries to hold a bed if the date of return is certain. If it is not certain, beneficiaries may pay.

Bench Mark/Medicare Advantage

See *Medicare Advantage Plans (MAP/ Common Features, section VI.B.*

Bend Point/Social Security

See also *Primary insurance amount (PIA)/Social Security; Average indexed monthly earnings (AIME)/Social Security.*

Bend points are successive earning levels of a worker's wage-indexed monthly earnings averaged over a working lifetime, as more fully described below:

Monthly retirement, disability and dependents' benefits and survivor benefits depend on a worker's primary insurance amount (PIA). The PIA figure is derived from a formula based on statutorily prescribed percentages, at successive earnings levels, of a "worker's wage-indexed monthly earnings," from "covered employment" (see *Covered employment/Social Security*) averaged over a working lifetime.

The worker's wage-indexed monthly earnings are determined by (a) averaging the worker's thirty-five (35) highest earning years that have been indexed to wage growth and (b) dividing by the number of months in those years. (Earning years are indexed by wage growth not inflation.) This number is called the average-indexed monthly earnings (AIME).

The successive earnings levels, to which statutory percentages apply, are referred to as bend points. Up to the first bend point, Social Security replaces ninety (90%) percent of AIME. Between the first and second bend point, Social Security replaces thirty-two (32%) percent of the worker's average indexed monthly earnings. Above the second bend point, Social Security replaces fifteen (15%) percent of AIME. The term "replacement rate" describes the amount of Social Security benefits received in the first year of retirement as a percentage of the amount of earnings in the last year of employment.

Beneficiary

A beneficiary is the individual or organization designated and entitled to receive the benefits of a will or insurance such as Medicare or a Medigap policy. In a general legal context, the beneficiary of a trust is the person for whose benefit the trust property is to be held or used by the trustee. Beneficial interests can be present or future rights, and vested or contingent.

Benefit Limit and Duration/LTCI

The maximum amount of benefits payable for covered services under LTCI. Although some policies are expressed in terms of a percentage of a reasonable charge defined by the insurer, LTCI policies usually state their benefits as a certain number of dollars per day. Policies may provide an indefinite amount of benefits during the period of time when the policy is in payment status. Typically, however, there will be a limitation on benefits: a maximum amount payable per home care visit; a maximum number of home care visits permitted per day and per year; and a maximum dollar amount payable for institutional care per year.

State insurance regulations usually define LTCI policies as policies that provide at least one or two years of benefits as a minimum benefit duration. Some policies___ offer lifetime benefits as an option. Usual choices by policyholders include durations of two (2), three (3), five (5) or six (6) years.

*Benefit Period/Medicare

The way that Original Medicare measures your use of hospital and skilled nursing facility (SNF) services. A benefit period begins the day you go into a hospital or skilled nursing facility. The benefit period ends when you haven't received any inpatient hospital care (or skilled care in a SNF) for 60 days in a row. If you go into a hospital or a skilled nursing facility after one benefit period has ended, a new benefit period begins. You must pay the inpatient hospital deductible for each benefit period. There is no limit to the number of benefit periods.

Benefit Periods, Part A/Medicare

See also *Part A/Medicare; Spell of illness/Medicare.*

Medicare Part A defines the length of benefits differently according to where care is provided, as set forth below:

> **Hospital.** Medicare covers ninety (90) days of medically necessary care in a Medicare-certified hospital during a single benefit period. If the beneficiary stays more than ninety (90) days in a benefit period, he/she can draw upon sixty (60) lifetime reserve days of Medicare coverage. (See also *Hospital benefit periods and copayments/Medicare*).

> **Skilled nursing facility.** Medicare provides for up to one-hundred (100) days of skilled nursing care in a benefit period if within thirty (30) days after a hospital stay of at least three (3) days. However, this statutorily authorized benefit is subject to the requirement that services be reasonable and necessary. As a result, the average number of days in a stay administratively authorized by Medicare is usually less than one-hundred (100) days. (See also *Skilled nursing facility/Medicare.*)

> **Home care.** Coverage for the services of skilled nurses and home health aides, on a part-time or intermittent basis (not full time), and the services of medical social workers and different kinds of therapists. (See also *Part-time/Medicare; Intermittent/Medicare.*)

> **Hospice.** Medicare covers a benefit period which consists of two periods of ninety (90) days each followed by an unlimited number of 60-day periods provided certain conditions are met. (See also *Hospice care/Medicare.*)

> **Psychiatric hospital.** A lifetime maximum of one-hundred ninety (190) days of inpatient care in a Medicare-participating psychiatric hospital is covered. Psychiatric care provided in a general hospital, however, is not subject to the one-hundred ninety- (190) day limit.

Benefits/Medigap
See *Medicare Supplemental Insurance – Medigap.*

Benefits/Supplemental Security Income (SSI)

Supplemental Security Income benefits generally come from two (2) sources, Federal and state governments. In many states, the two amounts are combined in a single check for the beneficiary. The Federal portion is determined by the status of the applicant, i.e., single or eligible spouse. The Federal benefit may be increased periodically by cost-of-living adjustments. A person can receive both Social Security and SSI benefits. In addition, a person can receive SSI benefits and Medicaid benefits. In many states a person who is eligible for SSI automatically is eligible for Medicaid.

Bequest

Provision in a will that designates personal property as a gift.

Bestower

A person who makes a gift or bequest or creates a trust.

Billing and Payment of Bills by Institutional Providers for Part A and Part B Services and Supplies/Medicare

Billing.
A request (bill) for payment is submitted to the fiscal intermediary by institutional providers (hospitals, skilled nursing facilities, home health agencies and hospices). It is not necessary for a patient to submit bills to Medicare in order for payment to them to be made for services. The provider in turn may bill the beneficiary for applicable coinsurance and deductibles.

Payment of Bills.
In the case of services rendered by institutional providers (skilled nursing facilities, home health agencies and hospices), payments are made by Medicare directly to the provider. The providers in turn may then charge the beneficiary for applicable deductibles and coinsurance payments.

Billing and Payment of Bills by Non-Hospital Providers for Part B Services and Supplies/Medicare
See also *Assignment/Medicare.*

Billing.
A claim (bill) for payment may be submitted to the carrier by the non-institutional provider (physician, practitioner, medical supplier) either on the provider's behalf for payment to the provider, or on behalf of the beneficiary for payment to him/her, depending upon, as set forth below, whether the provider has entered into a participation agreement with Medicare to accept assignment by the beneficiary or not. (A provider who agrees to assignment is known as a participating provider.)

Where provider has accepted assignment. The beneficiary, by signing an assignment statement, will assign to a provider his/her right to payment for services rendered and supplies provided, and authorize payment by Medicare to the provider. Medicare will pay eighty (80%) percent of the Medicare-approved (allowed) charges to the provider.

By accepting assignment, the provider agrees to accept the amount approved by Medicare as the full charge for the services and items rendered and supplied.

Where provider has not accepted assignment of services. Although payment is made to the beneficiary, the provider is responsible for handling, on the beneficiary's behalf, the paper work of claims to Medicare for payment. The provider will bill and seek payment from the beneficiary on the basis of an itemized bill. This method of billing is known as balance billing. Payment will be made by Medicare to the beneficiary for eighty (80%) percent of the Medicare-approved charge. The beneficiary is responsible for paying the bill which amount may not legally exceed one-hundred fifteen (115%) percent of the Medicare-approved charge. This approved charge is known as the limiting charge or actual charge. Several states by statute have prohibited (or limited) balance billing, and thus in effect have mandated assignment.

Payment of Bills.

In the case of services or supplies rendered under Part B by an institutional provider (e.g., home health agency), payments are made by Medicare directly to the provider. The provider in turn may then charge the beneficiary for applicable deductibles and coinsurance payments.

In the case of services or supplies rendered under Part B by physicians, practitioners, or durable equipment suppliers, payment may be made by Medicare to the physician or other providers only if the right to payment is assigned to them by the beneficiary and if they agree to be paid according to the rules of assignment (as set forth above).

Block Grants
See *Social services (Title XX) block grants.*

*Blood/Medicare

In most cases, the provider gets blood from a blood bank at no charge, and you won't have to pay for it or replace it. However, you will pay a copayment for the blood processing and handling services for every unit of blood you get, and the Part B deductible applies. If the provider has to buy blood for you, you must either pay the provider costs for the first 3 units of blood you get in a calendar year or have the blood donated by you or someone else.

You pay a copayment for additional units of blood you get as an outpatient (after the first 3), and the Part B deductible applies.

Blood/Medicare

Medicare Part A helps pay for blood (whole blood or units of packed red cells), blood components and the cost of blood processing and administration. If a person receives blood as an inpatient of a hospital or skilled nursing facility, Medicare will pay for these blood costs after the annual three- (3) pint deductible has been met. A patient is responsible for the non-replacement fees for the first three (3) pints or units of blood furnished by a hospital or skilled nursing facility in any calendar year. The non-replacement fee is the charge that some hospitals and skilled nursing facilities make for blood which is not replaced. If a patient has already paid for or replaced blood under Medicare Part B during the calendar year, he/she does not have to meet those costs again under Medicare Part A. Under Medicare Part B, the first three (3) pints of blood used in any calendar year must be paid for by the patient as a deductible. Medicare Part B will pay eighty (80%) percent of the approved charge for any subsequent pints of blood. The patient must pay the balance of twenty (20%) percent, plus any excess charges.

Board-and-Care Home
See also *Alternative Living Facilities.*

Typically, a board-and-care home is a large house in which several ambulatory seniors, who do not need medical care and who can manage their own medications with little or no assistance, live together. They often have their own bedrooms and share the common areas. There is usually live-in staff or a family that prepares meals and monitors, but does not administer the taking of medications. Laundry and housekeeping may or may not be included.

The term can also sometimes refer to a small facility, frequently having 6-12 beds for seniors who need or desire extra or special assistance. Such a facility is licensed by many but not all states. Generally, levels of activity and supervision differ, as do quality and price. Medicaid may be available for eligible residents.

Board-and-care homes are sometimes called adult homes, adult care homes, adult foster homes, residential care homes, domiciliary care homes, congregate housing and personal care homes.

*Bone Mass Measurement (Bone Density)/Medicare

Helps to see if you're at risk for broken bones. This service is covered once every 24 months (more often if medically necessary) for people who have certain medical conditions or meet certain criteria. Starting January 1, 2011, you pay nothing for this test if the doctor accepts assignment.

Bone Mass Measurement/Medicare

Medicare Part B covers bone mass measurement for women over age 65 who are at high risk for osteoporosis and for beneficiaries with vertebral abnormalities and certain bone defects. These measurements will be covered if at least twenty-three (23) months have elapsed since the last measurement or more frequently if they are determined to be medically necessary.

*Braces (arm/leg/neck)/Medicare

Included among the prosthetic/orthotic items covered by Medicare. In order for Medicare to cover your prosthetic or orthotic, you must go to a supplier that is enrolled in Medicare. You pay 20% of the Medicare-approved amount, and the Part B deductible applies.

Breast Cancer Screening/Medicare
See *Mammography/Medicare.*

Budget Neutrality/Medicare

A method of adjusting Medicare payment rates to providers when laws or rules change so that expenditures under new laws or rules will be the same as they would have been prior to the change.

Budget Period/Medicaid
See also *Spend down/Medicaid.*

The prospective period during which an applicant must spend down his/her income to become eligible for Medicaid as medically needy is called the budget period. It usually varies up to six (6) months for persons living at home and one month for institutionalized persons.

Bundled Payment

A single predetermined payment for a group of health services.

Burial Fund
See also *Exempt resources/Medicaid.*

Medicaid and other government benefit programs do not count in determining an applicant's eligibility as a financial resource, an individual's separate fund of money and/or life insurance policy set aside to pay for his/her burial so long as their combined value is under $1,500.

Buy-in Programs/Medicare/Medicaid

A person who is age 65 or over and who is not eligible for Medicare is able to obtain, that is, buy-in, Medicare Part A coverage by paying monthly premiums fixed by the government. People who obtain Medicare Part A coverage may enroll in and pay Medicare premiums for Part B.

Within the Medicaid program, there are several sub-programs known as buy-in programs or medical savings programs. They assist low-income Medicare beneficiaries to pay some or all of the deductibles and coinsurance under Medicare Part A and Part B, and payment of some or all of the premiums under Medicare Part B. There are several categories of low-income individuals – namely, Qualified Medicare Beneficiaries, Specified Low-Income Medicare Beneficiaries, Qualified Disabled and Working Individuals, and Low-Income Qualified Individuals (QI). (See entries under these named groups.) These beneficiaries may buy-in to the sub-programs without applying for full Medicaid coverage. The payments are made by state Medicaid agencies.

Bypass Trust
See also *Unified credit.*

This trust, also known as a unified credit trust, bypasses taxation in both the decedent's and surviving spouse's estate by use of the decedent's unified credit.

(continued on next page)

C

Cane/Medicare

See also *Durable medical equipment/Medicare.*

A stick used as an aid in walking. It is covered by Medicare if reasonable and necessary for a disabled person eligible for Medicare.

Capitation/Medicare

This payment by Medicare to a health care provider (see *Provider/Medicare*) consists of a fixed, per capita amount for each person served without regard to the actual number or nature of care and services provided to each person. Providers of such services and care do not receive extra payment even though the cost of the services and care exceed the fixed amount. Capitation is in contrast to the fee-for-service method of payment.

*Cardiac Rehabilitation/Medicare

Medicare covers comprehensive programs that include exercise, education, and counseling for patients who meet certain conditions. Medicare also covers intensive cardiac rehabilitation programs that are typically more rigorous or more intense than regular cardiac rehabilitation programs. You pay the doctor 20% of the Medicare-approved amount if you get the services in a doctor's office. In a hospital outpatient setting, you also pay the hospital copayment.

*Cardiovascular Screenings/Medicare

Blood tests that help detect conditions that may lead to a heart attack or stroke. This service is covered every 5 years to test your cholesterol, lipid, and triglyceride levels. You pay nothing for the tests, but you generally have to pay 20% of the Medicare-approved amount for the doctor's visit.

All entries preceded by an asterisk (*) are culled or copied from the official U.S. government **Medicare** handbook (*Medicare & You 2011*).

Care, home health
See *Home health care services; Home Care (Introduction).*

Care, intermittent
See *Intermittent care/Medicare.*

Care, long-term
See *Long-term care.*

Care, medically oriented home
See *Home care services.*

Care, non-medical home
See *Home care services.*

Care, personal
See *Custodial care, personal care/Medicaid; Personal care services/Home Care.*

Care, primary
See *Primary care doctor/Medicare; Primary care/Managed Care.*

Care, respite
See *Respite care.*

Care, subacute
See *Subacute care*

Care Recipient

An older person who requires some level of care and help from another person such as a relative, friend, health professional or home health aide.

Caregiver
See also *Home Care; Home care services; Home health care services/Medicare Long-distance caregiver; Primary caregiver.*

A generic term referring to a person, either paid or voluntary, who helps an older person with the activities of daily living, health care, financial matters, guidance, companionship and social interaction. A caregiver can provide more than one aspect of care. Most often the term refers to a family member or friend who aids the older person. Such caregivers are considered informal caregivers, to differentiate them from a formal or paid caregiver such as a home health aide or other personal care worker.

An organized home care program can be provided through a combination of: (i) informal caregivers, especially family members; (ii) formal caregivers who are medical or other trained persons, such as doctors, nurses, home health aides, therapists, geriatric care managers and social workers; and (iii) non-medical persons, such as personal care aides, community volunteers and city or state personnel. Under the direction of a physician, the care can be oriented to a patient's needs. It may be similar to the level of skilled care provided in a skilled nursing facility (e.g., nursing nutritional services, physical occupational and speech therapy), and more often than not it can be unskilled care in the nature of custodial or personal care.

Family members and friends are the largest single source of support and care for older persons who continue to live at home, but are limited in one or more activities of daily living (ADL). ADLs consist of activities usually performed for oneself in the course of a normal day and are usually considered to be mobility (e.g., transfer from, or to a bed or chair), dressing, bathing, eating and toileting. Assistance to a person limited in his or her ADLs is customarily performed by a family member, home-health aide or attendant (or a nurse's aide in a nursing facility). The assistance is of a non-medical nature (physical) commonly characterized as personal care, or custodial. Assistance provided in a home setting goes beyond ADLs to non-medical activities commonly referred to as instrumental activities of daily living (IADL). These include housekeeping and homemaker's chores (e.g., cleaning, cooking, laundry and shopping).

Carrier/Medicare
See also *Qualified independent contractors/Medicare.*

A private insurance organization which contracts with the Federal government to handle claims from doctors and suppliers of services covered by Medicare Part B supplemental medical insurance.

Carve-out Coverage
See *Coordination of coverage/Medicare.*

Case Management

Case management, also called care management, is the process of planning, coordinating and monitoring needed medical, social, educational and other care services provided by social workers, nurses and others to an older person. Case management can be performed by trained professional case managers who are employed by or under contract to government agencies, such as Medicaid, by home health agencies or by patients and their families. Case managers include geriatric care managers, nurses, social workers and hospital discharge planners.

Formal case management includes assessment as well as planning and ongoing monitoring of the elderly person's medical and nonmedical needs. It is an integral part of long-term care.

States can make these services available through Medicaid community-based waivers, through Medicaid's targeted case management option or through a mandatory Medicaid managed care entity (see *Medicaid mandatory managed care*). For the most part, Medicare does not cover case management.

Cash Balance Pension Plan
See also *Defined benefit plan; Defined contribution plan.*

Some employers replace the traditional defined benefit pension plan with a cash balance pension plan. Compared to a traditional defined benefit plan, the cash balance plan has a front loaded accrual pattern, like that of a defined contribution plan. This means that younger employees will generally accrue more benefits during the early years of employment under a cash balance plan than under the more traditional defined benefit plan. Thus, employees who terminate early will leave their employ with greater benefits than they would have earned under a traditional defined benefit plan. Conversely, employees with a long tenure of employment will leave their employ with fewer benefits than they would have earned under the traditional defined benefit plans.

CAT Scan

Computed tomography (CT), also known as computed axial tomography (CAT), is a painless, sophisticated x-ray procedure. Multiple images are taken during a CT or a CAT scan, and a computer compiles them into complete, cross-sectional pictures ("slices") of soft tissue, bone, and blood vessels.

A CT scan obtains images of parts of the body that cannot be seen on a standard x-ray. Therefore, these scans often result in earlier diagnosis and more successful treatment of many diseases.

*Cataract/Medicare
See *Eyeglasses/Medicare*

*Catastrophic Coverage/Medicare Part D Drug Coverage

Once you reach your drug plan's out-of-pocket limit, you automatically get "catastrophic coverage." Catastrophic coverage assures that once you have spent up to your plan's out-of-pocket limit for covered drugs, you only pay a small coinsurance amount or copayment for the drug for the rest of the year.

If you get Extra Help paying your drug costs, you won't have a coverage gap and will pay only a small or no copayment once you reach catastrophic coverage.

Catastrophic Drug Coverage/Medicare Part D Drug Coverage
See also *Out-of-pocket threshold; Doughnut hole/Medicare Part D Drug Coverage.*

Once an individual has reached out-of-pocket drug threshold has and paid for the drug costs of the coverage gap, known as the doughnut hole costs, the individual, for the rest of the year, only pays a small copayment (called catastrophic drug coverage) for Part D drugs.

Catastrophic Health Insurance

An insurance plan that features low-premium payments and a very high deductible and is designed to cover expensive and lengthy medical treatment. Catastrophic coverage insures against a financial catastrophe caused by very high medical bills in connection with a lengthy illness or disability.

Catastrophic Illness

An illness, generally involving significant cost, which is usually considered to be life-threatening or with the threat of serious continuing disability.

Categorically Needy/Medicaid

All states must provide Medicaid coverage to persons who are in the categorically needy group. This is one of the three main groups of potential Medicaid-eligible persons (i.e., categorically needy, optional categorically needy and medically needy). The classification describes individuals who satisfy the categorical requirements of age 65 or over or are blind or disabled, and in addition satisfy a state's Medicaid financial eligibility requirements of having assets or income below state-determined levels.

In most states an individual who receives SSI is automatically considered to be within this group. A categorically needy individual is not allowed to spend down.

Catered Living Facility
See *Assisted Living Facility.*

Catheters/Medicare
See *Medical supplies/Medicare.*

Centers for Medicaid and Medicare Services (CMS)

This Federal agency is part of the U.S. Department of Health and Human Services and is responsible for Medicare and Medicaid administration and regulations.

Certificate Holder/LTCI
See also *Group long-term care insurance.*

In a group medical insurance policy, a group such as an employer, corporation or charitable organization owns the policy and receives notices from the insurer. Each individual person covered under the group policy receives a certificate or card to evidence participation in the group and is called a certificate holder.

Certified Facility

A facility that meets the minimum standards set for Medicare and/or Medicaid and has agreed to accept Medicare and/or Medicaid patients.

Certified Home Health Agency (CHHA)
See *Home health agency.*

Certified Nurse

A registered nurse who has obtained certification credentials in a specialty such as anesthesiology or intensive care.

Channeling

Refers to an experimental program where providers provide both case management and actual home care services. The term has become associated with several specific Federal projects which have now ended.

Charge for Elective Surgery/Medicare

Medicare requires that for all elective surgical procedures costing more than $500 the physician must provide to the patient a written disclosure of estimated cost. Failure by the physician to give such notice may result in the physician reimbursing the patient the difference between Medicare's approved charge and the physician's charge.

Charge Limit/Medicare
See also *Balance billing/Medicare; Assignment/Medicare.*

The most that a doctor who has not taken "assignment" can charge a patient is one-hundred fifteen (115%) percent of the Medicare-approved amount.

Charitable Foundation

A corporation, usually not-for-profit, or a trust that is created for charitable purposes exclusively. Gifts to such an entity are free of any gift tax and, subject to certain limitations, reduce a decedent's estate for estate tax purposes. Gifts that individuals make to the entity are deductible for income tax purposes subject to certain limitations.

Charitable Lead Trust

A trust that initially provides for payments to a charity, usually for a term of years. When the charity's right to payment ceases, the trust assets are then either distributed outright or continue in trust for named individuals. The value of the gift to the individuals named in the trust is discounted for gift or estate tax purposes, since the receipt is delayed until the flow of payment to the charity ceases. This payment flow has an actuarial value.

Charitable Remainder Trust

This term generally refers to two types of trusts – annuity trust and unitrust – that first benefit a non-charitable beneficiary for life or a term of years and subsequently a charity. The two trusts differ in their methods of calculating payouts. With an annuity trust, payments are based on a fixed percentage of the initial fair market value of the trust. A unitrust pays a fixed percentage of the trust value that is determined annually. The grantor of a charitable remainder trust is entitled to an income, gift or estate tax deduction for the actuarial value of the charity's interest.

Children's Benefits/Social Security

See *Social Security program, sections VII.B and D.*

*Chiropractic Services/Medicare

Helps correct a subluxation (when one or more of the bones of our spine move out of position) using manipulation of the spine. You pay 20% of the Medicare-approved amount, and the Part B deductible applies. You pay all costs for any other services or tests ordered by a chiropractor.

Chiropractor's Services/Medicare

Medicare Part B helps pay for only one kind of treatment furnished by a licensed chiropractor: manual manipulation of the spine to correct a subluxation (i.e., partial dislocation). Medicare Part B does not pay for any other diagnostic or therapeutic services, including x-rays, furnished by a chiropractor.

The Balanced Budget Act of 1997 eliminated a previous requirement for a subluxation to be demonstrated by an x-ray before Medicare would pay for correction of the subluxation. The Secretary of HHS is required to develop and implement utilization guidelines for chiropractor services when a subluxation is not demonstrated by an x-ray to exist.

Chore Service

Help with repairs and non-medical chores inside and outside of a house or apartment. Chore services are often provided through the local area agency on aging, volunteer programs or youth groups to help older people live safely and comfortably in their own homes. Such services are not covered by Medicare.

Chronic Care

Care needed over a long period for a condition or illness from which an individual may not recover, as opposed to acute care needed to treat a relatively brief episode of illness or accident.

Claimant/Social Security

Someone who has filed a claim or application for Social Security benefits.

*Claims/Medicare

If you get a Medicare-covered service, you will get a Medicare Summary Notice (MSN) in the mail every 3 months. The MSN shows all of your services or supplies that providers and suppliers billed to Medicare during the 3-month period, what Medicare paid, and what you owe the provider.

Claims for Services/Medicare
See also *Waiver of liability/Medicare*

Under Medicare Part A it is not necessary for a patient to submit bills to Medicare in order for payment to be made. The provider of the service will submit the patient's claim to Medicare for payment. A Medicare claim determination will indicate the services provided and the coverage determinations.

In the case of claims covered by Medicare Part B, a doctor or supplier must submit a request that Medicare Part B payment be made for covered services, whether or not assignment is taken. The doctor or supplier should fully complete a formal request and send it to the proper Medicare carrier.

If an individual is enrolled in a Medicare Advantage plan, a claim will seldom need to be submitted on a patient's behalf. Medicare pays the Medicare Advantage organization a set amount (capitation) each month to cover services rendered to an enrollee by a provider in the organization's network.

If the claim of the beneficiary is for the rental of durable medical equipment, a doctor's prescription must be included with the claim. The prescription must show the equipment the patient's needs, the medical reason for the need and an estimate of how long the equipment will be medically necessary.

Cleaning Services

These services are not covered by Medicare.

Clinic

A facility, or part of one, for diagnosis and treatment of outpatients. It may be a freestanding building or within a hospital.

*Clinical Laboratory Services/Medicare

Includes certain blood tests, urinalysis, some screening tests, and more. You pay nothing for these services, but you generally have to pay 20% of the Medicare-approved amount for the doctor's visit.

Clinical Laboratory Tests/Medicare

Medicare will generally pay the full cost of these tests, which are those usually performed on body fluids such as blood or urine. Both independent labs and doctors must bill Medicare directly for one-hundred (100%) percent of the cost of covered lab services and cannot bill the patient for any deductible or copayment of any kind.

Clinical Nurse Specialist (CNS)/Medicare

A clinical nurse specialist is a registered nurse licensed to practice nursing in the state in which the services are performed and holds a Master's degree in a defined clinical area of nursing from an accredited nursing institution.

Historically, Medicare paid separately for CNS services only when provided in collaboration with a physician and only in a nursing home or a rural area setting. Under the Balanced Budget Act of 1997, CNSs became eligible for separate Part B payments if they provide physician-type services in any setting, but only as long as Medicare does not pay the facility or provider for their services. The CNS is paid eighty (80%) percent of the lesser of either the actual charge or eighty-five (85%) percent of the fee prescribed by the Medicare physician fee schedule.

Cluster Care

This is a cost-effective model of homemaker services for several senior residents living in a multi-unit housing complex. Traditionally, an individual contracts with an agency to provide the services of an aide for a minimum number of hours. With the cluster care model, one or more aides will service the needs of all home care recipients in one building, and thereby eliminate the need for an individual to pay for a minimum number of hours, and also allow an aide to revisit residents more than once a day if necessary.

COBRA Health Care Continuation Benefits
See *Consolidated Omnibus Budget Reconciliation Act (COBRA) of 1985*

COBRA Widow (Widower)

The Social Security Act was amended to provide disabled widows or widowers with increased disability benefits. As a result, many within this group lost their Medicaid coverage because their increased income put them over the SSI level.

To offset this result, the Consolidated Omnibus Budget Reconciliation Act of 1985 (COBRA) extended coverage of these individuals by granting to categorically needy widows or widowers all Medicaid benefits, which they otherwise would have had except for the increase of their disability benefits.

Cognitive Impairment Trigger/LTCI
See also *Long-term care insurance, tax status.*

A provision in a LTCI policy that will furnish insurance benefits based on documentation that the covered person suffers from memory impairment, impaired ability to reason, or loss of orientation to person, place and time, and therefore requires supervision. This provision or trigger is useful for persons such as Alzheimer's patients who are mobile and in good physical health, but cannot be left alone safely.

For a LTCI policy issued after January 1, 1997 to be tax-qualified – that is, for a portion of its premiums to be eligible for treatment as a medical deduction on income taxes – it must have a cognitive impairment trigger that is not linked to any ADL triggers.

Coinsurance, Part A/Medicare

The amount or percentage of the Medicare-approved charge which a patient must pay over and above that which Medicare will pay for inpatient care at a hospital, for care at a skilled nursing facility and for durable medical equipment (outpatient) is called coinsurance, also sometimes termed copayment. Specifically these amounts or percentages are as follows:

Hospital. The first day of the first sixty (60) days, a patient pays the deductible of $1,156 (2012). For days 61-90, the patient must pay $289 (2012) a day. For days 91-150, the patient pays $578 (2012) a day. (See also *Lifetime reserve days/Medicare*.)

Skilled Nursing Facility. Medicare eligibles pay nothing for the first twenty (20) days. For the 21st through the 100th days, the patient must pay $144.50 (2012), with Medicare paying the balance.

Durable Medical Equipment. Medicare pays eighty (80%) percent of the approved charge, and the patient pays the remaining twenty (20%) percent.

Coinsurance, Part B/Medicare

The Medicare beneficiary must share (cost sharing) in the payment of most Medicare services and durable medical equipment under Medicare Part B. The coinsurance by the beneficiary is normally twenty (20%) percent, with Medicare paying eighty (80%) percent, of the applicable Medicare approved charge. For clinical diagnostic laboratory tests provided by a laboratory or physician accepting Medicare assignment, Medicare will pay one-hundred (100%) percent. For non-hospital treatment of mental illnesses, the beneficiary must pay thirty-seven and one-half (37.5%) percent, and Medicare will pay sixty-two and one-half (62.5%) percent of Medicare-approved charges.

Coinsurance represents a so-called gap in Medicare coverage. To fill the gaps (i.e., the difference between the amount paid by Medicare and the Medicare-approved charges), Medicare-eligibles may obtain private Medigap insurance policies to protect against these areas in which the Medicare program is deficient in coverage.

*Colonoscopy/Medicare

Colonoscopy is a test that allows your doctor to look at the inner lining of your large intestine (rectum and colon). A colonoscopy helps find ulcers, colon polyps, tumors, and areas of inflammation or bleeding. This exam is generally conducted once every 120 months (high risk every 24 months) or 48 months after a previous flexible sigmoidoscopy. No minimum age. Starting January 1, 2011, you pay nothing for this test if the doctor accepts assignment.

*Colorectal Cancer Screenings/Medicare

To help find precancerous growths or find cancer early, when treatment is most effective.

Fecal Occult Blood Test – Once every 12 months if 50 or older. You pay nothing for the test, but you generally have to pay 20% of the Medicare-approved amount for the doctor's visit.

Flexible Sigmoidoscopy – Generally, once every 48 months if 50 or older, or 120 months after a previous screening colonoscopy for those not at high risk. Starting January 1, 2011, you pay nothing for this test if the doctor accepts assignment.

Colonoscopy – Generally once every 120 months (high risk every 24 months) or 48 months after a previous flexible sigmoidoscopy. No minimum age. Starting January 1, 2011, you pay nothing for this test if the doctor accepts assignment.

Barium Enema – Once every 48 months if 50 or older (high risk every 24 months) when used instead of a sigmoidoscopy or colonoscopy. You pay 20% of the Medicare-approved amount for the doctor's services. In a hospital outpatient setting, you also pay the hospital a copayment.

Colorectal Screening/Medicare

Medicare Part B covers fecal-occult blood tests every twelve (12) months, flexible sigmoidoscopies every four (4) years for average-risk beneficiaries age 50 or over, and colonoscopies every two (2) years for those at high risk. At the attending physician's discretion, a screening barium enema may be substituted for either the screening flexible sigmoidoscopy or the screening colonoscopy, but payment may not be made for both a screening barium enema and one of the other procedures during the specified time interval. Coverage for these tests is subject to the Medicare Part B deductible and the twenty- (20%) percent copayment.

*Community-Based Programs/Medicare

If you're already eligible for Medicaid (or, in some states, would be eligible for Medicaid coverage in a nursing home), you or your family members may be able to get help with the costs of services that help you stay in your home instead of moving to a nursing home. Examples include homemaker services, personal care, and respite care.

Community-Based Care

See also *Older Americans Act; Waivered services/Medicaid.*

In-home care offered by community-based agencies consists of support services that are frequently needed to complement other home care services. They may include:

> Adult social day care;
>
> Advocacy assistance;
>
> Transportation;
>
> Home maintenance tasks;
>
> Housing improvement;
>
> Personal emergency response system (PERS);
>
> Telephone reassurance for the patient; and
>
> Respite care for stressed family members.

The sources of Federal public funding are: Social Services Block Grants, the Older Americans Act, and various Medicaid waiver programs. In addition to Federal programs, many states offer some benefits to augment the services provided in the community.

Community Nursing Organization (CNO)/Medicare

CNOs are Federal demonstration projects designed to test a prepaid capitated payment, under the Medicare program, for community nursing and some ambulatory care furnished to Medicare beneficiaries in a nurse-care managed model. Several sites, each having multiple clinics or satellites, have been awarded contracts. They represent different types of health providers including a home health agency, hospital-based system and multi-specialty clinic. The Balanced Budget Act of 1997 expanded the program to include additional projects.

The more salient features of the CNO program are:

> Each CNO receives a monthly payment for each enrollee, which is equivalent to ninety-five (95%) percent of the anticipated cost for providing CNO services. In addition, each CNO receives $22 per month per enrollee for care management services.

CNO services consist of the following: part-time or intermittent nursing care; therapy (physical, occupational or speech); social related services supportive of a plan of ambulatory care; part-time or intermittent services of a home health aide; and durable medical equipment.

Each CNO utilizes a primary nurse provider to assess patients and the type and amount of services needed and to coordinate services.

Community Rating Policy/Medigap

See *Medicare Supplemental Insurance – Medigap.*

Community Spouse/Medicaid

See also *Spousal impoverishment/Medicaid; Waivered services/Medicaid.*

An individual who resides in the community and is the spouse of an institutionalized person. The term is used in the context of Medicaid eligibility-related income and resource protections for the community spouse. States can also apply such protections to spouses of people receiving waivered home care services.

Community Spouse Excess Income/Medicaid

Income owned by the community spouse of a nursing home patient receiving Medicaid assistance that is above the amount required by law to be set aside for the spouse. None of the spouse's income, whether it is protected or excess, is considered available to Medicaid to pay for nursing home care in determining the Medicaid recipient's eligibility for Medicaid.

Community Spouse Refusal/Medicaid

See *Spousal refusal/Medicaid.*

Community Spouse's Excess Resources/Medicaid

See *Spousal refusal/Medicaid*

Community Spouse's Income Allowance/Medicaid

See also *Minimum monthly maintenance needs allowance/Medicaid; Spousal impoverishment/Medicaid.*

Also called a minimum monthly maintenance needs allowance, this term refers to the amount of income which states are required to permit an institutionalized individual, who is married and receiving Medicaid assistance, to contribute to his/her spouse remaining in the community in order to bring that spouse's income to the minimum monthly allowance. Alternatively, states may also allow resources to be retained by the community spouse in sufficient amount to generate income to raise his/her income to the level of the minimum monthly needs allowance.

The amount allowed to the community spouse can be increased above the statutorily defined cap by court order or at a fair hearing when either spouse can show that exceptional circumstances resulting in significant financial duress require the provision of additional income.

Community Spouse's Resource Allowance (CSRA)/Medicaid

See also *Minimum monthly maintenance needs allowance/Medicaid; Income- first rule/Medicaid.*

The CSRA is an amount of resources that states must protect for the spouse (community spouse) of an institutionalized person seeking Medicaid coverage. It is determined by application of the formula set forth below, or, as explained below, through a fair hearing, or by court order. The CSRA may not be counted in determining the eligibility of an individual seeking Medicaid.

The CSRA is determined as follows:

> All non-exempt resources belonging to either member of the married couple will be pooled together regardless of who owns them, and regardless of martial property laws (e.g., equitable distribution laws, community property laws).

> The community spouse is entitled to an amount (community resource allowance) equal to one-half of the couple's assessed total countable resources, but not less than the minimum community spouse resource allowance, and not more than the maximum community spouse resource allowance permitted under Federal law - $22,728 (2012) and $113,640 (2012), respectively.

> The CSRA is determined as of the beginning of the most recent continuous period of institutionalization of the institutionalized spouse. Either the community spouse or the institutionalized spouse may ask the Medicaid agency to make the determination. "Continuous period of institutionalization" means at least thirty (30) consecutive days of institutional care in a medical institution and/or nursing facility, or receipt of home and community-based waiver

services, or a combination of institutional and home and community-based waiver services.

A state may establish a dollar amount that is both the minimum and maximum resources amount. Thus, a state, by opting to use the maximum resource amount, can establish that amount as both maximum and minimum.

The CSRA can be increased in two ways:

Either spouse can request a fair hearing in which to demonstrate that a larger amount of resources must be protected (i.e., transferred to the community spouse from the institutionalized spouse) to generate income needed to bring the community spouse's income up to the minimum monthly maintenance needs allowance; or

A court order granting a larger amount of resources for the community spouse may be obtained; the order must be honored by the Medicaid agency.

Companion

A person who helps an elderly individual only with daily living activities. A companion has no nursing responsibilities.

Comparability/Medicaid

According to this Medicaid concept, states must use comparable standards for financial eligibility both within the categorically needy and medically needy groups (termed vertical comparability), and between groups within the categorically needed and within the medically needy (called horizontal comparability). The current requirements for comparability are as follows:

Comparability of services is required between different categorically needy groups. Services may not be less in amount, duration and scope than those available to other categorically needy groups.

Services for the categorically needy cannot be less than those for the medically needy

Income and resource eligibility determination must be comparable between the categorically needy and the medically needy.

Competitive Bidding/Medicare Advantage

See *Medicare Advantage Plans (MAP) – Common Features, section V.*

Competitive Medical Plan

See also *Medicare risk contract/Managed Care.*

A health plan that provides a full range of health care coverage in exchange for a monthly fixed fee and that is eligible for a Medicare risk contract.

Comprehensive Outpatient Rehabilitation Facility (CORF)

A CORF is primarily engaged in providing (by or under the supervision of physicians) diagnostic, therapeutic and restorative outpatient services for the rehabilitation of injured, disabled or sick persons.

The CORF includes the following items and services furnished by a physician or other qualified professional personnel to CORF outpatients under a plan established and periodically reviewed by a physician:

> Physician's services;
>
> Physical therapy, occupational therapy, speech-language pathology services and respiratory therapy;
>
> Prosthetic and orthotic devices, including testing, fitting or training in the use of prosthetic and orthotic devices;
>
> Social and psychological services;
>
> Nursing care provided by or under the supervision of a registered professional nurse;
>
> Drugs and biologicals which cannot, as determined in accordance with regulations, be self-administered; and
>
> Supplies and durable medical equipment.

Conditions of Participation/Medicare, Medicaid

The requirements, in statute and regulation, that certain providers must meet in order to receive payment from Medicare or Medicaid. Under the Federal nursing home reform law, what were formerly called "conditions of participation" are now called   simply   "requirements."

Congregate Housing

One of the earliest defined types of housing with services. Congregate housing consists of a planned group environment offering the elderly who are functionally impaired or socially deprived, but not otherwise ill, the residential accommodations and support services they need to maintain or return to an independent lifestyle and prevent premature or unnecessary institutionalization as they grow older.

Congregate housing generally consists of individual apartments, in a managed multi-unit rental facility, with areas for group socializing and dining. Such housing caters to persons who are generally self-sufficient and mobile, who require no special care, but who choose to have certain services provided (e.g., meals, periodic housekeeping, transportation, social amenities and activities) that encourage and promote independence.

Congregate housing facilities usually provide more extensive professional services than either board-and-care homes or shared housing arrangements. They are most often built with Federal, state and/or local government financing, and range in size from smaller projects containing twenty-five (25) to thirty (30) units to complexes with some three-hundred (300) apartments. Licensure for this housing type varies by state.

Congregate Housing Services Program
See *Federal housing programs for the elderly.*

Conservator

A person appointed by a court, after a hearing, to supervise the financial affairs of a person who is incapable of financial self-management.

Consolidated Omnibus Budget Reconciliation Act (COBRA) of 1985

This legislation requires that an employer must continue to provide medical insurance for a specified time to an employee, after the employee has left his/her employment. This so-called COBRA coverage is for the medical insurance that the employer then has in effect and is at the employee's sole expense.

The opportunity to elect COBRA coverage is also open to qualified beneficiaries – spouses and dependent children of former employees; and retirees and the dependents or surviving spouse(s) of former employees whose previous employer files a petition for bankruptcy under Chapter 11 of the U.S. Code.

Eligibility to elect COBRA continuation coverage arises upon the occurrence of a qualifying event. COBRA defines a qualifying event as one which would normally result in the loss of coverage by a qualified beneficiary. The statute enumerates six (6) possible qualifying events:

> the death of the covered employee;
>
> the termination (other than for gross misconduct) or reduction in hours of the covered employee's employment;
>
> the divorce or legal separation of the covered employee from the employee's spouse;
>
> the covered employee's entitlement to Medicare;
>
> a dependent child's loss of dependent status; or
>
> the filing for Chapter 11 bankruptcy by a retiree's former employer. In this case, termination of employment can be voluntary (i.e., retirement or resignation) or involuntary (i.e., firing or reduction in force).

The maximum duration of time that the COBRA coverage will remain in effect for a qualified beneficiary depends on the qualifying event. If termination or reduction in hours is the qualifying event, COBRA coverage must last at least eighteen (18) months. For other qualifying events, the period of coverage is thirty-six (36) months. Coverage for retirees who become qualified beneficiaries because the employer filed a Chapter 11 bankruptcy extends for the lifetime of the retiree.

Contemplation of Death

This is an estate tax rule whereby a transfer made within three (3) years preceding death is presumed to be part of the estate of the decedent and therefore subject to estate tax.

Continuing Care

Skilled nursing care, intermediate care, and other levels of care provided to patients in various settings (such as hospitals or nursing homes) over an extended period of time.

Continuing Care Retirement Community (CCRC)
See also *Alternative housing facilities, sections I, II and III).*

This type of housing alternative, sometimes called a life care community, generally requires that an individual be able to live independently upon becoming a resident in the community. As a resident begins to need more assistance, specific additional services are made available. Most CCRCs offer three (3) basic levels of housing on an as-needed basis: fully independent living, assisted living (personal care services) and skilled nursing care.

The basic idea of a CCRC is that once an individual becomes a resident, he/she never has to move again because any housing type and personal care services he/she will probably ever need are provided within the single campus setting. A CCRC guarantees housing and care across the continuum in that one community.

Generally, a CCRC will charge an entrance fee as well as a monthly payment for its residential, leisure and nursing services. In some cases, health care and personal care services can be paid for on an as-needed basis. The entrance fee, formerly non-refundable, now is generally refundable on departure under a variety of specified conditions.

Basically, there are three types of CCRC contracts:

> ***Extensive contract*** covers shelter and residential services, amenities (e.g., swimming pool, possibly tennis courts and other types of recreation facilities) and unlimited long-term nursing care. The entrance fees and the monthly costs are usually higher than those under modified or fee-for-service contracts.

> ***Modified or fee-for-service contract*** provides shelter, residential services and amenities, plus a specified amount of nursing care, which the resident can obtain on an unlimited basis provided he/she pays for it at a daily or monthly nursing care rate.

> ***Fee-for-service continuing care contract*** covers shelter, meals, residential services and amenities, and in addition, emergency and short-term nursing care. Access to long-term nursing care is provided only upon a daily nursing care rate.

Continuous Period of Eligibility/Medicare Part D Drug Coverage

Continuous period of eligibility for a Part D-eligible individual begins on the first day the individual is eligible to enroll in a PDP and ends with the individual's death.

Continuous Period of Institutionalization/Medicaid
See also *Community spouse's resource allowance (CSRA)/Medicaid.*

A period of institutionalization in a medical institution or nursing facility that is expected to last for at least thirty (30) consecutive days. This term is relevant to Medicaid in determining institutionalization for purposes of spousal impoverishment protections. Only individuals in a continuous period of institutionalization are entitled to protect income and resources for a community spouse.

Continuously Covered/Medigap
See *Preexisting conditions, guaranteed issue/Medigap.*

Continuum of Care

The full range of services meeting the different levels of care needed by the elderly, ranging from minor chore assistance through medical and non-medical home care, from specialized housing for the elderly through institutionalization in a nursing home.

*Contract (private)/Medicare

A "private contract" is a written agreement between you and a doctor or other health care provider who has decided not to provide services to anyone through Medicare. The private contract only applies to the services provided by the doctor or other provider who asked you to sign it. You don't have to sign a private contract. You can always go to another provider who gives services through Medicare. If you sign a private contract with your doctor or other provider, the following rules apply:

Medicare won't pay any amount for the services you get from this doctor or provider.

You will have to pay the full amount of whatever this provider charges you for the services you get.

110

If you have a Medigap (Medicare Supplement Insurance) policy, it won't pay anything for the services you get. Call your Medigap insurance company before you get the service if you have questions.

Your provider must tell you if Medicare would pay for the service if you got it from another provider who accepts Medicare.

Your provider must tell you if he or she has been excluded from Medicare.

Conversion Factor/Medicare
See also *Fee schedule charge/Medicare.*

A dollar value that when multiplied by the relative value scale for specific medical, surgical, laboratory and radiology services determines the Medicare-covered fee schedule. The conversion factor is updated annually, by statutory formula, based upon the Medicare Economic Index.

Convertible trust
See *Trigger trust.*

Coordinated Care Plans/Medicare Advantage
See also *Medicare Advantage (MA) Coordinated Care Plans – Common Features.*

The Medicare Prescription Drug Improvement and Modernization Act of 2003 (MMA), which replaced the Balanced Budget Act of 1997 (BBA), provides (as did the BBA) to every individual entitled to Medicare Part A and enrolled under Part B (except individuals with end-stage renal disease) Medicare benefits through several alternative Medicare Advantage plans, in lieu of traditional fee-for-service Medicare.

A MA coordinated care plan (CCP) is offered by an MA organization and includes a network of providers that are under contract or arrangement with the organization to deliver at least the benefit package authorized by CMS. The network of providers must be approved by CMS to ensure that all applicable requirements are met, including access and availability standards, service area requirements, and quality standards. CMS has promulgated the following rules relating to access standards:

> **Provider Network**. The organization must maintain a network of appropriate providers.

PCP Panel. A panel of primary care physicians (PCPs) must be established by the organization from which the enrollee may select a PCP. If an enrollee desires to change his/her PCP, the enrollee can request the plan for the names of the other plan doctors in the plan area. There is no requirement that a treatment plan be updated by a PCP; any health professional or team of health professionals may develop the treatment plan. If a specialist develops a treatment plan, he/she should be the one to update it.

Enrollees in CCP plans, other than HMOs or PSOs, do not need a referral to a specialist.

Serious Medical Conditions. The organization must ensure it has in effect CMS-approved procedures which (i) identify individuals with complex or serious medical conditions; (ii) assess and monitor those conditions; and (iii) establish a treatment plan which includes an adequate number of direct access visits to a specialist.

Specialty Care. The organization must provide or arrange for necessary specialty care, and in particular for women enrollees the option of direct access to a women's health specialist within the network for routine and prevention health care services. The CMS regulations do not prohibit the organization limiting the number of direct visits to the specialist, as long as the number is adequate and consistent with the treatment plan.

Hours of Operation. Plan services must be made available by the organization twenty-four (24) hours a day, seven (7) days a week, when medically necessary.

Initial Assessment. The organization must make a best effort attempt to conduct an initial assessment of each enrollee's health needs.

Enrollees in most coordinated care plans are not required to pay the plan any premiums for Medicare basic benefits (Medicare Part A/B).

A physician or other provider who does not have a contract establishing payment amounts for services furnished to an enrollee of one of the CCP organizations is required to accept as payment in full for covered services amounts that physicians or other providers could collect if the individual were not enrolled in such organization (i.e., the amount that Original Medicare fee-for-services would have paid to an enrollee, if enrolled in Original Medicare).

A physician or other provider of services who has a contract with the plan establishing payment amounts for services furnished to an enrollee of a CCP organization is required to accept as payment in full for covered services the amount set forth in the plan's fee schedule.

A Medicare eligible may choose from among a variety of CCPs. They include, but are not limited to: health maintenance organization (HMO) plans (with or without point-of-service options), plans offered by local preferred provider organizations (PPOs), provider-sponsored organizations (PSOs), regional preferred provider organizations, religious fraternal benefits (RFB) plans, and specialized MA plans for special needs beneficiaries (SNPs).

Except in the case of a PSO (granted a waiver of state licensing requirements), all organizations offering the CCP must meet the state licensure requirements. Thus, the CCP must be offered by an entity that is (i) appropriately licensed as a risk-bearing entity by the state, and (ii) eligible to offer health insurance or health benefit coverage, in each state in which it offers an MA plan. The coverage that the entity provides may be on an indemnity basis, as in the case of PPO, or a pre-capitated basis, as in the case of an HMO. The entity does not need to be licensed specifically as an HMO, PSO or PPO to offer a CCP.

*Coordination of Benefits/Medicare

*When you have other insurance (like employer group health coverage), there are rules that decide whether Medicare or your other insurance pays first. The insurance that pays first is called the **"primary payer"** and pays up to the limits of its coverage. The one that pays second, called the **"secondary payer,"** only pays if there are costs left uncovered by the primary coverage. The secondary payer may not pay all of the uncovered costs. These rules apply for employer or union group health plan coverage:*

If you have retiree coverage, Medicare pays first.

If your group health plan coverage is based on your or a family member's current employment, who pays first depends on your age, the size of the employer, and whether you have Medicare based on age, disability, or End-Stage Renal Disease (ESRD).

If you're under 65 and disabled and you or your family member is still working, your plan pays first if the employer has 100 or more employees or at least one employer in a multiple employer plan has more than 100 employees. If you're over 65 and you or your spouse is still working, the plan pays first if the employer has 20 or more employees or at least one employer in a multiple employer plan has more than 20 employees.

If you have Medicare because of ESRD, your group health plan will pay first for the first 30 months after you become eligible for Medicare. These types of coverage usually pay first for services related to each type:

No-fault insurance (including automobile insurance)

Liability (including automobile insurance)

Black lung benefits

Workers' compensation

Coordination of Coverage/Medicare

Many companies provide health insurance benefits to their Medicare-eligible retirees as part of the company retirement package. In order to avoid a duplication or overlapping between benefits of a company plan and Medicare, the plans often coordinate the two sets of benefits by provision in the company plan for carve-out coverage, wrap-around coverage, coordination of benefits coverage and exclusion coverage, as described below.

> **Carve-out Coverage.** The plan deducts the amount that Medicare pays for services from a scheduled amount set forth in the plan representing a charge for the same services, and the plan pays the difference.

> **Wrap-around Coverage.** This is somewhat like Medigap insurance and will typically cover Medicare cost-sharing requirements and supplemental benefits, such as prescription drugs, preventive care and dental care.

> **Coordination-of-benefits Coverage.** This plan in most cases will pay the difference between the actual charge and the Medicare-allowed charge up to an amount scheduled in the plan. The effect of

this coverage is that Medicare will pay for Medicare-covered services, and to the extent that Medicare does not cover, the services will be subject to the plan's coinsurance requirements.

Exclusion Coverage. Medicare payments are subtracted from the actual charge for services, and the plan will pay the balance subject to the beneficiary's responsibility for the plan's cost-sharing and deductible provisions.

Copayment
See also *Coinsurance, Part A/Medicare; Coinsurance, Part B/Medicare.*

In a health insurance policy (private and Medicare), copayment is a form of cost-sharing in which a fixed amount of money, or a fixed percentage of a charge, is paid by the insured and the balance by the insurer or Medicare for each health service provided. This term is sometimes used interchangeably with coinsurance.

Copayment/Medicare Advantage

The Balanced Budget Act of 1997 permits copayments to Medicare Advantage organizations in the same manner as they are permitted in a fee-for-service arrangement.

Copayment and deductibles/Medicaid
See *Medicaid, section VI.*

Corpus
See *Principal.*

Cosmetic Surgery/Medicare

This service is not covered by Medicare Part B, unless it is necessary due to accidental injury or to improve the function of a malformed part of the body.

Cost-basis HMO/Managed Care
See *Medicare cost contract/Managed Care; Medicare Health Maintenance Organization (HMO).*

Cost-of-living adjustment (COLA)/Social Security

Usually referred to as COLA. Social Security and SSI benefits received in January are increased annually by the increase in inflation. The COLA is based on changes in the consumer price index.

Cost-sharing/Medicare

This term refers to the deductibles, coinsurance and copayments for which Medicare beneficiaries are liable.

Cost-sharing/Medicare Part D Drug Coverage

This term refers to the requirement that an enrollee of a prescription drug plan must pay part of the drug cost. The term includes: deductibles (a fixed amount of drug cost paid before the insurance company begins to pay any drug costs); the enrollee's co-pay (a percent of drug costs); and the coverage gap or doughnut hole.

Countable Income/Medicaid
See *Income/Medicaid.*

Countable Income/Supplementary Security Income (SSI)

In order to be eligible to receive SSI, a person cannot have countable income above a specified level which fluctuates annually. Countable income includes: one-half of earned income each month after the first $65 which is not counted; unearned income, except the first $20 each month, from such sources as pensions and Social Security; and certain in-kind assistance from a third party, for example payment for food, clothing or shelter.

Countable Resources/Medicaid
See also *Availability of income and resources/Medicaid; Exempt resources/Medicaid.*

Resources that are counted (i.e., available and not excluded) as income by Medicaid in determining financial eligibility of a Medicaid applicant.

The terms "assets" and "resources" sometimes are used interchangeably by people in regard to Medicaid. In fact, each has a special meaning defined by law. For Medicaid eligibility purposes, resources are such things as real estate, cars, life insurance, household possessions, bank accounts, stocks, bonds and certificates of deposit. In the context of Medicaid transfer penalty rules, the term "assets" has a different application than the term "resources." (See *Assets/Medicaid.*)

Countable Resources/Supplementary Security Income (SSI)

To qualify for SSI, an unmarried individual may not have resources that exceed $2,000 in countable assets. A married couple's resources, whether or not one or both are eligible for SSI, may not exceed $3,000 if they are living together.

Countable resources include:

Cash on hand;

Stocks and bonds;

Mutual fund shares;

Bank accounts (including joint accounts);

Pension funds;

Retirement funds;

Real property (other than a homestead); and

Deemed property (i.e., property in a spouse's sole name or the joint name of both spouses).

Resources that are not counted include:

An individual's home (including co-op or condominium) where he/she resides;

Household and personal effects up to a value of $2,000; and

An automobile of unlimited value, if it is required for transportation to work, medical treatment or other essential daily activities, or if modified for handicapped use (if not so required, the automobile's value must be under $4,500).

*Coverage Determination/Medicare Part D Drug Coverage

If you have Medicare prescription drug coverage (Part D), you have the right to do all of the following:

Get a written explanation (called a "coverage determination") from your Medicare drug plan. A coverage determination is the first decision made by your

117

*Medicare drug plan (not the pharmacy) about your benefits, including whether a certain drug is covered, whether you've met the requirements to get a requested drug, how much you pay for a drug, and whether to make an **Exception** to a plan rule when you request it.*

*Ask for an **Exception** if you or your prescriber (your doctor or other health care provider who is legally allowed to write prescriptions), believes you need a drug that isn't on your plan's formulary.*

*Ask for an **Exception** if you or your prescriber believes that a coverage rule (such as prior authorization) should be waived.*

*Ask for an **Exception** if you think you should pay less for a higher tier (more expensive) drug because you or your prescriber believes you can't take any of the lower tier (less expensive) drugs for the same condition. You or your prescriber must contact your plan to ask for a coverage determination or an **Exception**. If your network pharmacy can't fill a prescription, the pharmacist will show you a notice that explains how to, contact your Medicare drug plan so you can make your request. If the pharmacist doesn't show you this notice, ask to see it.*

*Coverage Gap/Medicare Part D Drug Coverage

Most Medicare drug plans have a coverage gap (also called the "donut hole"). This means that after you and your drug plan have spent a certain amount of money for covered drugs, you have to pay all costs out-of-pocket for your prescriptions up to a yearly limit. Not everyone will reach the coverage gap. Your yearly deductible, your coinsurance or copayments, and what you pay in the coverage gap all count toward this out-of-pocket limit. The limit doesn't include the drug plan premiums you pay or what you pay for drugs that aren't covered.

There are plans that offer some coverage during the gap, like for generic drugs. However, plans with gap coverage may charge a higher monthly premium.

If you reach the coverage gap in 2010, (and you aren't already getting Extra Help), you will get a one-time $250 rebate check to help you with your drug costs.

If you reach the coverage gap in 2011, you will get a 50% discount on covered brand-name prescription drugs at the time you buy them. There will be additional savings for you in the coverage gap each year through 2020 when you will have full coverage in the gap.

Coverage Gap/Medicare Part D Drug Coverage

See also *Initial coverage limit/Medicare Part D Drug Coverage; Out-of-pocket threshold/Medicare Part D Drug Coverage.*

This is the gap in coverage when the enrollee of a prescription drug plan must pay one-hundred (100%) percent of the discounted price of the drug cost. It is the period after an enrollee's drug spending exceeds the initial coverage limit and before the enrollee's out-of-pocket expenses reach the out-of-pocket threshold. This is referred to as the doughnut hole or coverage gap.

Coverage/LTCI

Long-term care insurance policies are available to cover: nursing home only; home care services only; both nursing home and home care; and the whole continuum of long-term care services including nursing home, assisted living, adult day care, Alzheimer freestanding units, respite care and home care.

Policies for the entire continuum of long-term care services are the newest type of policy from which the beneficiary may draw on a fixed pool of funds, contractually agreed upon with the insurer, for any combination of services needed by the beneficiary.

According to the Health Insurance Portability and Accountability Act, LTCI policies issued beginning in 1997 must offer coverage for adult day care if they are to qualify for the tax benefits conferred by the legislation.

Coverage Groups/Medicaid

Groups of people defined by age, disability or family status, or by income or resource, for purposes of determining entitlement to Medicaid. Some groups must be covered in state programs, while some may, at state option, be covered.

Covered Employment/Social Security

Generally, any type of work, including self-employment, part-time work and employment as a domestic worker, entitles an individual to Social Security benefits so long as the employee has complied with reporting requirements and has paid Social Security taxes for the employee. Frequently domestic employees are ineligible for benefits because their work has not been credited to them by their employers. Responsibility for withholding Social Security taxes and paying them lies with the employer, who is subject to criminal penalties if the required taxes are not collected and paid by the employer.

Covered Services/Medicare
See also *Medicare.*

The services for which Medicare will make payment are referred to as covered services. Under Medicare Part A, payment is available for four services: inpatient hospital services; inpatient care in a skilled nursing facility; limited home health care services; and hospice care. Each of these services is subject to eligibility requirements and limitations for length of care.

Under Medicare Part B, payment is available for medical care necessary as a supplement to Part A, particularly physician services and durable medical equipment. Not all services important to the elderly are covered (e.g., custodial care, dental services).

Credit Shelter Trust
See *Unified credit trust.*

Creditable Coverage/Medigap
See *Preexisting condition, waiting period/Medigap*

*Creditable Prescription Drug Coverage/Medicare (Part D Drugs)

Prescription drug coverage (for example, from an employer or union) that is expected to pay, on average, at least as much as Medicare's standard prescription drug coverage. People who have this kind of coverage when they become eligible for Medicare can generally keep that coverage without, paying a penalty, if they decide to enroll in Medicare prescription drug coverage later.

Creditable Prescription Drug Coverage/Medicare Part D Drug Coverage

Creditable prescription drug coverage means a beneficiary has coverage under a prescription drug plan (PDP) or MA-PD plan, Medicaid, group health plan, state pharmaceutical assistance program, the VA, Medigap plan with prescription drug coverage, the military or other coverage as deemed appropriate by CMS.

Such coverage pays, on average, at least as much as Medicare's standard prescription drug coverage. Individuals who have this coverage when they become eligible for Medicare can generally keep that coverage without paying a penalty, if they decide to enroll in Medicare prescription drug coverage later.

Credit/Social Security
See *Work credit/Social Security.*

Critical Access Hospital

A small facility that offers outpatient services, and inpatient services on a limited basis, to individuals in rural areas.

Cross-over Patient
See also *Dual eligible.*

An individual who is eligible for and has both Medicare and Medicaid coverage.

Crummey Power

A provision in a trust under which the grantor of the trust grants to the trust's beneficiary the right to withdraw an amount not exceeding the annual gift tax exclusion applicable to the year in which the grantor made the gift or established the trust.

Currently Insured/Social Security

For a determination of eligibility for certain Social Security benefits, a person is currently insured if he/she had at least six (6) quarters of covered employment during the thirteen (13) quarters before that person dies, becomes disabled or is entitled to Social Security benefits.

Custodial Care

The term refers to personal care that supplements or replaces an elderly person's self-care and does not require professional skills. Custodial care consists of a level of care that can be provided by a layperson and includes, for example, assisting a patient in activities of daily living or administering routine medication or routine care. Custodial care is expressly excluded by statute from Medicare coverage.

Customary Charge/Medicare

See also *Fee schedule charge/Medicare; Lesser of cost or charge principle/ Medicare.*

The uniform amount charged by an individual physician in the majority of his/her cases for a particular service. The term customary charge, historically, was part of the following phrase used in Medicare's determination of a reasonable charge: "the lower of the actual charge, customary charge, and prevailing charge." Medicare has replaced use of this phrase by converting to a fee-schedule basis in order to determine a charge for services. The term customary charge, however, continues to be used by Medicare in applying the lesser of cost or charge principle.

Customary, Prevailing and Reasonable Charge/Medicare

See *Fee schedule charge/Medicare.*

(continued on next page)

D

Deductible/LTCI
See also *Elimination period/LTCI.*

A deductible in LTCI is usually called the elimination period and expressed as a number of days an individual must pay for covered services prior to the insurer making any payment.

Deductible/Medicare, Medigap
See also *Annual deductible/Medicare; Medigap high-deductible policy.*

The amount of money a beneficiary of an insurance policy must pay for covered services before the insurer will make any payment. With respect to a variety of Medicare-covered services, the Medicare beneficiary is required to pay certain payments before Medicare will make any payment. These payments are designated as deductibles or sometimes as copayments. In the case of home health services, Medicare does not require payment of a deductible, nor are copayments required except in the case of durable medical equipment.

The deductibles and copayments represent a gap in Medicare coverage. To fill this gap (i.e., the difference between the amount paid by Medicare and the Medicare-approved amount), senior citizens may obtain private Medigap insurance policies to protect against the areas in which the Medicare program is deficient.

Deductible/Medicare Part D Drug Coverage
See also *Standard coverage/Medicare Part D Drug Coverage.*

This is the amount of spending on covered drugs by a Part D-eligible individual that is required before a Part D plan pays any insurance benefits. For standard coverage, an enrollee must pay a $320 deductible (2012) before the plan begins to pay for drugs.

Deeming/Medicaid

All entries preceded by an asterisk (*) are culled or copied from the official U.S. government **Medicare** handbook (*Medicare & You 2011*).

See also *Medicaid, section II.C.4(a).*

A concept used in public benefits eligibility determinations where the income and resources of one person are considered available to an applicant for benefits, regardless of whether they are actually contributed. Under Medicaid, income and resources are deemed from spouse to spouse (and from parent to dependent child). Both the income (earned and unearned) and the resources, excluding exempt resources, of each spouse are deemed to be available to the other spouse in calculating a spouse's Medicaid eligibility. According to Federal Medicaid law, financial responsibility of other relatives is excluded from this concept.

Under the rule of deeming, since the income and resources of a spouse who is not applying for Medicaid are added to those of the applicant spouse, deeming may result in an applicant's ineligibility. Once spouses stop living together, deeming ceases as of the end of the month that the couple separates.

Deferral, tax

The right of an estate to defer payment of taxes until a later date.

Deferred compensation

Under the provisions of an employment agreement, for a term of years, an employee can accumulate, beginning at a certain age, a stated sum of money for each year of his/her employment. The accumulated amounts are then paid over a stated period of years. The individual is not currently taxed on the accumulated amount but is taxed, if and when he/she receives the money.

Defined Benefit Plan
See also *Private pension.*

This is a private pension plan that establishes a definite pension payment for each employee. Under this type of plan, participants do not have an individual account; a single account is maintained for all participants. An actuary will determine an amount to fund the plan so that each participant will be able upon retirement to receive the retirement benefits described in the plan.

The size of the defined benefits will depend upon a variety of things such as an employee's age at retirement, number of years of service and salary paid. This type of plan is insured by Pension Benefit Guaranty Corporation, a Federal agency.

A beneficiary of a pension plan can move a lump-sum retirement payment from the plan into an IRA.

Defined Contribution Plan
See also *Private pension.*

This is a private pension plan provided to employees by an employer who maintains a pension plan. Under this type of plan, each employee has his/her own account. The employer will make a contribution to the account of the employee each year as required by the plan terms. The contribution may be in amounts specified in the plan or in the form of a percentage of the employee's salary. When an employee leaves his/her employment, he/she is entitled to a vested pension.

Participants frequently may be given a choice of several types of investments for the monies in their account such as stocks, bonds or guaranteed investment contracts. The amount of retirement benefits will depend upon the plan's investment success.

Delayed Retirement Credit/Social Security

When workers age 65 through 69 defer applying for Social Security benefits or have benefits withheld because of the earnings limit, the amount of future checks is increased by a delayed retirement credit. Individual workers and spouses who reached the age of 65 in 1996 or 1997 were entitled to a delayed retirement credit of five (5%) percent for every year benefits are deferred, with lesser percentage increases for individuals who became 65 in earlier years. The delayed retirement credit increased by one-half (0.5%) percent in subsequent even years until 2008 when the credit eventually reached eight (8%) percent per year.

Demand Billing/Medicare
See also *Home health agency advance beneficiary notice/Medicare.*

A recipient of home health care services cannot appeal an adverse initial determination made by the fiscal intermediary regarding these services unless a home health agency has submitted a claim for services actually rendered. This results in a denial to the patient of the right to appeal. However, if the patient pays for the services and the home health agency provides the requested care, the patient has the right to compel the home health agency to submit to the intermediary what is called a demand billing or no-payment billing, the denial of which by the intermediary can be appealed.

Dementia

A clinical term used to describe a group of brain disorders that disrupt and impair cognitive functions, namely thinking, memory, judgment, mood, personality and social functioning. Dementia is not considered a part of the normal aging process.

Denial Notices/Medicare
See *Medicare/Denial Notices.*

Denial of Benefits/Medicare

This is an official Medicare decision that services will not be approved for Medicare payment.

De Novo Hearing/Medicaid
See *Appeals/Medicaid, section III.*

Dental Services/Medicare

Medicare Part B generally does not pay for care in connection with the treatment, filling, removal or replacement of teeth; root canal therapy; surgery for impacted teeth; and other surgical procedures involving the teeth or structures directly supporting the teeth. Dentist bills for jaw or facial bone surgery, whether required because of accident or disease, are covered. Also covered are hospital stays provided by a dentist which would be covered under current law if provided by a physician.

Department of Health and Human Services/Medicare

In 1965, Medicare (Title XVIII of the Social Security Act) was enacted by Congress into law. Medicare is the country's only national insurance program. The Centers for Medicare and Medicaid Services (CMS), a division of HHS, directly manages and administers the Medicare program.

Medicaid (Title XIX of the Social Security Act) was also enacted by Congress. It is a shared state-Federal program paid in part by both entities, unlike Medicare which is entirely a Federal program with benefits paid entirely by Federal sources.

Dependent Benefits/Social Security

See also *Primary insurance amount (PIA)/Social Security; Early retirement reductions/Social Security; Family maximum/Social Security.*

Dependents who are entitled to Social Security benefits, based upon the work history of a fully insured wage earner, are the spouses, children and parents of the worker. The amount of a dependent's benefits is statutorily fixed as a percentage of the worker's primary insurance amount for each category of dependent. Subject to the family maximum and to early retirement reductions, dependents are eligible to receive the following percentages of the worker's primary insurance amount:

Spouse and/or divorced spouse...50%
Child of retired or disabled worker..50%
Child of deceased worker 75%
Mother/father with child-in-care 75%
Widow, widower, surviving divorced spouse 100%
Dependent parent of deceased worker..82.5%
Two dependent parents of deceased worker (each)...........................75%

Dependent Care Tax Credit

Deductible income tax credits are available for some home care and adult day care services.

Dependent Home Health Care Services/Medicare

See also *Qualifying skilled services/Medicare; Medicare, section 4.A.*

This term encompasses the following five (5) home health services: Medicare social services; durable medical equipment; Medicare supplies; services of interns and residents; and intermittent or part-time home health aide services. The services mentioned above are termed dependent services since coverage by Medicare depends upon the condition that a beneficiary must need at least one qualifying skilled service (e.g., skilled nursing) and must meet Medicare-qualifying criteria for home health care (e.g., be homebound).

*Depression/Medicare

See **Mental Health Care/Medicare*

Devise

A provision in a will gifting real property.

*Diabetes/Medicare

Medicare covers these screenings if you have any of the following risk factors: high blood pressure (hypertension), history of abnormal cholesterol and triglyceride levels (dyslipidemia), obesity, or a history of high blood sugar (glucose). Tests may also be covered if you meet other requirements, like being overweight and having a family history of diabetes.

Based on the results of these tests, you may be eligible for up to two diabetes screenings every year. You pay nothing for the test, but you generally have to pay 20% of the Medicare-approved amount for the doctor's visit.

Diabetes/Medicare

Medicare Part B will cover training services in an ambulatory setting for diabetes outpatient self-management, if recommended by a physician. Also covered are a blood glucose monitor and tests scripts for diabetes.

*Diabetes/Medicare Self-management Training

Medicare covers a program to help people cope with and manage diabetes. The program may include tips for eating healthy, being active, monitoring blood sugar, taking medication, and reducing risks. You must have diabetes and a written order from your doctor or other health care provider. You pay 20% of the Medicare-approved amount, and the Part B deductible applies.

Diagnosis-Related Group (DRG)/Medicare
See also *Medicare/Prospective Payment System.*

A prospective payment system, mandated by the Social Security Amendment of 1983, is used to reimburse acute care hospitals and to contain health costs. Under this system a standard flat rate per hospital admission is prospectively established by and paid for by Medicare regardless of the hospital's cost of providing that care.

Patients' illnesses or injuries are classified according to a list of DRGs or payment categories. Each DRG is assessed a numerical value which is used to calculate the payment due hospitals for treating specific illnesses or injuries.

Diagnostic Tests/Medicare

Diagnostic x-ray tests, diagnostic laboratory tests and other diagnostic tests are covered by Medicare Part B and are not subject to the payment of a deductible or coinsurance. Diagnostic tests must be ordered by the physician who is treating the beneficiary.

In this connection, qualified non-physician practitioners – clinical nurse specialists, clinical psychologists, clinical social workers, nurse-midwives, nurse practitioners and physician assistants – who furnish services that would be physician services if furnished by a physician, who are operating within the scope of their authority under state law and within the scope of Medicare statutory benefit, are treated the same as physicians.

*Dialysis (Kidney Dialysis)/Medicare

For people with End-Stage Renal Disease (ESRD). Medicare covers dialysis either in a facility or at home when your doctor orders it. You pay 20% of the Medicare-approved amount per session, and the Part B deductible applies.

Disability/Social Security

An impairment or combination of impairments, so severe that an individual is unable to engage in any substantial gainful activity, which has lasted or is expected to last at least twelve (12) months or result in death. This definition is very specific to the Social Security and SSI programs and may differ with other definitions of disability commonly used.

Disability Benefit Entitlement/Social Security
See also *Disability insured/Social Security; Fully insured/Social Security*

Social Security benefits are payable to workers who have been disabled for five (5) consecutive months and who were both fully insured and disability insured. A worker disabled due to blindness does not need to be disability insured in order to be entitled to disability benefits.

Disabled widows and widowers of workers are eligible for Social Security benefits if they are at least age 50, if they meet a very restrictive test for disability, and if the disability began within seven (7) years of a spouse's death or within seven (7) years of being eligible for benefits as a mother. Spouses and children of disabled workers are also eligible for benefits. (See also *Dependent benefits/Social Security.*)

Disability Insured/Social Security

To be disability-insured requires twenty (20) quarters of coverage, known as Social Security work credits, during the forty (40) quarters (ten years) ending with the quarter an individual becomes disabled. Individuals who become disabled prior to age 21 need credits in at least half the quarters after the quarter they attained age 21, in other words a minimum of six (6) quarters of coverage.

Disability Period/Social Security

A period of disability is a period of time during which a worker meets the test of disability in a continuous disability-insured status. The period begins on the date the disabling impairment commenced and ends on the last day of one of the following months, whichever comes first:

> The second month after the month in which the disability ceases;
>
> The month before the month in which the worker reaches age 65; or
>
> The month in which the worker dies.

Discharge Planning

This service is usually performed by a social worker or staff in connection with a discharge of a patient from a hospital, nursing home or like institution. Discharge planning involves the social worker assessing the patient's level of functioning and needs following his/her discharge, including a smooth transition in moving from one level of care to another, for example from a hospital to a nursing home or from a hospital to home care. The discharge planner also contacts home health agencies to assist the patient in connection with his/her home care.

Disclaiming

Renouncing a gift of a donor, whether under a will, trust or survivorship interest such as insurance or joint tenancy. The disclaimer is treated as if the beneficiary of the gift predeceased the donor or the event that would otherwise entitle him/her to the gift.

Discount for Minority Interests

When a person holds a minority interest (less than fifty (50%) percent) in a corporation or a partnership, the individual may be entitled to a discount in valuing that interest for gift tax and estate tax purposes. This is so because a prospective buyer who seeks to buy the minority interest is likely to pay a lower price than if the purchaser were to acquire a majority (controlling) interest.

*Disenroll/Medicare Part D Drug Coverage

If you want to drop your Medicare drug plan and don't want to join a new plan, you can do so during one of the following times:

When you're first eligible for Medicare (the 7-month period that begins 3 months before the month you turn 65, includes the month you turn 65, and ends 3 months after the month you turn 65).

If you get Medicare due to a disability, you can join during the 3 months before to 3 months after your 25th month of disability. You will have another chance to join 3 months before the month you turn 65 to 3 months after the month you turn 65.

Between November 15 – December 31 in 2010. Your coverage will begin on January 1, 2011, as long as the plan gets your enrollment request by December 31.

Any time, if you qualify for Extra Help.

If you move out of your plan's service area.

If you lose other creditable prescription drug coverage.

If you live in an institution (like a nursing home).

You can disenroll by calling 1-800-MEDICARE. You can also send a letter to the plan to tell them you want to disenroll. If you drop your plan and want to join another Medicare drug plan later, you have to wait for an enrollment period. You may have to pay a late enrollment penalty. If your Medicare Advantage Plan includes prescription drug coverage and you join a Medicare Prescription Drug Plan, you will be disenrolled from your Medicare Advantage Plan and returned to Original Medicare.

Dishwashing/Medicare

This service generally is not covered by Medicare.

Disproportionate Share of Payments/Medicaid

Hospitals serving a disproportionate share of low-income individuals are entitled to enhanced reimbursement, so-called disproportionate share payments.

Disregards/Medicaid
See also *Income/Medicaid; Section 209(b) states/Medicaid.*

Amounts that are not considered in determining an individual's income to establish his/her eligibility for a public benefits program. In SSI, and thus in Medicaid, because Medicaid relies primarily on SSI rules for determining eligibility for older or disabled individuals, certain amounts of money, such as the first $20 per month of unearned income and the first $65 of earned income, are deducted or disregarded from income. These deductions are known as SSI disregards, since they are mandatory in SSI states. Some 209(b) states use this SSI methodology as well.

Divorced Medicare Recipient

When a beneficiary's Medicare Part A coverage is based on a spouse's work record, coverage will end in the event of a divorce during the first ten (10) years of marriage. If the beneficiary is covered by Medicare based on his/her own work record, then coverage will continue as long as he/she lives.

Divorced Spouse/Social Security
See also *Currently insured/Social Security; Fully insured/Social Security.*

A divorced spouse who was married for at least ten (10) years is eligible for dependent benefits on the earnings record of the other spouse. More than one spouse or divorced spouse may receive benefits on the earnings record of one worker. A surviving divorced spouse of a currently or fully insured worker is eligible for survivor benefits if caring for the worker's child under age 16.

Domiciliary Care Home
See *Assisted living facility.*

Doughnut Hole/Medicare Part D Drug Coverage
See also *Initial coverage limit/Medicare Part D Drug Coverage; Out-of-pocket threshold/Medicare Part D Drug Coverage.*

When a Part D plan enrollee must pay one-hundred (100%) percent of the price for drugs purchased. It is the period after an enrollee's drug spending exceeds the initial coverage limit and before the enrollee's out-of-pocket expenses reach the out-of-pocket threshold.

Do-not-resuscitate (DNR) Order

An order by an attending physician, with patient consent (or possibly, by surrogate consent) that directs hospital personnel not to revive the patient if cardiopulmonary arrest occurs.

Dose Restrictions/Medicare Part D Drug Coverage

A drug formulary may limit the number of doses available on a particular drug in a Medicare prescription drug plan even if the prescription calls for more doses. A formulary with dose restrictions limits the number of tablets (or other dosage forms) that may be dispensed by a pharmacy to a beneficiary during a specific amount of time.

Dressing/Medicare

Assistance with putting on or removing clothes is a service generally not covered by Medicare.

Drug Formulary
See *Formulary/Medicare Part D Drug Coverage.*

*Drug Plan/Medicare Part D Drug Coverage

Medicare offers prescription drug coverage to everyone with Medicare. To get Medicare prescription drug coverage, you must join a plan run by an insurance company or other private company approved by Medicare. Each plan can vary in cost and drugs covered. If you decide not to join a Medicare drug plan when you're first eligible, and you don't have other creditable prescription drug coverage, you will likely pay a late enrollment penalty.

There are two ways to get Medicare prescription drug coverage:

Medicare Prescription Drug Plans. These plans (sometimes called "PDPs") add drug coverage to Original Medicare, some Medicare Cost Plans, some Medicare Private Fee-for-Service (PFFS) Plans, and Medicare Medical Savings Account (MSA) Plans.

Medicare Advantage Plans (like an HMO or PPO) or other Medicare health plans that offer Medicare prescription drug coverage. You get all of your Part A and Part B coverage, and prescription drug coverage (Part D), through these plans. Medicare Advantage Plans with prescription drug coverage are sometimes called "MA-PDs".

To join a Medicare Prescription Drug Plan, you must have Medicare Part A or Part B. You must also live in the service area of the Medicare drug plan you want to join.

You can join, switch, or drop a Medicare drug plan at these times:

When you're first eligible for Medicare (the 7-month period that begins 3 months before the month you turn 65, includes the month you turn 65, and ends 3 months after the month you turn 65).

If you get Medicare due to a disability, you can join during the 3 months before to 3 months after your 25th month of disability. You will have another chance to join 3 months before the month you turn 65 to 3 months after the month you turn 65.

Between November 15 – December 31, 2010. Your coverage will begin on January 1, 2011, as long as the plan gets your enrollment request by December 31.

Any time, if you qualify for Extra Help.

In most cases, you must stay enrolled for that calendar year starting the date your coverage begins. However, in certain situations, you may be able to join, switch, or drop Medicare drug plans at other times. Some of these situations include the following:

If you move out of your plan's service area.

If you lose other creditable prescription drug coverage.

If you live in an institution (like a nursing home).

If you have limited income and resources, you may qualify for Extra Help to pay for Medicare prescription drug coverage.

Once you choose a Medicare drug plan, you may be able to join by completing a paper application, calling the plan, or enrolling on the plan's web site or at www.medicare.gov. You can also enroll by calling 1-800-MEDICARE (1-800-633-4227). TTY users should call 1-877-486-2048. When you join a Medicare drug plan, you will have to provide your Medicare number and the date your Part A and/or Part B coverage started.

You can switch to a new Medicare drug plan simply by joining another drug plan. You don't need to cancel your old Medicare drug plan or send them anything. Your old Medicare drug plan coverage will end when your new drug plan begins. You should get a letter from your new Medicare drug plan telling you when your coverage begins.

If you want to drop your Medicare drug plan and don't want to join a new plan, you can do so. You can disenroll by calling 1-800-MEDICARE. You can also send a letter to the plan to tell them you want to disenroll. If you drop your plan and want to join another Medicare drug plan later, you have to wait for an enrollment period. You may have to pay a late enrollment penalty.

If your Medicare Advantage Plan includes prescription drug coverage and you join a Medicare Prescription Drug Plan, you will be disenrolled from your Medicare Advantage Plan and returned to Original Medicare.

Descriptions of the payments you make throughout the year in a Medicare drug plan are described below. Your actual drug plan costs will vary depending on the prescriptions you use, the plan you choose, whether you go to a pharmacy in your plan's network, whether your drugs are on your plan's formulary (drug list), and whether you get Extra Help paying your Part D costs.

Most drug plans charge a monthly fee (premium) that varies by plan. *You pay this in addition to the Part B premium. If you belong to a Medicare Advantage Plan (like an HMO or PPO) or a Medicare Cost Plan that includes Medicare prescription drug coverage, the monthly premium you pay to your plan may include an amount for prescription drug coverage.*

Starting January 1, 2011, your Part D monthly premium could be higher based on your income. This includes Part D coverage you get from a Medicare Prescription Drug Plan, or a Medicare Advantage Plan or Medicare Cost Plan that includes Medicare prescription drug coverage. If your modified adjusted gross income as reported on your IRS tax return from 2 years ago (the most recent tax return information provided to Social Security by the IRS) is above a certain amount, you will pay a higher monthly premium.

Generally, you must pay before your drug plan begins to pay its share of your covered drugs. Some drug plans don't have a deductible.

You must pay copayments or coinsurance at the pharmacy for your covered prescriptions after the deductible (if the plan has one). You pay your share, and your drug plan pays its share for covered drugs.

*Drugs (outpatient)/Medicare

Includes a limited number of drugs such as injections you get in a doctor's office, certain oral cancer drugs, drugs used with some types of durable medical equipment (like a nebulizer or external infusion pump) and under very limited circumstances, certain drugs you get in a hospital outpatient setting. You pay 20% of the Medicare-approved amount for these covered drugs.

If the covered drugs you get in a hospital outpatient setting are part of your outpatient services, you pay the copayment for the services. However, if you get other types of drugs in a hospital outpatient setting (sometimes called "self-administered drugs" or drugs you would normally take on your own), what you pay depends on whether you have Part D or other prescription drug coverage, whether your drug plan covers the drug, and whether the hospital's pharmacy is in your drug plan plan's network.

Other than the examples above, you pay 100% for most prescription drugs, unless you have Part D or other drug coverage.

Drugs/Medicare

Other than in certain limited examples (see below), a Medicare beneficiary just pays one-hundred (100%) percent for most prescription drugs, unless he/she has Part D or other drug coverage.

Medicare Part A covers all prescription drugs for Medicare-covered inpatient care that are ordinarily furnished by a hospital or CAH for the treatment of an inpatient. This may include a limited supply for a few days' use outside the hospital or CAH by the beneficiary until he/she can obtain a regular supply.

Medicare Part B coverage of outpatient prescription drugs is limited to the following:

> Hepatitis B vaccine for beneficiaries considered at high or intermediate risk of contracting the disease; the beneficiary is subject to Part B deductible and coinsurance.

> Pneumococcal pneumonia vaccine, one shot during a beneficiary's lifetime; no deductible or coinsurance is required.

> Influenza immunization vaccines during the fall of each year; the beneficiary is not subject to any deductible or coinsurance.

> Injectable drug approved for the treatment of a bone fracture related to post-menopausal osteoporosis under the following conditions: the patient's attending physician certifies the patient is unable to learn the skills needed to self-administer, or is physically or mentally incapable of self-administering the drug; and the patient meets the requirements for Medicare coverage of home health services.

> Immunosuppressive therapy prescription drugs in the first three (3) years after transplantation, plus up to an additional eight months of coverage. The beneficiary is subject to Part B deductible and coinsurance.

> A limited number of drugs such as certain oral cancer drugs, drugs used with some types of durable medical equipment (like a nebulizer or external infusion pump). The beneficiary is subject to Part B deductible and coinsurance.

> Prescription drugs for hemophilia patients competent to use blood clotting factors for the control of bleeding. These drugs are covered without a deductible or coinsurance.

> Home IV drug therapy, including nursing, pharmacy and related services, is covered without a deductible or coinsurance.

With Medicare Part D, eligible outpatients can add drug coverage by joining a Medicare prescription drug plan (see *Medicare/Outpatient Prescription Drug Program (Medicare Part D)*).

Dry Trust

This is a trust without any assets that contemplates funding should the creator of the trust become incompetent.

Dual Eligibles/Medicare

See also *Qualified Medicare beneficiary (QMB)/Medicare, Medicaid; Federal poverty level (FPL)*.

Individuals whose income is below one-hundred (100%) percent of the Federal poverty level and have low assets are eligible for full coverage under both Medicare and Medicaid. These so-called dual eligibles are exempt from mandatory enrollment in Medicaid managed care. Virtually all individuals receiving Medicaid who are age 65 or over are entitled to Medicare Part B at least. State Medicaid programs pay the Medicare Part B premiums for dual eligibles and should also pay Medicare Part A premiums for those not entitled to Part A by virtue of receiving Social Security retirement benefits. All dual eligibles are qualified Medicare beneficiaries (QMB), but not all QMBs are dually eligible.

Dual Eligibles/Medicare Part D Drug Coverage

These are individuals who are eligible for Medicare, and for full benefits under Medicaid. Historically, Medicaid paid for drugs for these individuals. They now receive their prescription drugs from a Part D plan. Their premiums and deductibles will be fully subsidized, and their copayments will be zero or nominal ($3 for brand/$1 for generic). (See also *Full benefit dual eligible.*)

*Durable Medical Equipment (like walkers)/Medicare

Items such as oxygen equipment and supplies, wheelchairs, walkers, and hospital beds ordered by a doctor or other health care provider enrolled in Medicare for use in the home. Some items must be rented. You pay 20% of the Medicare-approved amount, and the Part B deductible applies. In all areas of the country, you must get your covered equipment or supplies and replacement or repair services from a Medicare-approved supplier for Medicare to pay.

Medicare is phasing in a new program called "competitive bidding" to help save you and Medicare money; ensure that you continue to get quality equipment, supplies, and services; and help limit fraud and abuse. In some areas of the country if you need certain items, you must use specific suppliers, or Medicare won't pay for the items and you likely will pay full price. It's important to see if you're affected by this new program to ensure Medicare payment and avoid any disruption of service. This program starts January 1, 2011, in the following states: CA, FL, IN, KS, KY, MO, NC, OH, PA, SC, TX. In certain areas in the states listed above, you need to use specific suppliers for Medicare to pay for the following items:

Oxygen supplies and equipment

Standard power wheelchair, scooter, and related accessories

Certain complex rehabilitative power wheelchairs and related accessories

Mail-order diabetes supplies

Enteral nutrients, equipment, and supplies

Hospital beds and related accessories

Continuous Positive Airway Pressure (CPAP) devices and Respiratory Assist Devices (RADs) and related supplies and accessories

Walkers and related accessories

Support surfaces including certain mattresses and overlays (Miami, Fort Lauderdale, and Pompano Beach only).

Durable Medical Equipment/Medicare
See also *Medicare/Durable Medical Equipment (DME).*

The rental or purchase of durable medical equipment for use in a patient's home is paid for under Medicare Part B, subject to a coinsurance payment by the patient.

The patient is required to pay twenty (20%) percent of the Medicare-approved charges as coinsurance payment if the provider accepts assignment. If the provider does not accept assignment, patients are required to pay the coinsurance and any amount above Medicare's approved amount, charged by the provider. Under certain conditions, patients may elect to purchase an item of equipment rather than rent it.

To be considered durable medical equipment, the equipment must be:

> prescribed by a doctor;
>
> re-usable by other patients;
>
> needed primarily for a medical purpose;
>
> appropriate for use in the patient's home; and
>
> necessary and reasonable for the treatment of the patient's illness or injury or to improve the functioning of the patient.

Iron lungs, canes, walkers, oxygen, hospital beds, wheelchairs and seat lift chairs are some common examples of this equipment.

Durable Power of Attorney
See also *Power of attorney; Springing power of attorney.*

A legal document signed by a person, known as a principal, giving another person, known as an attorney-in-fact or agent, authority, which the principal may revoke at any time, over all his/her transactions or personal actions, or only over those transactions specified in the document. The power granted under the document becomes effective on the date of execution and continues in effect unless revoked, notwithstanding the principal's mental competence. This is in contrast to a springing power of attorney, which becomes effective only upon the principal's disability or incompetency.

Durable Power of Attorney for Health Care
See also *Advance directive; Living will.*

A power of attorney which names an agent to make health care decisions, including but not limited to decisions about life-sustaining medical procedures, if the individual signing thereafter becomes incapable of making or communicating decisions. This legal device is sometimes called a health care proxy.

(continued on next page)

E

Early Retirement/Social Security

Workers and spouses can receive retirement benefits beginning at age 62. Surviving spouses are eligible to receive benefits beginning at age 60, or age 50 if disabled. Benefits for early retirees, including disabled widows or widowers, are subject to early "retirement reductions."

Early Retirement Reductions/Social Security
See also *Normal retirement age/Social Security.*

Retirement benefits are reduced for each month that benefits are paid prior to the month in which the retiree reaches normal retirement age. Early retirement reductions vary for workers, spouses, widows and widowers. The percentage reduction for each month of early retirement is:

> Worker – 5/9 of 1% for each month up to 36 months, and 5/12 of 1% for each additional month;

> Spouse or disabled spouse – 25/36 of 1% for each month for 36 months and 5/12 of 1% for each additional month up to 47 months;

> Widow and widower (age 60 to full retirement age, called a reduction period) – The benefit payable at age 60 will be reduced by 28½%. The amount of the reduction for each month in the reduction period will range proportionately between 28½% at the month of attainment of age 60 and 0% at the month of attainment of full retirement.

Earned Income/Medicaid

This is income received as a result of working, including but not limited to wages, salaries, tips, commissions, bonuses, in-kind income and income from self-employment or a small business. The definition of income for Medicaid purposes generally is found in the SSI law.

All entries preceded by an asterisk (*) are culled or copied from the official U.S. government **Medicare** handbook (*Medicare & You 2011*).

Earned Income/Supplementary Security Income (SSI)
See *Supplemental Security Income, section II.*

Earning Limit/Social Security

A law effective January 1, 2000 allows all Social Security beneficiaries who have reached full retirement age to work without their benefits being reduced because of the amount of their annual earnings.

For Social Security beneficiaries under the full retirement age and who continue to work, an earnings limit is imposed. In calendar years prior to the year the beneficiary attains normal retirement age, the beneficiary may earn up to $14,460 (2012) ($1,205 per month). In the calendar year the beneficiary attains normal retirement age, the beneficiary may earn $38,880 (2012) ($3,240 per month). In calendar years after the beneficiary attains normal retirement age the beneficiary may earn unlimited amounts. These figures are adjusted annually for inflation.

*EKGs/Medicare

Medicare covers a one-time screening EKG if ordered by your doctor as part of your one-time "Welcome to Medicare" physical exam. You pay the doctor 20% of the Medicare-approved amount, and the Part B deductible applies. An EKG is also covered as a diagnostic test. If you have the test at a hospital or a hospital-owned clinic, you also pay the hospital a copayment.

Elder Abuse

A general term for the mistreatment of the elderly, which may include physical, psychological or sexual abuse; financial exploitation; or abandonment by a family caregiver, other family members, hired or volunteer aides or companions. Such abuse may occur in either a home or institutional setting.

Elder Cottage Housing Opportunity (ECHO) Unit

Sometimes called a granny flat or in-law apartment, this unit is a small, manufactured home that can be installed in the back or side of a single-family residence and removed when it is no longer needed. It is designed specifically for older persons and persons with disabilities and is intended to enable them to live close to their family or younger friends, who will provide the support necessary for the older adult to live independently. The addition of an ECHO unit to an existing house or property is contingent upon local zoning regulations.

Elder Foster Home
See *Alternative housing facilities.*

Elder Law

The specific laws and the legal specialty that deal with the rights and issues related to the health, finances and well-being of the elderly.

*Electronic Prescribing/Medicare

An electronic way for your prescribers (your doctor or other health care provider who is legally allowed to write prescriptions) to send your prescriptions directly to your pharmacy.

Eldercare

Incorporated in this term is a wide array of allied topics – such as housing, home care, pensions, Social Security, long-term care, health insurance and elder law – relating to the rights and needs of the elderly and to the fostering of their well-being. Eldercare broadly embraces public and private programs, formal and informal support systems, government policies and regulations and funding mechanisms, all collectively concerned with contributing to the care of older persons.

Eldercare Locator

A national guide to help older people and their families find sources of information about services and assistance in the communities where they live. The phone number is 1-800-677-1116, Monday – Friday, 9 a.m. – 8 p.m. EST.

Elective Surgery
See *Charge for elective surgery/Medicare.*

ELIGIBILITY AND ENROLLMENT/MEDICARE

INTRODUCTION

The eligibility criteria and enrollment process of Medicare Part A and Part B are described below (see sections I and II). For cancellation of coverage under Parts A and B of Medicare, see III below.

(See also *Enrollment/Medicare; Eligibility for and election of plans/Medicare Advantage (MA)*)

I. PART A (HOSPITAL INSURANCE).

Eligible Persons.

Seven (7) groups of persons are eligible for Medicare Part A benefits.

Persons age 65 and over, entitled to receive either Social Security or Railroad Retirement benefits. Also eligible are spouses or former spouses of these persons who qualify for Social Security benefits as dependents and who have attained 65 years of age.

Note: Persons who elect retirement at age 62 are not eligible for Medicare until they turn 65. Persons who elect to postpone Social Security retirement benefits and continue working after age 65 can begin receiving Medicare benefits at age 65.

Note: Employers with twenty (20) or more employees must offer employees over age 65 the option of receiving the same private health insurance package that they offer other employees in lieu of, or in addition to, receiving Medicare.

Persons under age 65 who have received Social Security or Railroad Retirement disability benefits for twenty-four (24) months. Eligibility begins on the twenty-fifth (25th) month. Medicare benefits will continue up to ninety-three (93) months after the individual has stopped receiving disability benefits because of successfully completing a nine- (9) month trial work period.

Transitional group of persons, not eligible for Social Security or Railroad Retirement benefits, who reached age 65 before 1968 or who became age 65 and had three (3) quarters of coverage for each year between 1967 and 1974.

Persons under age 65 with end-stage renal disease who require dialysis or a kidney transplant (if fully insured or currently insured or if wife or dependent child of such insured person). Most of these persons are eligible for Medicare benefits after a three- (3) month waiting period. The waiting period does not apply to transplant candidates, provided their surgery takes place before the third month or to individuals who participate in a self-care training program before the beginning of the third month.

Persons diagnosed with Amyotrophic Lateral Sclerosis who receive either Social Security or Railroad Retirement disability benefits.

Employees of the Federal government from 1983 on, as well as state and local government employees hired after March 1986. In each case these government employees must have the required work credits (quarters of coverage) under the Social Security program and meet several other technical requirements. Dependents and survivors of these workers are also covered.

Voluntary enrollees who: (a) attained age 65; (b) are not eligible for either Social Security or Railroad Retirement benefits; (c) are residents of the United States; and (d) are either citizens of the United States or aliens lawfully admitted for permanent residence (who have continuously resided in the United States for not less than five (5) years immediately before the month in which application for enrollment is made). These individuals may purchase Medicare coverage by payment of a monthly premium that CMS determines annually. In order for a voluntary enrollee to receive coverage in Medicare Part A, he/she must enroll in Medicare Part B.

Automatic Enrollment.

Enrollment is automatic for most persons age 65 or older who are entitled to and are receiving Social Security or Railroad Retirement benefits. Application by these persons for these benefits is considered to be an application for Medicare Part A and Part B (unless they indicate they do not want Part B), and automatically triggers the enrollment process without the necessity of a separate application.

Enrollment is also automatic for a person, irrespective of age, who has been a disability patient receiving benefits under the Social Security Act or Railroad Retirement Act for twenty-four (24) months. Such patient will automatically receive his/her Medicare card for Part A and Part B benefits.

Should a person be eligible for Social Security or Railroad Retirement benefits but not be receiving those benefits, then eligibility for Medicare Part A is not automatic, and he/she must file an application.

Application for Enrollment.

All Medicare-eligible persons who are not automatically enrolled must apply for enrollment during one of three (3) enrollment periods.

Enrollment Periods.

There are three (3) enrollment periods – initial enrollment period, general (annual) enrollment period and special enrollment period – as set forth below:

Initial enrollment period. This is a period of seven (7) months. It begins with the third month prior to the month when the prospective enrollee reaches age 65 and continues for three (3) months after the month of his/her 65th birthday. If an individual does not file during the initial enrollment period, then he/she can file during the general enrollment period.

Enrollment during the first three (3) months of the initial enrollment period will result in coverage the first day of the month the individual attains age 65. Enrollment after the first three (3) months will cause a delay in coverage. Enrollment in the month when the beneficiary reaches age 65 will result in coverage on the first day of the second month after the applicant enrolls. If the applicant enrolls during the last three (3) months of the initial enrollment period, there may be a delay in coverage of one (1) to three (3) months.

Should a voluntary enrollee file an application after the initial enrollment period, a Part A and Part B penalty surcharge will be imposed. Should other Medicare-eligible persons file an application after the initial enrollment period, no Part A penalty will be imposed. However, such individuals, except those specified in the special enrollment period (see below), will be subject to a Part B penalty surcharge.

General (annual) enrollment period. This is held during the period January 1 through March 31 of each year. Coverage begins on July 1 after the application is filed.

Special enrollment period. This period relates to working individuals age 65 or over who are covered by an employer group health plan covering twenty (20) or more employees whether it be their own or that of a spouse. These persons have the option to enroll in Medicare after age 65. The enrollment period begins on the first day of the month in which the person is no longer enrolled in an employer group plan and ends eight (8) months later. Enrollment will not result in any penalty payment of late enrollment charges.

II.   PART B (SUPPLEMENTAL MEDICAL INSURANCE).

Eligible Persons.

Medicare Part B is a voluntary program for eligible individuals who enroll in the program and pay a premium quarterly, or by having it deducted from their monthly Social Security check. Eligibility for Part B does not depend on Part A eligibility, although all individuals over 65 eligible for a Part A are automatically entitled to Part B. An individual age 65 or over is eligible for enrollment for Part B if he/she is either entitled to hospital insurance under Part A or is a United States resident who is either an American citizen or a permanent resident alien who has resided in the United States for the five (5) years immediately before the month of application for enrollment.

Automatic Enrollment.

Persons age 65 or older who are entitled to Social Security or Railroad Retirement benefits and are receiving such benefits are automatically eligible for Medicare Part B. As in the case of Medicare Part A, a separate Medicare enrollment for Part B is unnecessary.

Application for Enrollment.

If a person is eligible for but not receiving Social Security or Railroad Retirement benefits, he/she must file an application for Medicare Part B benefits. As in the case of Medicare Part A coverage, the application for Medicare Part B coverage should be filed during the initial enrollment period.

Should an individual fail to file an application during the initial enrollment period, then he/she will be subject to a late enrollment charge and will not be able to enroll until the next general enrollment period (January 1-March 31). If a person enrolls for Part B benefits during the general enrollment period, coverage will not begin until July of that year.

As in the case of Medicare Part A benefits, a person age 65 or over who is a U.S. citizen or a permanent resident alien residing in the United States for at least five (5) years immediately prior to application, can purchase Medicare Part B benefits by filing an application and paying monthly premiums which CMS fixes annually.

III. CANCELLATION OF MEDICARE COVERAGE.

Medicare Part A coverage will cease in the following instances:

When a beneficiary's Medicare hospital insurance (Part A) is based on a spouse's work record, coverage will end if the beneficiary and his/her spouse are divorced during the first ten (10) years of their marriage. If the beneficiary is covered by Part A based on his/her own work record, coverage will continue as long as he/she lives.

If the beneficiary has purchased Medicare Part A by paying monthly premiums, he/she will lose it upon cancellation of Medicare Part B or non-payment of the monthly premium.

Medicare Part B coverage will cease in the following instances:

If the beneficiary fails to make required monthly premiums;

If a beneficiary cancels Part B coverage and then later decides to re-enroll, he/she will have to wait for a general enrollment period (January 1 – March 31 of each year).

_____

(continued on next page)

ELIGIBILITY AND ENROLLMENT/MEDICARE PART C

INTRODUCTION

(See *Medicare Advantage Plans (MAP) Common Features, sections II and III*)

I.   ELIGIBLE PERSONS.

Beneficiaries entitled to Medicare Part A and Part B are eligible to elect a Medicare Advantage plan, except those with ESRD. (However, an individual who develops ESRD if enrolled in a Medicare Advantage plan is entitled to continue such enrollment.)

Certain limitations exist in enrolling in a medical savings account (MSA) plan, one of the MA plans.

Certain low-income Medicare beneficiaries are not eligible to participate in an MSA plan; namely, Qualified Medicare Beneficiaries, Qualified Disabled Working Individuals, Specified Low-income Medicare Beneficiaries, or individuals otherwise entitled to Medicaid cost-sharing assistance under the Medicaid program.

> In addition, certain other classes of Medicare beneficiaries are not eligible to choose an MSA plan:
>
> - Beneficiaries who have coverage benefits under high-deductible policies, including an employer's group plan that provides this coverage.
>
> - Beneficiaries who are retired Federal government employees and part of the Federal Employee Health Benefits Program.
>
> - Individuals who are retired Department of Defense or Department of Veterans Affairs employees.

A beneficiary's choice of Medicare Advantage plan coverage is deemed to continue until: (a) the beneficiary changes his/her election; (b) the Medicare Advantage plan is discontinued; or (c) the Medicare Advantage plan no longer serves the geographic area where the beneficiary resides.

II. ENROLLMENT PERIODS (ELECTION OF PLANS).

The periods during which elections may be made by individuals are set forth below:

Initial Enrollment (Initial Coverage Election) Period.

Upon attaining eligibility for Medicare, individuals have a choice between original fee-for-service Medicare (Medicare FFS) or any Medicare Advantage plans available in their area. Any individual failing to make an election during the initial election year will be deemed to have chosen the Original Medicare FFS option. An election becomes effective on the date a beneficiary becomes entitled to benefits under Part A and enrolls in Part B.

The initial election period of seven (7) months begins one month before the month that the beneficiary is first entitled to both Parts A and B and ends on the last day of the individual's Part B initial enrollment period. As instructively rephrased in the CMS handbook *Medicare and You 2012: When you first become eligible for Medicare, you can join a Medicare Advantage plan during the 7-month period that begins 3 months before the month you turn 65, includes the month you turn 65, and ends 3 months after the month you turn 65.*

Open Enrollment Period.

Between October 15 and December 7 of each year (open enrollment period), an individual can join, switch, or drop a Medicare Advantage plan. Coverage will begin on January 1, as long as the plan gets the individual's request by December 7. The election made during an open enrollment period will become effective on the first day of the first month after enrollment.

A Medicare Advantage organization must accept eligible beneficiaries who elect that organization's plan during an open enrollment period without restrictions, waiting period, or pre-existing medical exclusion.

A beneficiary can elect an MSA plan only during the initial enrollment period or the annual coordinated election period.

Annual Coordinated Election Period.
If an individual does not enroll for Part A and/or Part B when first eligible, he/she may enroll, subject to a late enrollment penalty, during the annual coordinated election period which runs from January 1 to March 31 each year.

During the annual coordinated election period, all Medicare beneficiaries are free to elect among all available options, including Original Medicare, MA plans, MA-prescription drug plans (MA-PDP), or prescription drug plans (PDPs). They may choose to enroll in an MA plan, change a default MA plan, or return to Original Medicare, and an above-stated enrollment is effective the following January.

Special Enrollment Periods (SEP).
An individual may disenroll from a Medicare Advantage plan, other than during the annual coordinated election period, and may make a new choice of plans, in certain events: (i) the individual's plan has been terminated (see below), or (ii) the individual has moved (i.e., changed place of residence, see below), or (iii) the organization has breached its contract or made material misrepresentations, or (iv) other special circumstances (e.g., for cause).

In cases of <u>termination or discontinuance of an organization</u>, the SEP begins when the organization is required to give notice to beneficiaries and ends three (3) months after the notification.

For a <u>beneficiary who has moved</u>, the SEP runs for three (3) months starting with the month prior to the permanent move and ending the month after the move. The beneficiary may choose an effective date of up to three (3) months after the month when the Medicare Advantage plan receives the beneficiary's completed enrollment form, but the effective date may not be prior to the date the beneficiary moved or the date the Medicare Advantage organization received the completed enrollment form.

In the <u>case of breach of contract or material misrepresentations by the organization</u>, the SEP begins once CMS agrees that a violation occurred. The length of the SEP depends on whether the beneficiary immediately elects a new Medicare Advantage plan on disenrollment from the original, or whether the beneficiary first elects Original Medicare before choosing a new Medicare Advantage plan.

5-Star Special Enrollment Period.

Medicare and You 2012 instructively explains this new enrollment period as follows:

Medicare uses information from member satisfaction surveys, plans, and health care providers to give overall performance star ratings to plans. A plan can get a rating between one and five stars. A 5-star rating is considered excellent. These ratings help you compare plans based on quality and performance. Starting December 8, 2011, you can switch to a 5-star Medicare Advantage plan at any time during the year. The overall plan star ratings are available at www.medicare.gov/find-a-plan. You can only join a 5-star Medicare Advantage plan if one is available in your area. You can only use this special enrollment period to switch to a 5-star plan one time each year. You can't use this period to join a Medicare cost plan.

Special Enrollment Periods for Employees.

There is a special enrollment period (SEP) available for individuals who elect their Medicare Advantage plans through their employers. The SEP may be used during the open enrollment period if the employer group health plan is not open for enrollment at the same time as the Medicare Advantage open enrollment. The SEP may also be used when the employer group health plan would permit a beneficiary to change elections based upon their election if they do so before December 15 of the year they make an election.

Change of Election.

An enrollee of a Medicare Advantage plan, in addition to the right to drop the plan during the open enrollment period (October 15 – December 7), may leave the plan and switch to Original Medicare between January 1 and February 14. As instructively stated in the CMS handbook *Medicare and You 2012:*

Between January 1 - February 14, if you're in a Medicare Advantage plan, you can leave your plan and switch to Original Medicare. If you switch to Original Medicare during this period, you will have until February 14 to also join a Medicare prescription drug plan to add drug coverage. Your coverage will begin the first day of the month after the plan gets your enrollment form.

(continued on next page)

ELIGIBILITY AND ENROLLMENT/MEDICARE PART D DRUG COVERAGE

I. ELIGIBILITY.

Prescription drug coverage benefits are available to Medicare eligibles under a newly enacted Medicare Part D Program of Title XVIII of the Social Security Act. (Section 101 of the Medicare Prescription Drug and Improvement Act of 2003 (Act)), also known as the Medicare Modernization Act (MMA).

The Centers for Medicare and Medicaid Services (CMS) has overall responsibility for implementing the Medicare Part D prescription drug benefits of the Act. An individual is eligible for the Medicare prescription drug program if he or she is entitled to Medicare Part A and/or enrolled in Medicare Part B.

The Act provides for premium and cost-sharing subsidies of prescription drug coverage for certain individuals with low income and resources. The purpose of the subsidy program is to assist Medicare beneficiaries with limited financial means to pay for Medicare prescription drug coverage under Medicare Part D. Individuals with low incomes and limited resources may be eligible for a subsidy (referred to as extra help subsidy) to help pay for monthly premiums, coinsurances and the annual deductible under Medicare Part D.

Medicare beneficiaries are able to obtain prescription drug coverage either through (i) a stand-alone prescription drug plan (PDP), available to enrollees in original Medicare fee for services, or (ii) a comprehensive Medicare Advantage plan (MA-PDP) available to Medicare eligibles who enroll in Medicare Advantage plans. The prescription drug coverage is operated through private insurance entities that contract with CMS.

II. ENROLLMENT.

A. Introduction.

Enrollment in Part D requires the beneficiary to take affirmative steps to enroll and get Part D coverage. The beneficiary must first choose a drug plan from the options available in his/her area. Then, the beneficiary must enroll through the plan that he/she chooses. If the beneficiary may be eligible for a low-income subsidy, he/she must file a second affirmation.

In order to be eligible to enroll in a PDP, the individual must reside in the plan's service area and cannot be enrolled in a MA plan (other than a medical savings account, or a private fee-for-service plan) that does not provide qualified prescription drug coverage.

PDP enrollees are locked in to their plan for the remainder of the calendar year, even though the plan in which they enroll may change the formulary of cost-sharing arrangements during the year. Enrollees in PDPs must wait until the next annual coordinated enrollment period to switch plans, with enrollment in the new plan becoming effective on January 1 of the following year.

B.   Enrollment Periods.

There are three (3) coverage enrollment periods: (i) the initial enrollment period; (ii) the annual coordinated election period; and (iii) special enrollment period, as set forth below:

> ***Initial Enrollment Period.*** The initial enrollment period for individuals who are first eligible to enroll in Part D, corresponds to the initial enrollment period for Part B, i.e., the seven- (7) month period running from three (3) months before the month when individual first becomes eligible and ending three (3) months after the first month of eligibility.

> ***Annual Coordinated Enrollment Period.*** The annual coordinated enrollment period corresponds to the annual coordinated enrollment period for Part C and runs from October 15 through December 7.

> ***Special Enrollment Period.*** Individuals may be eligible for a special enrollment period if:

>> they did not enroll in Part D during their initial enrollment because they had other prescription drug coverage deemed to be "creditable coverage," (as defined in G.7 below) and they lose the creditable coverage;

they were given incorrect information concerning the status of their other prescription drug coverage as creditable coverage;

they were given incorrect information about enrollment by a Federal employee;

they have Medicare and full Medicaid coverage or a Medicare savings program (MSP);

they move out of a plan's service area;

their PDP's contract with Medicare is terminated;

they enrolled in a Medicare Advantage plan with prescription drug coverage (MA-PDP) during the first year of eligibility and want to return to traditional Medicare and a PDP; or

they move into or out of a nursing home.

C. Effective Date of Enrollment.

Part D coverage becomes effective:

the same month that Part A and/or Part B coverage becomes effective for individuals who enroll before their month of entitlement to Part A or enrollment in Part B; the first day of the next calendar month after enrollment for individuals who enroll after the first month of entitlement for Part A or enrollment in Part B;

the following January 1, for individuals who enroll during the annual coordinated enrollment period; and

at the time specified by CMS for individuals who enroll during a special enrollment period.

D. Involuntary Disenrollment.

An individual may be involuntarily disenrolled from a drug plan for one of several reasons. These include no longer living in the plan's service area, loss of eligibility for Part D, death of the individual, termination of the PDP, failure to pay premiums on a timely basis, and/or engaging in disruptive behavior that substantially impairs the ability of the plan to arrange for or provide services.

E. Ability to Change Plans Mid-Year.

Between October 15 and December 7 (open enrollment period), an individual with a MA plan may switch his/her plan without drug coverage to a MA plan that offers drug coverage. Conversely, an individual with a MA plan with drug coverage may switch to a plan with drug coverage without drug coverage.

During the open enrollment period, an individual may switch from one Medicare prescription drug plan to another. Such individual may also drop his/her Medicare PDP.

From January 1 to February 14, an individual who during this period has switched to original Medicare will have until February 14 to also join a Medicare PDP and thereby add drug coverage. His/her prescription drug coverage will begin the first day of the month after the plan obtains the individual's enrollment form.

During the period January 1 to February 14, individuals cannot switch from original Medicare to a MA plan, nor switch from one Medicare PDP to another.

F. Enrollment Process for Individuals Who Are Full-Benefit Dual Eligible.

A full-benefit dual eligible individual means an individual who is determined eligible by the state for (i) medical assistance for full-benefits under Title XIX of the Social Security Act, under any eligibility category covered under a state plan; or (ii) medical assistance under the Act authorized for the medical need, or permitted by states that use more restrictive eligibility criteria than are used by the SSI program.

The MMA established an enrollment process involving automatic assignment into drug plans for individuals who are full-benefit dual eligibles, who are eligible for Medicare and Medicaid and who do not choose their own PDP or MA-PDP during their initial enrollment period. Full-benefit dual eligibles are automatically eligible for a continuous special enrollment period and therefore are not ever locked into a prescription drug plan. CMS must automatically enroll full-benefit dual eligible individuals who fail to enroll in Part D plan into a PDP offering basic prescription drug coverage in the area where the individuals reside that has a monthly beneficiary premium that does not exceed the low-income premium subsidy amount.

Nothing prevents a full-benefit dual eligible individual from: (i) affirmatively declining enrollment in Part D; or (ii) disenrolling from the Part D plan in which the individual is enrolled and electing to enroll in another Part D plan during the special enrollment period.

Enrollment of full-benefit dual eligible individuals is effective as follows: (i) the first day of the month the individual is eligible for Part D for individuals who are Medicaid eligible and subsequently become newly eligible for Part D; and (ii) for individuals who are eligible for Part D and subsequently become newly eligible for Medicaid after January 1, 2006. (Enrollment is effective as soon as practicable after being identified as a newly full-benefit dual eligible individual.)

G.   Failure to Enroll on a Timely Basis.

A beneficiary who does not enroll in a Part D plan within sixty-three (63) days of his/her initial enrollment period, and who does not have other creditable prescription drug coverage, must pay a late penalty if he/she subsequently enrolls in a Part D plan. Creditable coverage is other coverage equivalent to Medicare basic drug benefit (e.g., VA coverage, Medigap coverage, and most employer- (or union) sponsored retiree plans). Should a beneficiary's existing drug coverage end or change and thus cease to be creditable, he/she has up to sixty-three (63) days to enroll in a Medicare drug plan.

The penalty is assessed at one (1%) percent of the national average premium for each month of delayed enrollment, for the remainder of the time in which the beneficiary is enrolled in a Part D plan. Thus, a beneficiary who first becomes eligible for Part D at age 65, but who delays enrolling until age 70 may be assessed a sixty- (60%) percent penalty on his/her premium (5 years x 12 months x 1%). Since the penalty is based on a percentage of the average premium each year, the dollar value of the penalty changes as the national average premium changes.

(continued on next page)

ELIGIBILITY FOR MEDICAID SERVICES

INTRODUCTION

Medicaid eligibility for services depends upon: (i) whether the Medicaid-eligible person resides in a Supplemental Security Income (SSI) or a Section 209(b) state (see I below); (ii) the status of the applicant (see II below); (iii) the financial circumstances of the applicant (see III below); and (iv) applicant's category of eligibility (see IV below).

I. SSI AND SECTION 209(B) STATES.
See also *SSI state/Medicaid; 209(b) states/Medicaid.*

In determining the applicable financial eligibility criteria for people who are aged, blind or disabled, a distinction is made between SSI and Section 209(b) states. Most states are SSI states. Persons in these states who meet the financial test to be eligible for Supplemental Security Income (SSI) are considered categorically needy for Medicaid purposes and are thus eligible for Medicaid.

Twelve (12) states classified as 209(b) states use what is currently referred to as the 209(b) option, which is named for the section of Public Law 92-603 which authorized the option. These states are Connecticut, Hawaii, Illinois, Indiana, Minnesota, Missouri, New Hampshire, North Carolina, North Dakota, Ohio, Oklahoma and Virginia. The option permits states to use eligibility standards that are more restrictive than those of the SSI program, as long as they are not more restrictive than what the state used in 1972.

Some 209(b) states use income levels (limits) for categorically needy individuals that are more restrictive than those in SSI states. However, 209(b) states must allow people with incomes above their more restrictive standard to become eligible for Medicaid if they spend down their excess income incurring medical bills. States that have chosen the 209(b) option can also have more restrictive definitions of blindness or disability than SSI uses, but they cannot use a different age standard.

II. STATUS TESTS.

Any elderly, disabled or blind person who is a United States citizen or among a limited category of qualified aliens (permanent resident alien status) is eligible to apply for Medicaid. The individual must be age 65 or older or meet the SSI definition of blindness or disability, or a state's more restrictive definition of blindness or disability if the person is in a 209(b) state.

According to the Personal Responsibility and Work Opportunity Act of 1996, aliens lawfully residing in the United States and receiving SSI on August 22, 1996 may continue to receive Medicaid medical assistance as if they were citizens. Likewise, aliens who lawfully resided in the United States on August 22, 1996 and who met the statutory definition of blind or disabled are also entitled to receive such benefits.

Legal immigrants arriving in the country after August 22, 1996 generally are barred (banned) from Medicaid medical assistance during the first five (5) years after their entry into the United States. However, certain categories of these immigrants are exempted from this ban:

> honorably discharged U.S. military veterans and active duty personnel, their spouses and unmarried dependents;
>
> individuals who singly or collectively with their spouse have worked forty (40) qualified quarters of Social Security coverage;
>
> current and future refugees;
>
> individuals granted political asylum; and,
>
> individuals granted status as Cuban, Haitian or Amerasian entrants.

All of these legal immigrants are eligible for Medicaid medical assistance for seven (7) years after their entry into this country.

III. INCOME AND RESOURCE TESTS.

To be eligible, individuals must have income and resources below prescribed standards. Generally speaking, these are related to either SSI standards or Federal income poverty guidelines. The particular standard applicable to an individual depends on the category into which he/she fits.

Certain resources known as exempt resources, such as an individual's primary residence, burial plot, an automobile of limited value, household and personal effects of limited value, a small amount of life insurance and, in some instances, a small amount of income-producing property, are not taken into account in determining eligibility. The amount of exempted resources is slightly more generous for an applicant in a nursing home who has a spouse continuing to live outside a nursing home, the so-called community spouse. Should a spouse (institutionalized spouse) enter a nursing home, Medicaid, upon request, will identify the value of the couple's joint resources (take a "snapshot" of them) to assure that a community spouse's resource allowance is allocated from the joint resources.

Certain income is disregarded, i.e., not counted, in determining an applicant's Medicaid eligibility. Also, some money received by an individual is not considered income – for example, certain veterans' benefits. (See *Disregards/Medicaid.*)

According to the rule of deeming, the income (earned and unearned) and resources (excluding those exempted) of the spouse not applying for Medicaid are added to those of the applicant spouse. This deeming may cause an applicant to be ineligible for Medicaid. However, when one spouse enters a nursing home, deeming of income and resources ceases at the end of the month the couple stops living together.

In addition to the basic rules about what income and resources are counted, special Medicaid rules for trusts determine whether the income or principal of trusts are considered "available," and therefore counted, in determining a Medicaid applicant's eligibility for Medicaid. (See *Trust, Medicaid eligibility rules.*)

IV. CATEGORIES OF ELIGIBILITY.

There are three (3) categories of SSI and Medicaid recipients: categorically needy, optional categorically needy, and medically needy.

SSI recipients in SSI states are categorically needy. These states are required to provide them Medicaid assistance and have the option of serving those in the other two categories. The medically needy group is optional to states. Thirty-seven (37) states and the District of Columbia have this category. It is for persons who meet the non-financial (age, disability) requirements for categorical assistance, but whose income and/or resources are over the categorical levels. Unlike the categorically needy or optional categorically needy, a medically needy person has the right to reduce his/her income to below state-prescribed levels through the deduction of incurred medical expenses, a process commonly referred to as "spending down." When incurred medical expenses reduce income to the state's medically needy income level, the individual is eligible for Medicaid.

The <u>optional categorically needy</u> group is comprised of many subgroups. States can choose among the subgroups. One subgroup important to aged, blind and disabled individuals permits states without a medically needy program (sometimes called 300% states) to provide nursing home care for people whose income and resources are a certain percentage above the SSI level. (For SSI purposes, the maximum allowed income is gross, not net, income.) Optional categorically needy individuals have no right of spend down.

In determining many of the services and entitlements available to a Medicaid-eligible person, there can be considerable variance depending upon the category into which the individual falls. Persons in the optional categorically needy group are entitled to all of the same services as the categorically needy.

Services for the medically needy cannot be greater in amount, duration and scope than those for the categorically or optional categorically needy.

(continued on next page)

Eligibility/Social Security
See *Social Security Program.*

Eligibility/Supplemental Security Income (SSI)
See also *Countable income, SSI; Countable resources, SSI.*

To be eligible for Supplemental Security Income (SSI), a person must be age 65 or over, blind or disabled and poor. The individual's or couple's income and assets cannot exceed certain levels for individuals and couples, respectively, which are established by Congress. The person must be a resident of the United States for 30 consecutive days and either a citizen of the United States or an alien (see below) who meets one of the exceptions to the general ban on SSI benefits for non-citizens.

Aliens lawfully residing in the United States and receiving SSI benefits on August 22, 1996 are entitled to continue enjoying such benefits. Other aliens exempted from the ban on non-citizens receiving SSI are:

> Honorably discharged U.S. military veterans and active duty personnel, their spouse and unmarried dependent children;

> Individuals who singly or collectively with their spouse have worked forty (40) qualified quarters of Social Security coverage; and

> Individuals granted political asylum, refugees, and individuals whose deportation is withheld (including Cuban and Haitian entrants, Amerasians, certain Native Americans from Canada and non-citizen children of a battered parent); this category of individuals may receive SSI benefits for the first seven (7) years after being granted applicable status.

It is not necessary for a person to be completely unable to work to qualify for SSI benefits. Some persons may be considered disabled even though they can do some types of work. It is also not necessary for a person to have no income to qualify for SSI, but such other income as the person has must be less than the SSI benefit income level.

Not all resources are counted in determining SSI eligibility. Some resources, such as a person's home, may be excluded. SSI recipients are entitled to retain a minimum monthly amount as a personal allowance.

Elimination Period/LTCI

This is equivalent to the deductible in other health policies. In LTCI policies it is expressed as a number of days. The elimination period is the length of time the individual must pay for covered services before the insurer will make any payment. Common elimination periods range from twenty (20) days to one-hundred (100) days. The longer the elimination period, the less the premium will be.

Emergency Care/Medicaid

Hospitals that participate in Medicaid are required by federal law to make available their emergency room to all Medicaid-eligible persons for examination to determine whether they have an emergency medical condition and to provide stabilizing treatment.

Emergency Care/Medicare

Federal law requires hospitals that participate in Medicare and have an emergency room to examine all persons seeking care in the emergency room to determine whether they have an emergency medical condition. If staff personnel determine that an emergency medical condition exists, they must provide stabilizing treatment, that is, requisite medical treatment, so that when the person is transferred from the hospital no material deterioration of the person's condition is likely to result.

*Emergency Department Services/Medicare

When you have an injury, a sudden illness, or an illness that quickly gets much worse. You pay a specified copayment for the hospital emergency department visit, and you pay 20% of the Medicare-approved amount for the doctor's services. The Part B deductible applies.

Emergency Medical Condition

A condition which acute symptoms which, without immediate medical attention, might result in seriously impairing a person's health, his/her bodily functions or a bodily organ.

Emergency Response System
See *Personal emergency response system (PERS).*

Employee Retirement Income Security Act (ERISA)
See also *Private pension.*

This 1974 law provides Federal protection to and defines rights of employees under pension plans. A plan that meets ERISA requirements and that is voluntarily provided by an employer is known as a qualified plan.

Employee's Election under Employer Health Plan/Medicare

Employer group health plans or Medicare group health plans of employers with twenty (20) or more employees are required to offer workers age 65 or over, and workers' spouses who are age 65 or over, the same health insurance benefits under the same conditions offered to younger workers and spouses. In such situations, the beneficiary and spouse have the option to accept or reject the employer's health plan. If an employee accepts the employer's health plan, it will pay first on the employee's health claims; Medicare will become the secondary payer. If the beneficiary rejects the employer's health plan, Medicare will remain the primary health insurance payer. If an employee elects Medicare to be the primary payer, the employer cannot offer coverage that supplements Medicare.

Employer Medical Insurance
See *Coordination of coverage/Medicare; Consolidated Omnibus Budget Rehabilitation Act (COBRA) of 1985.*

Employer-sponsored Drug Benefit Programs for Retirees

Qualified retirees' prescription drug plans have been made available to employer-sponsors to prompt them through special subsidy payments to continue to provide retirees' drug benefits. The plans must provide an actuarial equivalence to standard coverage. Some employer-sponsored health plans help retirees pay medical expenses which are not covered by Medicare. Those expenses could include copayments and deductibles, the catastrophic costs of severe illness and the cost of preventive care and prescription drugs, beyond what Medicare might pay. Individuals who have drug coverage through their former employers will lose the company's coverage (and possibly their individual insurance coverage) if they sign up for Part D.

End-Stage Renal Disease (ESRD)
Kidney disease requiring lifetime dialysis or a kidney transplant. ESRD patients are eligible for Medicare and may be eligible for Social Security payments if found to be disabled. They are not eligible to enroll in MA plans.

Energy Assistance

Assistance programs are available in many states to help low-income persons with home-energy matters and expenses. Financial assistance may be available even if heat and utilities are included in the rent.

Enhanced Alternative Coverage/Medicare Part D Drug Coverage
See also *Medicare/Outpatient Prescription Drug Program (Medicare – Part D), section V.*

This coverage provides standard prescription drug coverage and supplemental benefits.

Enrollment/Medicare
See *Eligibility and enrollment/Medicare.*

*Enrollment/Medicare – Parts A, B, and C

I.   **PART A AND PART B.**

    A.   Automatic **Enrollment for Some Medicare Eligibles.**

In most cases, if you're already getting benefits from Social Security or the Railroad Retirement Board (RRB), you will automatically get Part A and Part B starting the first day of the month you turn 65. If your birthday is on the first day of the month, Part A and Part B will start the first day of the prior month.

    B.   **Enrollment of Medicare Eligibles Who Are Not Entitled to Automatic Enrollment.**

If you aren't getting Social Security or RRB benefits (for instance, because you're still working) and you want Part A or Part B, you will need to sign up. You should contact Social Security three months before you turn 65. If you worked for a railroad, contact the RRB to sign up. Call Social Security at 1-800-772-1213 about your Medicare eligibility and to sign up for Part A and/or Part B. You can also apply for Part A and Part B online at www.socialsecurity.gov/retirement. *If you get RRB benefits, call the RRB at 1-877-772-5772.*

C.   Initial Enrollment Period.

You can sign up when you're first eligible for Part B. If you're eligible for Part B when you turn 65, this (the Initial Enrollment Period) is a 7-month period that begins 3 months before the month you turn 65, includes the month you turn 65, and ends 3 months after the month you turn 65.

To get Part B coverage the month you turn 65, you must sign up during the first 3 months before the month you turn 65. If you wait until the four months of your Initial Enrollment Period to sign up for Part B, your start date for coverage will be delayed.

If you enroll in Part B during the first three months of your Initial Enrollment Period, your coverage start date will depend on your birthday:

- *If your birthday **isn't** on the first day of the month, your Part B coverage starts the first day of your birthday month. For example, your 65th birthday is July 20, 2011. If you enroll in April, May or June, your coverage will start on July 1, 2011.*

- *If your birthday **is** on the first day of the month, your coverage will start the first day of the prior month. For example, your 65th birthday is July 1, 2011. If you enroll in March, April or May, your coverage will start on June 1, 2011. To read the chart correctly, use the month **before** your birthday as "the month you turn 65."*

If you enroll in Part B the month you turn 65 or during the last 3 months of your Initial Enrollment Period, your Part B start date will be delayed. For example, if you turn 65 in July, when your coverage starts depends on the month you enroll.

Month You Enroll	*Month Coverage Starts*
July	*August 1*
August	*October 1*
September	*December 1*
October	*January 1*

D.   General Enrollment Period.

If you didn't sign up for Part A and/or Part B when you were first eligible, you can sign up between <u>January 1 – March 31 each year</u>. <u>Your coverage will begin July 1</u>.

If you sign up during these months	*Your coverage will begin on*
January	
February	*July 1*
March	

E.   Special Enrollment Period.

If you didn't sign up for Part A and/or Part B when you were first eligible because you're covered under a group health plan based on current employment, you can sign up for Part A and/or Part B as follows:

Anytime that you or your spouse (or family member if you're disabled) are working, and you're covered by a group health plan through the employer or union based on that work	***Or***	**During the 8-month period that begins the month after the employment ends or the group health plan coverage ends, whichever happens first**

Usually, you don't pay a late enrollment penalty if you sign up during a Special Enrollment Period. This Special Enrollment Period doesn't apply to people with End-Stage Renal Disease (ESRD). You may also qualify for a Special Enrollment Period if you're a volunteer serving in a foreign country.

If you have COBRA coverage or a retiree health plan, you're not eligible for a Special Enrollment Period when that coverage ends.

II.   PART C.

You can join a Medicare Part C Plan when you first become eligible for Medicare (the 7-month period that begins 3 months before the month you turn 65, includes the month you turn 65, and ends 3 months after the month you turn 65). If you get Medicare due to a disability, you can join during the 3 months before the 3 months after your 25ᵗʰ month of disability. You will have another chance to join 3 months before the month you turn 65 to 3 months after the month you turn 65 between November 15 – December 31 in 2010. Your coverage will begin on January 1, 2011, as long as the plan gets your enrollment request by December 31; any time, if you qualify for Extra Help.

You are able to join by completing a paper application (i.e., filing an election form with the plan's sponsoring organization), calling the plan, or enrolling on the plan's web site or on **www.medicare.gov***. You can also enroll by calling 1-800-MEDICARE (1-800-633-4227). When you join a Medicare Advantage Plan, you will have to provide your Medicare number and the date your Part A and/or Part B coverage started.*

Enrollment/Medicare Part D Drug Coverage

This is a seven- (7) month initial enrollment period that begins three (3) months before the month an individual first meets the eligibility requirements for Medicare, and ends three (3) months after that first month of eligibility. The initial enrollment period runs from November 15 until December 7 of each year, when a Medicare beneficiary may switch from original Medicare to a Medicare Advantage plan, or enroll in a stand-alone plan if he/she so chooses.

Entry Age/LTCI

The age at which a person first purchases a LTCI policy. LTCI policies are usually level-premium policies based on the purchaser's age at the time of purchase. Premiums can and often do increase when there are class-wide increases; for example, rates go up for all 75-year-olds.

Equipment
See *Durable medical equipment/Medicare.*

Established Trust
See *Trust, Medicaid eligibility rules.*

Estate/Medicaid
See also *Robert Wood Johnson Long-Term Care Program/LTCI.*

The term refers to all real and personal property and other assets included within an individual's estate under state probate law. Medicaid, in connection with its recovery program, permits states to use a broader definition of the term to include, whether or not the asset is the subject of probate, any real or personal property and other assets in which an individual had an interest at the time of death such as an interest in jointly owned property.

Excess Charge/Medicare

The difference between a doctor's or other health care provider's actual charge and the Medicare-approved charge.

Excess Shelter Allowance/Medicaid

See *Minimum monthly maintenance needs allowance/Medicaid.*

*Exception/Medicare Part D Drug Coverage

If you have Medicare prescription drug coverage (Part D), you have the right to do all of the following:

Get a written explanation (called a "coverage determination") from your Medicare drug plan. A coverage determination is the first decision made by your Medicare drug plan (not the pharmacy) about your benefits, including whether a certain drug is covered, whether you've met the requirements to get a requested drug, how much you pay for a drug, and whether to make an exception to a plan rule when you request it.

Ask for an exception if you or your prescriber (your doctor or other health care provider who is legally allowed to write prescriptions), believes you need a drug that isn't on your plan's formulary.

Ask for an exception if you or your prescriber believes that a coverage rule (such as prior authorization) should be waived.

Ask for an exception if you think you should pay less for a higher tier (more expensive) drug because you or your prescriber believes you can't take any of the lower tier (less expensive) drugs for the same condition.

You or your prescriber must contact your plan to ask for a coverage determination or an exception. If your network pharmacy can't fill a prescription, the pharmacist will show you a notice that explains how to contact your Medicare drug plan so you can make your request. If the pharmacist doesn't show you this notice, ask to see it.

You or your prescriber may make a standard request by phone or in writing, if you're asking for prescription drug benefits you haven't received yet. If you're asking to get paid back for prescription drugs you already bought, you or your prescriber must make the standard request in writing.

You or your prescriber can call or write your plan for an expedited (fast) request. Your request will be expedited if you haven't received the prescription and your plan determines, or your prescriber tells your plan, that your life or health may be at risk by waiting.

If you're requesting an exception, your prescriber must provide a statement explaining the medical reason why the exception should be approved.

If you disagree with your Medicare drug plan's coverage determination or exception decision, *you can appeal. There are five levels of appeal. The first level is appealing to your plan. Once your Medicare drug plan gets your appeal, it has 7 days (for a standard appeal) or 72 hours (for an expedited appeal) to notify you of its decision. If you disagree with the plan's decision, you can ask for an independent review of your case. The notice you get with the plan's decision will explain the next level of appeal.*

Exclusion Coverage/Medicare
See *Coordination of coverage/Medicare.*

Exclusion Period/Medigap
See also *Preexisting condition, waiting period/Medigap.*

A period of time of up to six (6) months when an insurance company can refuse to cover a preexisting existing condition. Sometimes also called a waiting period.

Exclusion Ratio/Annuity
See also *Annuity.*

The formula given in the Internal Revenue Code for determining the portion of an annuity payment that will be taxable, and the portion that will be received tax-free.

Exclusions/LTCI

Conditions or circumstances under which benefits will not be payable under long-term care insurance policies:

Mental or emotional conditions;

Consequences of war;

Effects of suicide attempts;

Care rendered by family members;

Treatment of preexisting conditions (this is not excluded in newer policies if disclosed on the application);

Care rendered outside the United States; and

Care furnished in a Veterans Administration or other Federal government facility.

Exclusions/Medicaid
See also *Home Care, section 4.*

To the extent applicable to home care, the following services are not covered by Medicaid: room and board, full-time nursing care, and care provided by family members.

Exclusions/Medicare
See also *Medicare Part A hospital benefits, section 3; Medicare Part B benefits, section 4; Reasonable and necessary/Medicare.*

The two largest Medicare exclusions that may affect most people are prescription drug coverage and long-term care, especially custodial care, in a nursing home or at home. Since most long-term care needs are custodial, Medicare does not cover most long-term care.

Medicare expressly excludes coverage of many services:

Full-time nursing care;

Routine foot care, or orthopedic shoes;

Meals delivered to the home;

Cosmetic surgery;

Homemaker chores (e.g., general housekeeping, meal preparation, shopping) unrelated to patient care;

Custodial care;

Transportation;

Services that would not be covered as inpatient hospital services;

Ambulance from home to a doctor's office or a dialysis facility;

Routine physical examinations and tests directly related to such examinations (except some Pap smears, mammograms and prostate cancer screening);

Eye or ear examinations to prescribe or fit eyeglasses or hearing aids;

Immunizations, except flu vaccinations, pneumococcal pneumonia and hepatitis B vaccinations, or immunizations required because of an injury or immediate risk of infection;

Acupuncture;

Most chiropractic services;

Dental care;

Private room, TV and radio in hospital;

Private nurse;

Services payable by workers compensation, auto insurance, employer health plan or other governmental programs; and

Services provided outside the United States.

In addition, Medicare generally excludes any services that are not reasonable and necessary for the diagnosis or treatment of illness or injury, or to improve the functioning of a malformed body organ.

Exclusions/Medigap

See *Medicare supplemental insurance – Medigap.*

Medigap coverage generally excludes the same items excluded by Medicare. However, some of the standardized policies will cover items not covered under Medicare such as foreign travel emergency, preventive screening and partial prescription coverage.

Exclusive Provider Organization (EPO)/Managed Care

An EPO is a variant type of an HMO and provides an exclusive hospital and physician network from which a member must obtain health care services. A member who selects a hospital or physician from outside the network bears the entire cost of such services.

Exempt Resources/Medicaid

Those resources that are not counted, that is considered as not available, by Medicaid in determining an applicant's eligibility. The rules relating to Medicaid-exempt resources are rooted in SSI law. States can be more generous than the Federal law in their exemptions, but cannot be more restrictive, except in Section 209(b) states. Generally, states must exempt the following:

> Home of any value as long as the individual lives there or intends to return there, or as long as a spouse or disabled or dependent children live there;
>
> Household goods and personal effects of limited value;
>
> Automobile of limited value;
>
> A burial space of unlimited value, or the value of an agreement to purchase a burial space;
>
> A separate identifiable burial fund, not more than $1,500;
>
> Life insurance policies with a face value of $1,500 or less regardless of cash surrender value. The combined value of the burial fund and face value of life insurance policies cannot exceed $1,500 in aggregate; and

Up to $6,000 equity in non-business property (personal and real estate) that produces net annual income of at least six (6%) percent of the amount of the protected property, for example farm equipment to grow an individual's own food.

Different exempt resource rules apply to married couples when one spouse is in nursing facility, and, in some states, when one is receiving waivered home care services. (See *Community spouse's resource allowance (CSRA)/Medicaid*).

Exempt (Penalty) Transfer/Medicaid
See also *Transfer penalty civil/Medicaid; Transfer penalty criminal/Medicaid.*

Certain transfers of assets are exempt from transfer penalty rules and therefore do not trigger a transfer penalty. These are:

Transfers for fair market value or where the individual intended to receive fair market value;

Transfers exclusively for a purpose other than qualifying for Medicaid eligibility;

Transfers to a child under age 21 or to a child of any age who is blind or disabled as defined by SSI, or to a trust established for that child's benefit;

Transfers to or from an individual's spouse or to a third party for the sole benefit of the individual's spouse, as well as transfers from the individual spouse to the other spouse for the sole benefit of the spouse;

Transfers of an individual's home, if transferred to:

- The individual's spouse;
- The individual's child who is under age 21, or who is blind or disabled;
- The sibling of an individual who had an equity in the home and resided in its for one year prior to the individual's institutionalization;
- An individual's child (other than a child who is under age 21, blind or disabled) who resided in the home at least two (2)

177

years prior to the individual's institutionalization and who provided services to the individual that delayed institutionalization;

Transfers to a trust for a disabled person under the age of 65 of that person's assets, established for his/her benefit by the person's parent, grandparent, legal guardian or court; upon the death of the disabled person, any funds remaining in the trust must be used to repay the state for the person's Medicaid assistance;

Transfers where the transferred assets have been returned; and

Transfers where the state determines that a penalty would result in undue hardship.

Exempt Trusts/Transfer Penalty/Medicaid

See *Trust, Medicaid eligibility rules; Trust transfer penalty rules/Medicaid.*

Expenses in Calculating Spend Down/Medicaid

See also *Spend down/Medicaid.*

These are medical and remedial expenses that are deducted from an individual's income in determining eligibility for Medicaid. Generally, states must include medical services and supplies recognized under state law whether or not they are included in the state's Medicaid program. The expenses need only be incurred, not paid.

Explanation of Medicare Benefits (EOMB)

See also *Summary notice/Medicare.*

A notice from the Medicare insurance carrier informing the patient how much it has paid for a service covered by Medicare Part B, the services covered and charges approved. For services for which a doctor or other provider has taken assignment, the carrier pays the doctor or other provider directly. For unassigned services, the carrier pays the patient, and he/she is responsible for paying the provider.

The Medicare summary notice has replaced the explanation of Medicare benefits.

Extended Care Facility

A term for what is now more commonly called a skilled nursing facility.

Extended Care Services/Medicare

Services provided in a skilled nursing facility for a limited time after a hospital stay and for the same condition as the hospital stay.

*Extra Help (Help Paying Medicare Drug Costs)/Medicare

A Medicare program to help people with limited income and resources pay Medicare prescription drug program costs, such as premiums, deductibles, and coinsurance.

Extra Help Subsidy/Medicare Part D Drug Coverage
See also *Low-income beneficiaries/Medicare Part D Drug Coverage.*

Individuals without SSI or who are not dual eligibles, but have low income and resources may be eligible for the low-income subsidy called extra help subsidy.

*Eyeglasses/Medicare

One pair of eyeglasses with standard frames (or one set of contact lenses) after cataract surgery that implants an intraocular lens. You pay 20% of the Medicare-approved amount, and the Part B deductible applies.

Eyeglasses/Medicare
See also *Optometrist services/Medicare.*

Medicare does not cover eyeglasses, except for one pair following cataract surgery. In some states Medicaid pays for eyeglasses.

(continued on next page)

F

Fair Hearing/Medicaid
See also *Appeals/Medicaid.*

A formal hearing for the benefit of an applicant for or recipient of Medicaid to challenge various determinations of the Medicaid agency. Because Medicaid coverage is so critical to program recipients, they have a constitutional right to a full and fair process, including access to their records, the right to bring witnesses to cross-examine the agency's witnesses and to present evidence. Fair hearings can be used to increase the community spouse's income and resource allowances.

Family Allowance/Medicaid
See also *Permitted deductions/Medicaid.*

A family allowance for each dependent family member is among the deductions taken from the income of a Medicaid recipient in determining the amount available that an individual must apply to the cost of nursing home care. The family allowance for each dependent family member is an amount equal to one-third of the difference between the family member's income and one-hundred fifty (150%) percent of the monthly Federal poverty standard for a two-person household.

Family Maximum/Social Security
See also *Primary insurance amount (PIA)/Social Security.*

The family maximum varies from ten (10%) percent to one-hundred eighty-eight (188%) percent of the worker's primary insurance amount (PIA) for retirement or survivor benefits and from ten (10%) percent to one-hundred (100%) percent of the PIA for disability benefits. The worker always receives the full benefit payable. If the family maximum is reached, each dependent receives a prorated share of the remainder. Benefits to a divorced spouse or to the surviving divorced spouse of a deceased worker are payable without regard to the family maximum and do not affect benefits to other eligible dependents.

All entries preceded by an asterisk (*) are culled or copied from the official U.S. government **Medicare** handbook (*Medicare & You 2011*).

Farmers Home Administration (FHA)

The Farmers Home Administration is a home financing agency within the United States Department of Agriculture. FHA programs are limited to jurisdictions with less than 20,000 residents. FHA sponsors various programs including mortgages for low- and moderate-income home buyers, home repair programs and low-interest mortgages for affordable multifamily rental developments. Some FHA multifamily rental developments are restricted to people who are at least 62 years of age or disabled.

*Fecal Occult Blood Test/Medicare

Once every 12 months if 50 or older. You pay nothing for the test, but you generally have to pay 20% of the Medicare-approved amount for the doctor's visit.

Federal Housing Programs for the Elderly

The Federal government provides a variety of housing and rental subsidy programs for seniors and/or non-elderly disabled persons who meet specific eligibility requirements. The basic structure and qualifying requirements for many of these programs have been significantly modified over the years to reflect changing federal priorities and resources and may differ by community and year enacted.

The Housing and Development Act of 1959, as amended, was the landmark legislation passed by Congress that established a Federal housing policy for senior citizens and created many of these prototype programs. To qualify for most Federal housing and/or subsidy programs, persons must be 62 years of age or older and have incomes that do not exceed eighty (80%) percent of the median income for that geographic area.

A few of the more popular Federal programs, commonly known by the relevant section number in the Housing and Urban Development Act, are described below. Some of these programs are no longer funded.

> **Section 202** provides one-hundred (100%) percent of the funds to community-based non-profit sponsors to construct and operate rental apartment housing for low-income older and/or handicapped persons. Generally provides for a rental subsidy for eligible residents.

> **Section 8 rental subsidy** has been the most frequently used rental subsidy program available and is widely used in public housing. Generally the

program provides owners of rental housing a direct subsidy to cover the difference between the rent collected from an income-eligible tenant and the actual cost to operate his/her apartment. For Section 202 buildings for elderly tenants constructed after 1990, the Section 8 subsidy program evolved into the project rental assistance (PRAC) program. Under both programs, eligible residents pay no more than thirty (30%) percent of their adjusted gross income, as defined by HUD, for rent.

Section 232 provides ability for HUD-approved lenders to make insured loans for the refurbishing, new construction and substantial rehability of resident care facilities, including skilled care nursing, intermediate care and assisted-living facilities.

Section 221(d) provided mortgage insurance and tax incentives for investors and non-profit organizations during the 1960s and early 1970s to develop rental housing for persons of low to moderate income.

Section 236 provided a significant mortgage subsidy, generally 1%, to developers and sponsors of rental apartments for low-to-moderate income persons. This program was most popular during the 1960s and 1970s and is no longer available.

Congregate Housing Services Program provides funding to sponsors of senior housing for the inclusion of certain support services for the residents of the housing project. Established in 1978 as a demonstration project, this program continues to be funded on a very limited basis.

Home Investment Partnerships Programs (HOME). The HOME program was created under Title 11 of the National Affordable Housing Act of 1990 to extend and strengthen partnerships among all levels of government and the private sector, including for-profit and non-profit organizations, in the production and operation of affordable housing. The HOME program provides funding and general guidelines to state and local governments, empowering them to design and tailor affordable housing strategies to address local needs and housing conditions.

Federal Poverty Level (FPL)

The FPL is used to determine the income standard for Medicaid eligibility for certain categories of beneficiaries. It is adjusted annually for inflation and published by the Department of Health and Human Services as poverty guidelines.

*Federally Qualified Health Center Services/Medicare

Includes many outpatient primary care and preventive services you get through certain community-based organizations. Generally, you pay 20% of the Medicare-approved amount.

Federally Qualified HMO

Such an HMO is authorized by law to enter into a contract with Medicare.

Fee-for-Service

An arrangement whereby a physician or health care provider is paid a fee for each service after it is performed. This is in contrast to a fixed fee prepayment, capitated arrangement with Medicare Advantage plans, which is without regard to the number of services actually used.

Fee-for-Service Continuing Care Contract
See *Continuing care retirement community (CCRC).*

Fee-for-Services Plans (PFFS)/Medicare Advantage
See *Medicare Advantage private fee-for-service (PFFS) plans.*

Fee Schedule
See also *Fee schedule charge/Medicare.*

A comprehensive listing of fees used by either a government or private health care plan to reimburse physicians and/or other providers on a fee-for-service basis.

Fee Schedule Charge/Medicare
See *Approved charge/Medicare; Conversion factor/Medicare; Resource-based relative value scale (RBRVS)/Medicare; Physician fee schedule/Medicare.*

The fee schedule charge replaces the customary, prevailing and reasonable charge that historically was the basis for Medicare reimbursement. The core of the fee schedule method is the computation system under which the Secretary of HHS assigns numerical values to all medical services. The government uses a monetary conversion factor to arrive at a price for a given service, multiplying the conversion factor and a geographic adjustment factor by the numerical value assigned to the service by the Secretary. The conversion factor is updated annually, by statutory formula, based upon the Medicare economic index.

Feeding/Medicare

Feeding by an aide is not covered by Medicare except in limited instances when prescribed by a doctor.

Financial Incentive Plans/Managed Care

Physicians in prepaid health care organizations generally receive fee-for-service payments, salary or capitation payment for their service. In addition, organizations may offer them financial incentives plans such as withholds, bonuses or unused capitation to encourage them to control referral services and to refer patients for treatment by specialists for inpatient hospital care only when medically necessary.

First-Dollar Coverage

Insurance coverage by a third-party payer, from the first dollar of expense for services incurred. The insured does not pay a deductible.

Fiscal Assessment/Medicaid
See also *Snapshot rule/Medicaid.*

A fiscal assessment by Medicaid is one of the steps in establishing an applicant's eligibility for Medicaid home care services by comparing the cost of needed home care to the cost of nursing home care.

Fiscal Intermediary/Medicare
See also *Intermediary/Medicare.*

A private company, also called an intermediary, that has a contract with Medicare to pay Part A (hospital) bills.

Fixed Annuity
See *Annuity.*

Flat Monthly Maintenance Allowance/Medicaid
See *Minimum monthly maintenance needs allowance/Medicaid.*

*Flexible Sigmoidoscopy/Medicare

Generally, once every 48 months if 50 or older, or 120 months after a previous screening colonoscopy for those not at high risk. Starting January 1, 2011, you pay nothing for this test if the doctor accepts assignment.

*Flu Shot/Medicare

Generally covered once per flu season in the fall or winter. You pay nothing for the flu shot if the doctor or other health care provider accepts assignment for giving the shot.

Flu Shot/Medicare

Medicare Part B helps to pay for this immunization each fall. No Part B deductible or coinsurance is required.

*Foot Exam/Medicare

If you have diabetes-related nerve damage and/or meet certain conditions. You pay the doctor 20% of the Medicare-approved amount, and the Part B deductible applies. In a hospital outpatient setting, you also pay the hospital a copayment.

Formal Caregiver

A trained volunteer or paid health care provider associated with a service system. Contrasts with informal caregiver.

*Formulary/Medicare Part D Drug Coverage

A list of prescription drugs covered by a prescription drug plan or another insurance plan offering prescription drug benefits.

Formulary/Medicare Part D Drug Coverage

A list of covered drugs available through the Part D plan. A Part D plan's formulary must include at least two (2) drugs in each therapeutic category and class. Money spent on medicines "on formulary" counts towards the out-of-pocket threshold; money spent on non-formulary drugs does not count towards the out-of-pocket threshold. A beneficiary's doctor or health professional may be able to help the beneficiary obtain an exception if a medicine he/she needs is not on formulary.

If the exception is approved, the patient's share of that drug's cost would then count towards out-of-pocket spending. (See *Out-of-pocket spending/Medicare Part D Drug Coverage*).

Forward Averaging

A technique for reducing the income tax on a lump-sum pension payout by treating it as if it had been received over five (5) years or ten years rather than a single year. Individuals who receive lump-sum distributions after December 31, 1999 no longer have an option of using five- (5) year forward averaging. However, ten- (10) year averaging will remain available to individuals born before 1936.

Foster Care

Placement of an older person in need of minimum assistance into a family environment in a state- or county-licensed home.

Free Look/Medigap

A period of time, usually thirty (30) days, during which an applicant can examine a Medigap policy. If he/she is dissatisfied with the policy or changes his/her mind about wanting the coverage, the policy can be canceled, and any payment made for the policy must be returned to the policy applicant.

Freedom of Choice Legislation
See *Any willing provider bill.*

Friendly Visitor

This person, who is also known as a senior companion, visits an elderly person at scheduled times to provide companionship and socialization.

Full-Benefit Dual Eligible/Medicare Part D Drug Coverage
See also *Dual eligibles/Medicare.*

Individuals who are entitled to full Medicaid status.

Full Subsidy/Medicare Part D Drug Coverage

All full-subsidy eligible individuals are entitled to the entire subsidy premium, elimination of the deductible, continuation of coverage through the doughnut hole, and elimination of all cost-sharing except as stated in next paragraph after they meet the out-of-pocket thresholds.

Copayments are paid by full-subsidy individuals as follows:

> no copay if institutionalized;

> for those with incomes up to one-hundred (100%) percent of FPL, not more than $1.10 for a generic or preferred brand or $3.30 non-preferred brand; and

> for the other full-subsidy individuals, $2.50 for a generic or preferred brand or $6.30 for a non-preferred brand, indexed annually to the cost of Part D drugs in 2010.

Full-Subsidy Eligible Individuals/Medicare Part D Drug Coverage

Full-subsidy eligible individuals are individuals with full Medicaid status (full-benefit dual eligibles), those with SSI but not Medicaid, those enrolled in one of three (3) medical savings account programs, and individuals with incomes below one-hundred thirty-five (135%) percent of the Federal poverty level and countable resources of not more than $8,440 (2012) for an individual and $13,410 (2012) for a couple.

Fully Insured/Social Security
See also *Social Security Program.*

For Social Security purposes, an individual is fully insured when he/she has the requisite quarters (now called work credits) of covered employment which generally is forty (40). For each year of birth prior to 1929, one less quarter of coverage is required. Fully insured status is required for entitlement to most Social Security benefits for workers.

(continued on next page)

G

Gag Rule/Managed Care
See *Health Maintenance Organization (HMO)*.

Gap/Medicare
See also *Deductible/Medicare, Medigap*.

Medicare does not pay in full for medical services although they are Medicare-approved. The difference between the charge for such services and the amount Medicare will pay is called a gap. Also, there are many medical services that Medicare does not cover which are generally called exclusions. When a gap or exclusion exists, the patient must pay out of pocket. Some help with these gaps and exclusions is available from private insurance companies through Medicare supplemental (Medigap) insurance and long-term care insurance.

Gatekeeper

The gatekeeper is a physician, usually a primary care doctor, responsible for the administration of a patient's treatment. This doctor coordinates and authorizes all medical services, laboratory studies, specialty referrals and hospitalizations. In the instance of HMOs, if an enrollee visits a specialist without prior authorization from his/her designated primary care physician, the medical services delivered by the specialist will have to be paid in full by the patient.

Gatekeeper Mechanism

In health care, an arrangement whereby a patient is assigned to or chooses from a selected group of primary care physicians, and the primary care physician (gatekeeper) assumes responsibility for and approves all health services of the patient. This mechanism entails a system such as a utilization review set up by the insurance carrier to ensure that benefits are paid only to those who qualify under the terms of the policy.

All entries preceded by an asterisk (*) are culled or copied from the official U.S. government **Medicare** handbook (*Medicare & You 2011*).

*General Enrollment Period/Medicare (Part A, Part B)

If you didn't sign up for Part A and/or Part B (for which you pay monthly premiums) when you were first eligible, you can sign up between January 1 – March 31 each year. Your coverage will begin July 1st. You may have to pay a higher premium for late enrollment.

General Enrollment Period/Medicare

See *Eligibility and enrollment/Medicare.*

General Power of Appointment

A power that allows the trustee, without the consent of the creator (grantor) of that power or any other party, to vest trust assets in himself, his estate, his creditors or the creditors of his estate. If the trustee dies holding a general power of appointment, trust assets subject to the power will be included in the trustee's taxable estate, even though the trustee has not exercised the power and the trustee's estate does not have access to trust property to pay the tax.

Generation Skipping Tax

This Federal transfer tax is imposed on transfers of property, testamentary or *inter vivos*, between parties separated by two (2) or more generations. The generation skipping tax (GST) prevents property from passing over a generation without being subject to estate tax. For example, when a grandparent bequeaths his/her property to a grandchild rather than to a living child, the tax on the passage of property to the grandchild, but for the GST, would be avoided.

Each time a generation skipping transfer takes place, the GST is levied at a rate equal to the then highest estate tax rate. Transfers subject to GST are: distributions from a generation skipping trust; the termination of the interest of a preceding generation; and direct transfers to grandchildren or later generations.

Each person is entitled to a cumulative $1 million lifetime exemption which may be allocated to any generation skipping transfer made by that person before the GST is imposed.

Generic Substitution/Medicare Part D Drug Coverage

The dispensing of a generic drug in place of a brand name drug. Generic drugs must contain the same active ingredients as the brand name drugs.

Geriatric Assessment

An evaluation of an older person's physical, psychological and social condition by a professional team of specialists in geriatrics and gerontology, who make recommendations to the older person, family and primary care doctor. Geriatric assessments are available in geriatric evaluation centers which are generally associated with hospitals.

Geriatric Care Manager

See also *Case management; Information and referral services.*

A geriatric care manger is a social service professional with expertise in devising, monitoring and coordinating care plans for older people. This manager may be retained privately by an older person and his/her family, although care management is frequently done by insurers or public agencies.

Geriatric Evaluation Center

See *Geriatric assessment.*

Geriatric Medicine

The branch of medicine dealing with the disorders and conditions, such as incontinence and Alzheimer's disease, associated with the aging process. Also known as geriatrics.

Geriatric Social Worker

A licensed professional who assists the elderly and their families in understanding and coping with the social, emotion and psychological aspects of aging. A geriatric social worker coordinates, directs and instructs in assessing elder care services.

Geriatrician

A physician who specializes in geriatric medicine.

Gerontology

The field of learning, applied research and social work relating to older people and the process of aging. The term usually applies broadly to the non-medical aspects of aging.

Gift Tax
See also *Annual gift tax exclusion.*

This is a Federal tax on the value of transferred property determined on the date of the transfer. A gift of a present interest in property qualifies for an annual exclusion. Thus, a gift in the year 2010 of up to $13,000 (adjusted for inflation annually) to a donee will qualify for a complete exclusion from the gift tax. Such exclusion is separately applicable for an unlimited number of donees.

*Glaucoma Test/Medicare

Covered once every 12 months for people at high risk for the eye disease glaucoma. You're at high risk if you have diabetes, a family history of glaucoma, are African-American and 50 or older, or are Hispanic and 65 or older. An eye doctor who is legally allowed by the state must do the tests. You pay the doctor 20% of the Medicare-approved amount, and the Part B deductible applies for the doctor's visit. In a hospital outpatient setting, you also pay the hospital copayment.

Grantor of a Trust

The grantor, also referred to as settlor, is the person who creates and funds a trust. However, if someone other than the grantor named in the trust instrument is the primary source of funding for the trust, this individual would be considered the grantor for tax purposes. If more than one person funds the trust, there will be multiple grantors for tax purposes.

Grantor Retained Annuity Trust (GRAT)
See also *Grantor retained income trust (GRIT).*

A GRAT is an estate tax-saving trust. It pays the trust creator (or grantor) a set annual amount for a specified period of time, and thereafter pays the trust beneficiaries. The value of the gift to the beneficiaries is determined by subtracting the total amount of payments to the creator from the principal of the trust. If the creator of the trust dies during the payment period, his/her estate for tax purposes would include part or all of the trust assets depending on how much of the estate assets are required to pay the remaining payments due to the creator of the trust.

Grantor Retained Income Trust (GRIT)

A GRIT (also called a house grit or, more often, QPRT or qualified personal residence trust) is an estate tax-saving trust involving a donor's gift of his/her personal residence regardless of whether it is the primary residence or a vacation home. The donor places the residence in trust but reserves the use of the residence for a specified number of years. After that period the donor's rights cease, and title to the residence passes to the trust beneficiaries. The value of the gift is actuarially determined so that the longer the donor retains use of the premises, the smaller is the value of the gift that is subject to estate tax. However, if the donor dies during the specified period he/she retains the right to use the residence, the entire value of the property is included in his/her estate for tax purposes.

Grantor Retained Unitrust (GRUT)

A GRUT is an estate tax-saving trust comparable to a GRAT. The difference is that the amount of the annual payment to the creator of a GRUT is not set as with a GRAT but changes from year to year if the value of the trust assets changes. The payments to the creator of the trust would be equal to a specified percentage of the trust assets re-determined each year.

Grievance Procedures/Medicare Advantage

Each MA organization must provide meaningful grievance procedures for the timely hearing and resolving of grievances between enrollees and the organization or any other entity or individual through which the organization provides health care services under any Medicare Advantage plan it offers.

Grievance means any complaint or dispute, other than one that constitutes an organization determination, expressing dissatisfaction with any aspect of an MA organization's or provider's operations, activities, or behavior, regardless of whether remedial action is requested.

Grievance procedures are distinct from appeal procedures, which address an organization determination. Upon receiving a complaint, an MA organization must promptly determine whether the complaint is subject to its appeal or grievance procedures. MA organization grievance procedures are also different from the quality improvement organization (QIO) complaint process where the QIO reviews beneficiaries' written complaints about quality of services they have received under the Medicare program. For quality of care issues, an enrollee may file a grievance with the MA organization, file a written complaint with the QIO, or both.

An enrollee must file his grievance with an MA organization, either orally or in writing, within sixty (60) days of the event that gives rise to the grievance. The MA organization must notify the enrollee of its decision as expeditiously as the case requires based on the enrollee's health, but no later than thirty (30) days after its receives the grievance. The organization may extend the thirty- (30) day timeframe by up to fourteen (14) days if the enrollee requests the extension or if the organization can show the delay is in the enrollee's best interest.

When an MA organization extends the deadline, it must inform the enrollee in writing of the reasons for the delay.

If the enrollee submits the grievance in writing, the MA organization must respond in writing. The MA organization must respond in writing to all grievances relating quality of care, regardless of how the grievance is filed. The response must include a description of the enrollee's right to file a written complaint with the QIO. For any complaint submitted to the QIO, the MA organization must cooperate with the QIO in resolving the compliant.

An MA organization must respond to an enrollee's grievance within twenty-four (24) hours if:

> The complaint involves an MA organization's decision to invoke an extension relating to an organization determination or reconsideration.

> The complaint involves an MA organization's refusal to grant an enrollee's request for an expedited organization determination or reconsideration.

An expedited grievance process provides important protections for enrollees who are unable (or prefer not) to obtain a physician's certification that when applying the standard time frame for appeals, would have adverse consequences for the enrollee. If an expedited grievance proceeds under these circumstances, the decision about the grievance would not be the organization determination, but the plan's appropriate use of its discretion to extend the time frame.

Gross Income

Gross income is all of a taxpayer's income from whatever source derived, whether in the form of money, property or services.

Group Home

A home occupied by a group of unrelated people who share in meal preparation, housekeeping, maintenance and financial activities.

Group Long-term Care Insurance

A contract between an employer or organization such as an association, and an insurance company that provides for stipulated long-term care benefits for the employees/members. Sometimes other family members such as spouses and parents may be offered coverage. Premiums may be paid solely by the employer or employee or shared by both. At present, coverage and terms of individual policies are generally more favorable to the consumer.

Guaranteed Issue/Medigap
See *Preexisting condition, Guaranteed issue/Medigap.*

Guaranteed Renewable Policy/LTCI

The insurer issuing a guaranteed renewable long-term care insurance policy cannot cancel the policy or refuse to renew it when it expires unless policy benefits have been exhausted or the insured person has failed to make timely premium payments. The insurer cannot increase a particular policyholder's or certificate holder's premiums because of his/her age or mental condition. However, the insurer can increase the premiums for an entire class of policyholders or certificate holders. According to the Health Insurance Portability and Accountability Act of 1996, all LTCI policies sold after January 1, 1997 must be guaranteed renewable in order to be eligible for the tax advantages allowed by the legislation.

Guardian of the Estate
See *Adult guardian.*

Guardian of the Person
See *Adult guardian.*

(continued on next page)

195

H

Health Care Financing Administration (HCFA)

This Federal agency now known as Centers for Medicaid and Medicare is part of the U.S. Department of Health and Human Services and is responsible for Medicare and Medicaid administration and regulations.

*Health Care Proxy/Medicare

A health care proxy (sometimes called a "durable power of attorney for health care") is used to name the person you wish to make health care decisions for you if you aren't able to make them yourself. Having a health care proxy is important because if you suddenly aren't able to make your own health care decisions, someone you trust will be able to make these decisions for you.

Health Care Proxy
See *Advance directive.*

Health Insurance Card/Medicare

Medicare-eligible persons receive a Medicare Health Service card in the mail following an application for Medicare or in certain cases automatically. The card is red, white and blue. It shows the name of the Medicare person, his/her Medicare claim number (Social Security number), entitlement to Hospital Insurance (Part A) and/or Supplemental Medical Insurance (Part B), and the effective date of each. If the Medicare eligible should lose or damage the Medicare health insurance card, he/she can order a new card online at *www.socialsecurity.gov* (selecting a number from the "subject" list) or by calling the Social Security Administration at 1-800-772-1213. Persons who are deaf, hard of hearing or have speech impairments can call 1-800-325-0778.

All entries preceded by an asterisk (*) are culled or copied from the official U.S. government **Medicare** handbook (*Medicare & You 2011*).

Health Insurance Claim Number/Medicare

This claim number appears on the Medicare card. It is the means by which all medical claims are identified.

Health Insurance Counseling and Assistance program (HICAP)

To help Medicare beneficiaries understand their health insurance coverage and options, CMS grants states funds to set up and operate this volunteer-based counseling program. Its name varies from state to state. In most states the area agencies on aging are the local administrators of HICAPs whose mission is to provide unbiased information not only about standard Medicare insurance and Medicare Advantage plans but also about Medigap policies, Medicaid and long-term care insurance options.

Health Insurance Plans, Private

Many commercial companies market a range of health insurance plans designed for seniors, including Medicare supplemental (Medigap) insurance, hospital indemnity insurance, major medical or catastrophic insurance and long-term care insurance. The terms of the policies and the rates are regulated by an insurance commission in each state. Consequently, policies differ from state to state.

Health Insuring Organization (HIO)/Medicaid
See also *Medicaid Mandatory Managed Care.*

HIOs are Medicaid managed care organizations that pay for the services of subcontracting providers and assume all financial risk in exchange for a premium. The HIO organizes the network of providers with preauthorization and utilization review to control the volume of services. Providers in the network serve as case managers and, in some HIOs, receive capitated payments. While HIOs function very much like independent practice associations, they include all physicians who are willing to abide by the specified contractual arrangements for all Medicaid beneficiaries who live in a designated area.

(continued on next page)

HEALTH MAINTENANCE ORGANIZATION (HMO)/MEDICARE, MEDICAID

INTRODUCTION

(See Managed care; Medicare Advantage (MA)/HMO plans; Medicare Advantage (MA) program, sections I. A and B, sections II. A–C.)

Health maintenance organizations (HMOs) are a type of managed care provided to participants (enrollees) under a medical benefits plan, featuring a network of doctors, hospitals and other health care providers. An individual may enroll in an HMO on his/her own, or as a participant of a group plan offered by an employer or an association. HMOs undertake to provide all of the care necessary for a given beneficiary, acting in essence as an insurer as well as a provider.

Prior to the Balanced Budget Act of 1997 (BBA), Medicare beneficiaries had the option of enrolling in Medicare HMOs instead of the traditional Medicare fee-for-service program. With the passage of the BBA, beneficiaries may enroll in a Medicare Advantage HMO, which has replaced the original Medicare HMO.

Many states are shifting recipients of Medicaid assistance into HMOs. (See *Medicaid mandatory managed care.*)

The salient features of an HMO are set forth below.

I.   MODELS OF HMOS.

HMOs are classified into three models:

Staff model. A single large HMO that employs physicians and pays them a salary to provide services exclusively to plan enrollees.

Group model. An HMO which contracts with groups of physicians to provide care to its plan enrollees typically for a capitated rate and with which physicians have an exclusive relationship.

Independent Practice Association (IPA). In contrast to the staff and group models, this type HMO contracts with an organization of physicians for only a portion of their practices. Physicians in the IPA provide care for the HMO's enrollees at a capitated rate or fee-for-service rate paid to the IPA which in turn pays the participating physicians. The physicians work in their own settings.

II.   PRIMARY CARE (GATEKEEPER).

HMO participants are assigned or choose a physician in the HMO network, sometimes called a gatekeeper, who renders primary care, determines a patient's need for a specialist to treat a particular illness or injury, and refers the patient to a designated specialist.

III.   CAPITATED FEE.

Medicare Advantage HMO enrollees pay a fixed periodic fee, known as a capitated fee, covering an agreed upon range of services, regardless of the extent to which these services are utilized.

IV.   ENROLLEES ARE LOCKED IN.

Enrollees are usually locked into an HMO plan. Only services provided through the HMO, with a few exceptions such as emergency care or urgent care, will be paid for by the HMO. Under the lock-in feature, patients desiring a physician or a specialist who is not part of the HMO network are liable for all payments in connection with services performed by such providers.

As enrollment in HMOs has expanded, states have increasingly focused on particular aspects of HMOs' procedures and practices. Several states have passed legislation affecting particular policies and practices of HMOs.

> **Any willing provider.** Several states have proposed or enacted legislation known as any willing provider bills or freedom of choice legislation which require HMO networks to accept any physician who has appropriate credentials and agrees to abide by contract terms and conditions.

Emergency Care. Several states have enacted legislation under which health networks must pay for emergency care services whenever a prudent layperson would consider a situation an emergency. The care may not be delayed to obtain the health care organization's approval.

Gag Rules. Legislation enacted in several states prohibits health organization networks from restricting the information which physicians may give to patients about care choices. The legislation is directed to "gag" clauses in contracts between an HMO and its participating physicians which limit their ability to counsel patients about a full range of medically necessary treatment options, regardless of their cost.

Withholds. Several states, such as Maryland, have enacted legislation which prohibits HMOs from holding back until the end of the financial year a set dollar amount or a portion of the physician's service fee, capitation or annual salary, depending on predetermined factors. Withholds are intended to be an incentive for a physician to keep the cost of the services below specific targets. The legislation has extended this ban to physicians in fee-for-service discount networks. The legislation continues to allow HMO to pay bonuses for keeping costs down. In such cases, patients, the state or both are required to be informed of financial incentives that health networks offer to physicians.

V.   FEDERAL POLICIES AND PROTECTIONS.

At the Federal level, CMS regulations protecting Medicare and Medicaid HMO enrollees in a fashion similar to state legislation discussed above first were expanded and then codified in the Balanced Budget Act of 1997. Key elements of the regulations and legislation are described below.

Gag Rules. HMOs are forbidden to insert gag clauses in contracts with participating physicians.

Prohibited Physician Payments. HMOs may not directly or indirectly make a payment to a physician or physician group under an incentive plan that directly or indirectly may have the effect of reducing or limiting medically necessary services covered under the organization's contract with an enrollee.

Stop-loss protection. In any incentive plans, HMOs may not subject a physician or physician group to substantial financial risk beyond a statutory maximum amount or threshold risk, if the risk is based on the cost or use of referral services such as those of specialists or hospitals. This is termed stop-loss protection. Amounts at risk based solely upon factors other than levels of referral services are not considered in determining what constitutes substantial financial risk.

Disclosure Requirements. HMOs with incentive plans must disclose to CMS information about these plans, including the amount of any bonus, withhold or capitation and the amount of stop-loss protection. Upon request, Medicare beneficiaries and Medicaid recipients must be provided a summary of the information supplied to CMS.

(continued on next page)

Health Maintenance Organization (HMO)/Medicare Advantage
See also *Health maintenance organization/Medicare, Medicaid.*

A Medicare Advantage HMO is one of the several types of Medicare Advantage coordinated care plans authorized by the Balanced Budget Act of 1997. (See *Coordinated care plans/Medicare Advantage.*) The HMO is a managed care arrangement between: (i) individual participants and the HMO, which provides to the participants through a network of doctors and other health providers an array of Medicare-covered medical services (physician services, and a range of laboratory, x-ray and ancillary services); and (ii) the HMO and Medicare which pays the HMO a fixed predetermined, periodic fee, known as a capitation fee.

The plan participants are locked into and may only use a network provider (except for emergency or urgent care). Services received by a participant, other than through the HMO network, will not be paid for by the HMO; the participant is personally liable for these out-of-network services. An HMO with a point-of-service option is available to Medicare Advantage plan enrollees – this type of managed service plan allows enrollees to use medical providers (e.g., doctors and hospitals) outside the plan for no additional costs.

An enrollee generally will be asked to choose a primary care doctor (commonly referred to as a gatekeeper). Should the enrollee seek a specialist, he/she needs a referral from the primary care doctor, except that generally a woman does not need a reference for a yearly screening mammogram, or in-network pap tests and pelvic exams (at least every other year), provided the specialist is in the network.

An enrollee who wants prescription drug coverage must get it from the HMO plan.

Health Plan Organization

An organization that acts as insurer for enrolled participants.

*Hearing Aids/Medicare

Medicare does not cover hearing aids. If you need a hearing aid or certain other services that Medicare doesn't cover, you will have to pay for them yourself unless you have other insurance to cover the costs. Even if Medicare covers a service or item, you generally have to pay deductibles, coinsurance and copayments.

Hearing Aid/Medicare

Not covered by Medicare, but in certain states Medicaid may cover.

203

Heart Transplant/Medicare

Under certain limited conditions, Medicare Part B helps pay for heart transplants.

HEDIS/Managed Care

To evaluate managed care plans according to a set of performance measures, the National Committee for Quality Assurance has developed the health plan employer data and information set (HEDIS). The HEDIS performance measures include the effectiveness of care, access/availability of care, satisfaction with care, the cost and the operational services of a health plan.

Hemophilia Clotting Factors/Medicare

Medicare Part B helps pay for blood-clotting factors and items related to their administration for hemophilia patients who are able to use them to control bleeding without medical or other supervision. The amount of clotting factors necessary to have on hand for a specific period is determined for each patient individually.

*Hepatitis B Shots/Medicare

Covered for people at high or medium risk for Hepatitis B. Your risk for Hepatitis B increases if you have hemophilia, End-Stage Renal Disease (ESRD), or certain conditions that increase your risk for infection. Other factors may increase your risk for Hepatitis B, so check with your doctor. You pay nothing for the shot if the doctor accepts assignment.

Hepatitis B Vaccine/Medicare

Medicare Part B helps pay for hepatic B vaccine administered to beneficiaries considered to be at high or intermediate risk of contracting the disease.

*HIV Screening/Medicare

Medicare covers HIV (Human Immunodeficiency Virus) screening for people with Medicare of any age who ask for the test, pregnant women, and people at increased risk for the infection. Medicare covers this test once every 12 months or up to 3 times during a pregnancy. You pay nothing for the test, but you generally have to pay the doctor 20% of the Medicare-approved amount for the doctor's visit.

Home and Community-Based Care Services
See also *Older Americans Act; Optional services/Medicaid.*

Home and Community-Based Waivers/Medicaid
See also *Waivered services/Medicaid.*

CMS grants waivers of certain requirements imposed by the Federal Medicaid program on state Medicaid plans, so that the states can provide Medicaid long-term care services in settings other than nursing homes, in order to prevent premature institutionalization. States generally serve small populations of either elderly or non-elderly disabled individuals under waiver programs. If they provided the same services without the waiver, as optional services, they would have to provide them to all people eligible under their general Medicaid program. Thus, the waiver allows states to limit their coverage substantially. Many of the benefits offered under the Medicaid waiver programs are also available through funding under the Older Americans Act.

The services that the states, at their option without a waiver, may provide include case management, personal care, adult day health, rehabilitation, respite care, transportation, in-home support services, meal services, special communication services, minor home modifications and adult day care.

Home Attendant
See also *Home health aide.*

An individual, sometimes also called a personal care aide, who performs unskilled personal care services, such as bathing, feeding and dressing a disabled person at home. A home attendant is distinct from a home health aide who performs more skilled tasks and has received in-service training through an approved program.

(continued on next page)

HOME CARE

INTRODUCTION

(See also *Medicare/Home Health Care, sections I, II and III*)

Home care services permit a physically impaired older person to live at home independently, in a familiar environment, rather than in the institutional setting of a nursing home, or in a board-and-care facility. As a general rule, any person who is not acutely ill can be adequately cared for in the home provided his/her resources, governmental assistance and/or community-based services are available.

An organized home care program can be provided through a combination of informal caregivers, especially family members, as well as formal caregivers such as a geriatric case manager and providers from a home health agency. Under the direction of a physician, the care can be oriented to a patient's needs. It may be similar to the level of skilled care provided in a skilled nursing facility (nursing, nutritional services, physical, occupational and speech therapy), and more often than not it can be unskilled care in the nature of custodial or personal care.

Home care is a broadly based term (see *Home care services*) whose meaning encompasses the more restrictive, medically oriented term "home health care." The two terms should not be confused. Medicare, on a limited basis, covers home health care and carefully defines home health care and the conditions for coverage.

I. PROVIDERS OF SERVICE.

Services may be provided by medical or other trained persons such as doctors, nurses, home health aides, therapists, geriatric care managers and social workers. Non-medical services may be provided by personal care aides, homemakers, family members, community volunteers and city or state agency personnel. Family members and friends are the largest single sources of support and care for older persons who continue to live at home but are limited in one or more activities of daily living.

II. RESOURCES.

Many resources provide information about or the actual delivery of home care and related services, including hospital discharge planners, home health agencies, public health and welfare departments, area agencies on aging, non-profit voluntary agencies (e.g., United Way), adult day care centers, senior centers and churches and synagogues.

Home health agencies are the major sources for obtaining home health services. They provide nursing services, home health aide services, medical supplies and equipment, physical, occupational and speech therapy, nutritional counseling and social work services.

III. TYPES OF SERVICE.

Home care services can be divided into four (4) major categories – medically oriented, non-medical, nutrition and case coordination. (See also *Home care services; Home health care services/Medicare.*)

IV. PAYMENT FOR SERVICES.

Home care services are covered in part, and funded in part, by Federal and state programs and by private sources such as long-term care insurance and the resources of older people and their families. Details about these sources of payment are set forth below.

A. Medicare.

Medicare home health care services represent a medically oriented category of service provided to Medicare beneficiaries. The services are furnished to them under the Hospital Insurance (Part A see below) and supplemental Medical Insurance (Part B see below) of the Medicare program.

1. Part A – Post-Institutional Home Health Services.

For beneficiaries enrolled in both Parts A and B, the Balanced Budget Act of 1997 changed Part A payment for Part A post-institutional home healthcare services. For these beneficiaries Medicare payments during a home health spell of illness were shifted from Part A to Part B for post-institutional home health services after the first one-hundred (100) home health visits. This shift was phased in between 1998 and December 31, 2002 according to a prescribed formula. Part A post-institutional home health services are those furnished to a Medicare beneficiary within fourteen (14) days after discharge from an inpatient hospital or rural primary hospital care stay of at least three (3) days or from a skilled nursing facility initiated within fourteen (14) days after discharge. A home health spell of illness begins when a patient first receives post-institutional home health services and ends when a beneficiary has not received inpatient care in a hospital, skilled nursing facility or home health services for sixty (60) days.

Hence, after an individual covered by Parts A and B has one-hundred (100) visits of Part A post-institutional home health services, Part B finances the balance of the home health spell of illness. To the extent that visits are not part of the first one-hundred (100) visits, following a stay in the hospital of at least three (3) days or in a skilled nursing facility, they are considered to be Part B home health services.

Beneficiaries who are enrolled only in Part A and qualify for Medicare home health care services (see *section A.2.1* below) will be covered for such services without regard to post-institutional limitations. If a beneficiary is enrolled only in Part B and qualifies for Medicare home health care services, then such services are covered under Part B.

2.   Part B – Qualifying Skilled Services.

Part B covers qualifying skilled services. These services are limited to intermittent skilled nursing care (except private duty nursing, which Medicare will not cover), physical and occupational therapy, and speech-language pathology. Occupational therapy is counted as a qualifying skilled service only if it is part of a care plan that also includes intermittent skilled nursing, physical therapy or speech-language pathology services.

Supportive dependent services are incidental to the qualifying skilled services and also are covered by Medicare only if one qualifying skilled service is required. Dependent services consist of the following: intermittent or part-time home health aide services; medical social services; intern and resident services; medical supplies (other than drugs and biological); and durable medical equipment.

2.1   Conditions to Qualify for Part B Home Health Care
       Services:

To qualify for home health care benefits set forth above, a
Medicare beneficiary must meet the Medicare reasonable and necessary
requirement, plus the following four conditions:

Be homebound;

Need one of the qualifying skilled services – intermittent
skilled nursing care, physical therapy, speech-language
pathology therapy or occupational therapy if part of a
plan including at least one of the other qualifying skilled
services;

Obtain the services from a home health agency certified
by Medicare; and

Obtain from his/her physician a plan of care prescribing
the needed services.

2.2   The following home care services are not covered by
       Medicare:

Personal (custodial) care, customarily rendered by a personal
care aide. This is an unskilled service that assists elderly persons with
activities of daily living such as bathing and eating. These services, to a
limited extent, may be covered by Medicare when performed by a home
health aide, if prescribed by the patient's physician, and only if incidental to
Medicare home health services.

Non-skilled services to assist with instrumental activities
of daily living, such as preparing meals, shopping and
light housework.

Community-based services such as homebound meals
("meals on wheels") or congregate meals.

Management and coordination of services such as case
management.

B.   Medicaid.

Because Medicaid, unlike Medicare, is a welfare program, not an insurance program, Medicaid assistance is provided only to low-income persons who meet certain financial criteria. Under Medicaid, unlike Medicare, the Medicaid-eligible person is not required to be homebound, nor is he/she required to need skilled care as a condition to obtaining unskilled care.

Certain home health care services provided to a person eligible for Medicaid are mandated by Medicaid such as nursing, home health aides and medical supplies and equipment for use in the home. Other home health care services are optional to states such as physical therapy, occupational therapy and speech-language therapy. In addition, non-medical oriented services are optional to states. These include home personal care services, care provided under Medicaid personal care options and Medicaid waivered services.

The qualifying conditions and the procedures for applying for Medicaid-assisted home health services vary from state to state. Usually a written application is made to a Medicaid state agency, a personal interview followed by a nursing assessment is necessary, and extensive financial documentation coupled with a fiscal analysis of the comments is needed to establish eligibility. To receive home personal care additional documentation must be completed, including medical information more extensive than a general application for Medicaid assistance.

C.   Older Americans Act.

Many of the home care needs of individuals age 60 or over who are frail and homebound may be met directly by the home and community-based services authorized by the act, such as home-delivered and congregate meals, adult day care, telephone reassurance, homemaker services, personal care and transportation. Priority is given to individuals with the greatest economic and social needs. Further, the Older Americans Act provides a framework for volunteer service by seniors for other seniors in the community at large.

D.   Block Grants.

Block grants by the Federal government to states represent one of the sources of Federal funding for non-medical home care. They are not so prominent a funding source of socially oriented and home and community-based services as is the federal funding provided under the Older Americans Act.

Block grants are directed at a number of community-based types of care: adult day care services; transportation services; information, referral and counseling services; preparation and delivery of meals; and management and maintenance of the home. There are few restrictions imposed on the states by the Federal government. Such matters as eligibility and coverage standards are determined by the states.

E.   Community and Non-profit Voluntary Agencies.

Most communities have agencies and organizations that provide information about where to obtain assistance and which also offer actual services.

Various social welfare or public agencies and departments perform a variety of services. These may include homemaker services to assist in light house cleaning or personal assistance, as well as services to assist with heavier household chores. Community pharmacies and grocery stores may provide delivery, often free within their service areas. Volunteers are often available to serve as home companions, run local errands, help with small household tasks, accompany an elderly person to a physician's office, and so forth. In addition, most communities offer transportation services at a reduced cost. In some communities door-to-door transportation services, as such as vans or minibuses which accommodate wheelchairs, walkers and other devices, are provided.

Some communities offer volunteer or for-pay respite services which provide short-term, temporary care for an impaired person to relieve family members who provide daily care to their relative. To reassure older persons living alone, many communities provide daily telephone contact, friendly visiting, the U.S. Postal Service's carrier alert program, and an emergency assistance program.

Non-profit voluntary organizations (e.g., United Way) within a community will provide their programs at little or no cost.

(continued on next page)

Home Care Services

Home care is a generic term that embraces several distinct types of services listed below with examples.

> **Medically oriented (home health) services.** Nursing care, medical supplies and equipment, therapy (occupational, physical and speech), audiology and psychosocial rehabilitation for mental illness.

> **Non-medical services.** Personal care services, homemaker chores (cleaning, cooking, laundry), shopping, transportation, electronic emergency response, bill payment and money management, respite care, adult day care and training in care provision for family members.

> **Nutrition services.** Meals on wheels.

> **Case Coordination**. Information and referral, case management and channeling.

Home-delivered Meals Program
See *Meals on wheels.*

Home Equity Conversion Plans
See also *Reverse mortgage.*

Through home equity conversion, a homeowner can use the equity of his/her home to provide a stream of income over a period of years while continuing to live in his/her home. Home equity conversion plans primarily consist of sale-leaseback plans or reverse mortgage plans.

> **Sale-leaseback.** Under a residential sale-leaseback, the owner of the home sells his/her home at a discounted price to a third-party buyer/investor who then leases it back to the owner for life or until he/she moves. As part of the transaction, the buyer pays a portion of the purchase price in cash, and the balance by a note payable to the homeowner-seller, secured by a mortgage on the property for a stated term. The periodic payments, usually monthly, from the buyer are greater than the monthly rental from the homeowner-seller. At closing the buyer can take out an annuity which will pay to the seller for his/her lifetime, upon expiration of the mortgage term, the same periodic payments as paid during the mortgage term.

Reverse Mortgage. With a reverse mortgage, a lender loans a homeowner a sum of money against the equity of his/her house. Repayment of the loan, plus interest and any associated costs such as settlement and service fees, does not have to be made until after the homeowner sells or moves away from his/her house. Unlike a sale-leaseback arrangement, a reverse mortgage allows the homeowner to retain title to his/her property as long as he/she lives in it. Most loans now provide a guarantee of lifetime tenancy. Payments from a reverse mortgage can be in the form of a single lump sum of cash, regular monthly advances or a line of credit.

Home Health Agency
See also *Medicare/Home Health Care, section I.B.4.*

A public or private organization that specializes in providing skilled nursing services, therapeutic services such as physical therapy, and home health aide services. A patient must receive these services from a certified home health agency in order for Medicare or Medicaid to cover them. To be certified, a home health agency must meet certain Medicare and Medicaid conditions of participation before it can receive payment from these programs. Among other conditions, certification requires an agency's compliance with patients' rights and with state and Federal law.

Home Health Agency Advance Beneficiary Notice/Medicare
See also *Demand billing/Medicare.*

Before a home health agency initiates or continues services, it is required to send a written notice to a beneficiary seeking services if it expects Medicare will deny payment for some or all some health care services. This notice is called a home health agency advance beneficiary notice.

The home health agency advance beneficiary notice is required each time and as soon as the agency determines that Medicare will not make payment for home health services or will cease to pay for home health services ordered by a beneficiary's physician. Medicare can deny the requested services because, among other reasons, they are not medically necessary and reasonable or are custodial or because the beneficiary is not homebound or does not require part-time or intermittent care.

A beneficiary must sign the advance beneficiary notice (ABN). This action makes the beneficiary liable to pay the home health agency out of pocket if Medicare denies payment. If an ABN is defective or not given to the beneficiary, the agency is not entitled to payment by Medicare or the beneficiary. If the fiscal intermediary determines the services are covered, the agency must refund the beneficiary or the third-party insurer for any payments made. If the intermediary determines that the services are not covered and that the agency did not provide the beneficiary with adequate notice, the agency must make appropriate refunds. If the intermediary denies coverage and the agency has provided a valid ABN, the agency may seek payment from the beneficiary.

If a beneficiary requests an official Medicare determination of an ABN, the agency must submit a bill (called demand billing) to the intermediary, indicating that the beneficiary believes the services to be covered. All demand bills are subject to medical review in a timely manner.

Home Health Aide
See also *Medicare/Home Health Care, section I.B.1.*

An individual who is trained to give semi-skilled health assistance to a disabled person at home, such as changing bandages or dressings. A home health aide has more training than a home attendant, or personal care aid, or homemaker, and may perform more skilled tasks. Every year a home health aide must receive twelve (12) hours of in-service training. For the services of a home health aide to be covered by Medicare, they must be obtained through a certified home health agency just as in the case of a nurse.

*Home Health Care Services/Medicare

Covers medically necessary part-time or intermittent skilled nursing care, or physical therapy, speech language pathology, or a continuing need for occupational therapy. A doctor or other health care provider enrolled in Medicare must order the care, and a Medicare-certified home health agency must provide it. Home health services may also include medical social services, part-time or intermittent home health aide services, durable medical equipment, and medical supplies for use at home. You must be homebound, which means that leaving home is a major effort. You pay nothing for covered home health services and for Medicare-covered durable medical equipment information.

Home Health Care Services/Medicare

Medicare home health care services are roughly divided into two basic categories – qualifying skilled service and dependent services – defined more fully under *Qualifying skilled service/Medicare,* and *Dependent services/Medicare.*

Home Health Spell of Illness/Medicare
See *Home Care, section I. A.*

Home Modification

Adaption and renovation of an older person's home, sometimes called retrofitting, to make living easier, comfortable, safe and secure. Many local, state, Federal and volunteer organizations provide special grants, loans and other assistance for home remodeling, repair and modification.

Homebound/Medicaid

Unlike Medicare, a Medicaid eligible is not required to be homebound in order to receive Medicaid home care services.

Homebound/Medicare

A homebound beneficiary is an individual confined to home, not necessarily bedridden, who has a condition due to an illness or injury that restricts his/her ability to leave the home without the aid of another person or supportive device, such as crutches, a cane, a wheelchair, a walker, or specialized transportation. A person's "home" is any place in which a beneficiary resides that does not meet the definition of a hospital, skilled nursing facility or rehabilitation facility. Services can be provided in an outpatient setting if: (a) equipment is required that could not be made available in a beneficiary's home, or (b) services were furnished while the beneficiary is at a facility to receive services requiring equipment that cannot be made available at home; and the outpatient setting is in an approved hospital, skilled nursing facility, or rehabilitation facility. Such sources may include medical services provided at adult day care centers.

The medical services and treatment provided to the homebound individual must be in accordance with a physician's order and are performed under the supervision of a licensed health professional for the purpose of diagnosis or treatment of an illness or injury.

An absence of an individual from home will not disqualify the individual from being considered confined to home if the absence is of an infrequent or relatively short duration; for example, a trip to the barber or an occasional drive. Absences to attend a religious service are considered to be absences of infrequent or short duration.

Homemaker Services

Non-medical services, such as bathing, shopping and cooking provided to homebound individuals. These services help the individual to preserve independent living and normal daily life. Receiving homemaker help with these simple but essential jobs can mean the difference between an older person being able to live at home or going into a nursing home. These services may be covered by Medicaid, Older Americans Act programs or Title XX block grants. They generally are not covered by Medicare.

Horizontal Comparability/Medicaid
See *Comparability/Medicaid.*

Hospice

Caring for the terminally ill to enable the patient to live as comfortably as possible. Inpatient facilities are provided to patients unable to be cared for at home. The hospice multi-disciplinary team includes physicians, nurses, social workers, chaplains, and volunteers.

*Hospice Care/Medicare

For people with a terminal illness. Your doctor must certify that you're expected to live 6 months or less. Coverage includes drugs for pain relief and symptom management; medical, nursing and social services; certain durable medical equipment and other covered services as well as services Medicare usually doesn't cover, such as spiritual and grief counseling. A Medicare-approved hospice usually gives hospice care in your home or other facility where you live like a nursing home.

Hospice care doesn't pay for your stay in a facility (room and board) unless the hospice medical team determines that you need short-term inpatient stays for pain and symptom management that can't be addressed at home. These stays must be in a Medicare-approved facility, such as a hospice facility, hospital, or skilled nursing facility which contracts with the hospice. Medicare also covers inpatient respite care, which is care you get in a Medicare-approved facility so that your usual caregiver can rest. You can stay up to 5 days each time you get respite care. Medicare will pay for covered services for health problems that aren't related to your terminal illness. You can continue to get hospice care as long as the hospice medical director or hospice doctor recertifies that you're terminally ill.

Hospice Care/Medicare
See *Medicare, section IV.A.4.*

Hospital Bed/Medicare
See also *Durable medical equipment/Medicare.*

A hospital bed is covered by Medicare.

*Hospital Care (Inpatient Coverage)/Medicare

*Hospital Care is covered under Medicare Part A and includes semi-private room, meals, general nursing, and drugs as part of your inpatient treatment, and other hospital services and supplies. This **doesn't** include private-duty nursing, a television or telephone in your room (if there is a separate charge for these items), or personal care items like razors or slipper socks. It also doesn't include a private room, unless medically necessary. If you have Part B, it covers the doctor's services you get while you're in a hospital.*

Staying overnight in a hospital doesn't always mean you're an inpatient. You're considered an inpatient the day a doctor formally admits you to a hospital with a doctor's order.

Hospital Indemnity Insurance

A type of insurance that pays a fixed amount (weekly or monthly) for each day of hospitalization, regardless of the expenses incurred or other insurance. While relatively inexpensive, these policies are not designed to keep up with the rising costs of hospital care, nor will they pay for non-hospital related expenses. Generally, if a person has Medicare Parts A and B and a Medicare supplemental or Medigap policy, hospital indemnity insurance or specific disease policies are not necessary.

Hospital Insurance/Medicare

There are two parts (A and B) to the traditional Medicare program of which Part A Medicare (Hospital Insurance) helps pay for inpatient hospital care, inpatient care in a skilled nursing facility, limited home health care, hospice care and care in a psychiatric hospital. Part B (Medicare Supplemental Insurance) helps pay for doctors services, other outpatient ambulatory services and, with the advent of the Balanced Budget Act of 1997, limited home health care.

(continued on next page)

I

Immediate Annuity
See *Annuity.*

Immunosuppressive Therapy Drugs/Medicare
See *Drugs/Medicare.*

Income/Medicare Part D Drug Coverage

For purposes of determining eligibility for Part D prescription drug programs, income includes earned wages, earnings from self-employment, royalties, annuity payments, pension payments, disability benefit payments, veterans compensation and pension, workmen's compensation payments, old age survivor and disability insurance benefit payments (including Social Security payments), unemployment insurance payments, prizes, support and alimony payments, inheritances, and earned rents or dividends. If married and living in the same household, the income of the individual and that of the spouse will be added together in determining whether a beneficiary is a subsidy-eligible individual.

Income, Earned/Medicaid
See *Earned income/Medicaid.*

Income, Unearned/Medicaid
See also *Earned income/Medicaid.*

This is income that is not received as compensation for work performed. It includes, but is not limited to, Social Security retirement or disability payments, pensions, benefits, dividends, interest, insurance compensation, income from roomers, boarders and lodgers and income from rental property. Income definitions used in Medicaid generally are found in the SSI statute and regulations.

All entries preceded by an asterisk (*) are culled or copied from the official U.S. government Medicare handbook (*Medicare & You 2011*).

Income and Resources Tests/Medicaid
See *Medicaid, section I.B.2.*

Income Cap States/Medicaid
See also *Medically needy/Medicaid; Optional categorically needed/Medicaid; Spend down/Medicaid.*

Several states, referred to as income cap states, do not have a medically needy program servicing nursing facility residents. In these states individuals are not allowed to spend down to the SSI income level (i.e., cap) to become eligible for Medicaid-covered nursing home care.

These states avail themselves of an optional Medicaid program termed the optional categorically needy program under which individuals are provided limited nursing facility coverage. Under this program individuals qualify for Medicaid nursing home coverage if their countable income does not exceed a cap of a prescribed percentage, usually three-hundred (300%) percent, of the SSI benefit for one person. The cap is categorically fixed and severe: one dollar of excess income above the cap will disqualify the individual. An individual is not permitted to spend down for medical expenses, nor can he/she forego collection of a pension, Social Security benefits or interest income in order to fall within the income cap.

A possible method for reducing the income of an individual seeking to qualify under the optional categorically needy program, also commonly referred to as the three-hundred (300%) percent program, is to obtain from a state court a qualified domestic relations order which allocates pension payments to the community spouse. The community spouse as the payee under such order arguably is the beneficiary of the pension, and payments to him/her would contribute to his/her income under the name-on-the-check rule, not income of the institutionalized spouse who was the original pensioner.

Another method of qualifying for the optional categorically needed program is available under the provisions of OBRA '93. With this law Congress allowed individuals in income cap states to become eligible for Medicaid nursing home assistance by putting their income (e.g., pension, Social Security benefits) into a so-called Miller trust. During the Medicaid recipient's lifetime, all but a small portion of the money in the trust must go toward paying the nursing home bill. If any money remains in the trust after the recipient's death, it must be paid to the state, up to the amount of Medicaid assistance that was rendered.

The income cap states are Alabama, Alaska, Colorado, Delaware, Idaho, Mississippi, Nevada, New Mexico, Ohio, South Dakota and Wyoming.

Income-First Rule/Medicaid
See also *Minimum monthly maintenance needs allowance/Medicaid; Spousal impoverishment/Medicaid.*

When a community spouse's monthly income is less than the minimum monthly maintenance needs allowance set by the state, then the community spouse, in order to bring this/her income up to the amount prescribed for this allowance, may apply at a fair hearing for an increase in the community spouse's resource allowance (CSRA) out of the resources of the institutionalized spouse.

Several states have taken the position that the community spouse may not resort to this fair hearing process so as to increase the CSRA, unless the institutionalized spouse has first made available to the community spouse out of his/her income an amount sufficient, if possible, to make up the deficiency. This requirement that the community spouse must first seek an income distribution from the institutionalized spouse equal to the deficiency prior to increasing his/her resource allowance is sometimes referred to as the income-first rule.

Income-Only Trust/Medicaid
See also *Trust, Medicaid eligibility rules.*

An *inter vivos* irrevocable trust established by an individual which provides that only income from the trust shall be paid to the grantor for life, but excludes distribution of the trust principal to the grantor.

The principal of the trust is not considered available to a grantor in determining his/her Medicaid eligibility since the principal cannot be distributed to or for the benefit of the grantor. The income of the trust, to the extent paid or payable to the grantor, is considered available in determining his/her Medicaid eligibility.

The principal of income-only trusts is subject to the trust transfer penalty rules. Thus, Medicaid will invoke a sixty- (60) month look-back period. The establishment of a trust will be treated as a transfer of assets for less than fair market value resulting in the Medicaid applicant being subject to a period of ineligibility for various long-term care services such as nursing facility care and waivered home care services. The length of the period of ineligibility depends on the value of the transferred assets.

Incontestability Period

This insurance term refers to a period of time (usually two (2) years from the policy's effective date) after which the insurer will be prevented from denying benefits for any reason other than deliberate and fraudulent misstatements made by the covered person when applying for the policy.

Indemnity Insurance

This is a type of health care insurance. Customarily indemnity insurance reimburses a provider's charges on a fee-for-service basis as contrasted to a prepaid plan. The indemnity insurance contract defines the maximum amount that will be paid for covered services. Some hospital and LTCI policies pay the insured individual an agreed upon per diem rate, once the individual meets the criteria for insured status, regardless of the actual cost of services.

Independent Laboratory Services/Medicare
See also *Assignment/Medicare.*

Medicare Part B pays the full approved charge for covered clinical diagnostic tests provided by independent laboratories approved to perform them. The laboratory must accept assignment for these tests. Not all laboratories are approved by Medicare.

Independent Living Retirement Community
See also *Alternative housing facilities, section III.*

Generally, this community is designed architecturally to be compatible with an older person's lifestyle, but offers no specific services beyond shelter, recreational activities and security. Most communities offer a variety of social activities and programs in an on-site clubhouse such as golf, tennis, swimming and other social amenities.

Structurally, an independent living retirement community can be built as single-family detached units, duplexes, mobile homes and other types of senior-oriented low-density developments, or it can include apartment buildings and condominiums designed for older persons. It typically does not provide meals or other basic services due to the proximity to nearby community services.

Communities vary from independent ownership of units to monthly rentals depending on the individual community. While most are composed of private pay market-rate units, some rental apartment buildings may be subsidized. (See also *Federal housing programs for the elderly.*)

Independent living retirement communities are also sometimes called retirement villages and communities, leisure or adult communities, residential apartments and residential villages.

Independent Practice Association (IPA)/Managed Care
See *Health maintenance organization (HMO).*

Indexing Year/Social Security

The indexing year is used when calculating an individual's Social Security benefit. It is the year that is two (2) years before a person either reaches age 62 or becomes disabled.

Individual Retirement Account (IRA)
See also *Private pension; Roth IRA.*

This is an individual's private retirement account, commonly referred to as an IRA, created by the individual to accumulate resources to support his/her retirement years. The individual may annually contribute limited amounts of money to the IRA, on a tax deductible basis, which may be invested by the IRA and together with the income earned on the investments accumulate tax free. Income tax will be imposed on the amounts in the IRA only upon distribution. However, if an individual who established an IRA should die before all IRA funds are distributed, continuing distributions by the IRA may be rolled over to a pension plan or IRA covering his/her surviving spouse without the imposition of any income tax. IRA payouts must begin by April 1 of the year after an individual reaches age 70½.

Induced Demand/LTCI

Also known as moral risk, induced demand is the circumstance of individuals seeking care because insurance benefits are available, when they would not seek the same care if they had to pay for it out of pocket.

Ineligibility Period/Medicaid
See *Period of ineligibility/Medicaid.*

Inflation Protection/LTCI
See also *Long-term care insurance, section II.F.*

The longer the time span between the purchase of an LTCI policy and collection of initial benefits, the more likely it is that the cost of long-term care will increase in the interim, and the larger the increase is likely to be. Therefore to protect against this inflation contingency, the insured person can either purchase a policy with a larger benefit than contemporary pricing requires or purchase a policy with an inflation protection rider.

Inflation protection can automatically increase policy benefits a certain amount each year, or the insured person can have the option to purchase additional insurance on a defined schedule, without further proof of insurability. Important variables are the way that inflation is defined, whether the inflation protection is compounded, and whether there is a maximum age to which inflation protection is available, such as to age 75 or age 80, or a maximum amount inflation protection, such as a limit of fifty (50%) of the original benefit.

According to the Health Insurance Portability and Accountability Act of 1996, LTCI policies issued after January 1, 1997 must offer purchasers the option to obtain inflation protection, if such policies are to be eligible for the tax advantages allowed by the legislation.

Influenza Immunization/Medicare
See *Flu shot/Medicare.*

Informal Caregiver
See also *Caregiver.*

Refers to an unpaid, often untrained, individual such as a family member or friend who provides care.

Information and Referral Services

This service is offered by government, community agencies, and other sources to answer questions of the elderly and their families relating to access to and delivery of health care and social services, and to make appropriate referrals to service providers.

In each state and locality, there are sources that provide information about home care and related services. Local Offices for the Aging are often a good source to obtain information about the services available in each locality. Other sources for information or referral include home health agencies, public health and welfare departments, non-profit voluntary agencies (such as United Way), adult day care centers, senior centers, churches and synagogues. The National Eldercare Locator, which can be reached at (800) 677-1116, provides contact information on the local office for the aging or a community-based family services organization in localities across the country.

Many people who require or desire to pay privately for home care – whether they do so through direct contracting or through a home health agency – will find it helpful to utilize the services of a geriatric care manager to obtain information about home care required and then to obtain, screen, monitor and coordinate all of the care services. Geriatric care managers are often needed when the patient lives far from family members or friends, who are therefore less capable of monitoring the care and ensuring that the patient's needs are met. Geriatric care managers are located in all states, and many are members of the National Association of Professional Geriatric Care Managers, which can be contacted at (520) 881-8008. Nutritional counseling may be obtained from home health agencies.

Informed Consent

A patient's agreement, or the agreement of the patient's representative in the event of the patient's incompetence, to a proposed medical treatment requires that the physician inform the patient or his/her representative of all the risks and benefits of the suggested treatment and of alternative treatments.

Initial Coverage Limit/Medicare Part D Drug Coverage
See also *Medicare/Outpatient Prescription Drug Programs (Medicare Part D), section IV.*

The amount which determines when cost sharing of covered drug costs ends. In standard coverage, it is the level of total prescription costs at which twenty-five (25%) percent of the coinsurance ends. Then, the beneficiary is required to pay one-hundred (100%) percent of the cost of Part D covered drugs, up to the out-of-pocket threshold limit. The initial coverage limit is $2,930 (2012) in total drug spending. The copay is $652.50 – twenty-five (25%) percent of the yearly drug cost representing the costs between the $320 (2012) annual deductible and the initial coverage limit of $2,930.

Initial Determination/Medicare
See also *Appeals/Medicare; Appeals/Social Security.*

Relates to and is the first stage of Medicare and Social Security appeals processes.

It is a determination, with respect to Medicare and Social Security claims, made by the fiscal intermediary or carrier after a home health agency or other provider submits a claim, and only after some care has actually been provided.

Initial Enrollment/Medicare Advantage
See *Medicare Advantage plans common features, section III.B; Initial coverage election period/Medicare Advantage.*

Initial Enrollment Period/Medicare
See also *Eligibility and enrollment/Medicare; Eligibility for and election of plans/Medicare Advantage (MA).*

This is a period of seven (7) months. It begins with the third month prior to the month when the prospective enrollee reaches age 65 and continues for three (3) months after the month of his/her 65th birthday. If an individual does not file during the general enrollment period (annual coordinated election period, January 1 – March 31), then he/she can file during the general enrollment period. Enrollment during the first three (3) months of the initial enrollment period will result in coverage the first day of the month the individual attains age 65. Enrollment after the first three (3) months will cause a delay in coverage. Enrollment in the month when the beneficiary reaches age 65 will result in coverage on the first day of the second month after the applicant enrolls. If the applicant enrolls during the last three (3) months of the initial enrollment period, there may be a delay in coverage of one (1) to three (3) months.

In-kind Income or Support/Medicaid

Generally contributions of goods and services from a third party to support a Medicaid recipient are not counted as income. The third party's contribution(s) must go directly to the vendor or service provider; if made to the Medicaid recipient, the contributions are counted as unearned income. Payment for a recipient's food, shelter and medical bills are examples of in-kind support which a third party can pay for a Medicaid recipient.

Inpatient

In general, a patient who is admitted to a hospital or skilled nursing facility and stays overnight during his/her treatment.

Inpatient Hospital Care/Medicare

Health services provided by a hospital to patients who have been admitted to the hospital. These services include bed and board, nursing services, diagnostic or therapeutic services, and medical or surgical services.

Inpatient Rehabilitation Facility

Hospital or part of a hospital that offers an intensive rehabilitation regimen to inpatients.

*Institution/Medicare

A facility that provides short-term or long-term care, such as a nursing home, skilled nursing facility (SNF), or rehabilitation hospital.

Institutional Care

Care in a nursing home or other facility as distinct from care in a person's home or on an outpatient basis.

Institutionalized Individual/Medicaid

A person receiving care in a Medicaid-covered nursing facility or an acute care hospital. In addition, states at their option can choose to apply the term to an individual receiving home community-based care under a Medicaid waiver.

Institutionalized Special Needs Individual/Medicare Advantage

An institutionalized special needs individual is an MA-eligible individual who continuously resides or is expected to continuously reside for ninety (90) days or longer in a long-term facility which is a skilled nursing facility; nursing facility; an intermediate care facility for the mentally retarded; or an inpatient psychiatric facility.

Institutionalized Spouse/Medicaid

Applies to a married person who is expected to remain in a medical institution or nursing home for a continuous period of at least thirty (30) days or who is receiving home care under a waiver and who applies for and/or has obtained Medicaid eligibility. Medicaid eligibility rules for an institutionalized spouse, generally speaking are different from those relevant to a married Medicaid applicant living in the community.

Instrumental Activities of Daily Living (IADL)
See also *Activities of daily living (ADL)*.

Those activities ancillary to activities of daily living. The term includes light housework, preparing meals, shopping, using the telephone, keeping track of money or bills and taking of medicines. Medicare does not cover these activities.

Insured Status/Social Security
See also *Social Security program, section 1*.

A worker's entitlement to Social Security benefits depends upon his/her insured status, among other factors. There are three (3) basic types of insured statuses: fully insured, currently insured and specially insured for disability benefits (disability insured). Each kind of insured status controls eligibility for a different type of Social Security benefit. For example, to qualify for retirement benefits a worker must be age 62 or over or must be fully insured. To qualify for disability benefits, a worker must meet the test of disability, be fully insured and be disability insured.

Integrated Health Systems
See *Managed Care, section 3*.

Integrated Policy/LTCI
See *Long-term care insurance, section II.B*.

Integration/Social Security

For pension purposes, the practice of reducing benefits under a pension plan by taking into account either the employer's share of Social Security taxes, or the Social Security benefits received by the employee after retirement.

Inter Vivos Trust

See *Trust, Medicaid eligibility rules.*

Intermediary/Medicare

A private insurance organization that contracts with the Federal government to handle, as a fiscal intermediary, Medicare Part A (hospital insurance) payment for services by hospitals, skilled nursing facilities and home health agencies.

Intermediate Care Facility (ICF)/Medicaid

A health care facility previously recognized under the Medicaid program and licensed under state law to provide, on a regular basis, health services to residents who do not require the degree of care provided by a hospital or skilled nursing facility, but who do require health services, beyond just board and lodging, that can be made available through an institutional facility.

Prior to 1990 nursing homes were classified by Federal Medicaid law as skilled nursing facilities and intermediate care facilities. Medicaid recognized two types of ICFs – a plan ICF and an ICF-MR (intermediate care facility for the mentally retarded). These two different ICFs were regulated under separate sets of rules. In 1990 the Medicaid program eliminated the distinction between a skilled nursing facility and plain ICF, instead subsuming them under the classification nursing facility. ICF-MRs continue to be recognized as a separate category of care facility.

Intermittent Care/Medicare

See also *Part-time/Medicare; Part-time or intermittent/Medicare.*

The need for skilled nursing care must be intermittent. The word "intermittent" as it relates to skilled nursing is used both as a condition of eligibility for home health services and as a coverage limitation as it relates to the duration of coverage.

As an eligibility requirement, the term "intermittent" determines health benefits of a patient because of his/her need for intermittent skilled nursing care. In this context, intermittent is defined by the Balanced Budget Act of 1997 (Act) to mean skilled nursing care that is needed for the following durations:

- fewer than seven (7) days each week; or

- fewer than eight (8) hours of each day for periods of twenty-one (21) days or less, with extensions in exceptional circumstances when the need for additional care is finite and predictable.

Intermittent is also part of the statutory terms "part-time or intermittent nursing care" and "part-time or intermittent services of a home health aide." In this context, intermittent constitutes a coverage limitation for the services. As such, intermittent relates to the duration of, as distinguished from eligibility for, a Medicare beneficiary's entitlement to skilled nursing care. As a coverage limitation, part-time or intermittent services are defined to mean skilled nursing and home health aide services (combined) for the following number of days per week:

- a number of days per week less than eight (8) hours a day, and twenty-eight (28) or fewer hours per week; or

- on a case-by-case basis, subject to review, need for care less than eight (8) hours a day and thirty-five (35) or fewer hours per week.

Intern and Resident Services/Medicare
See also *Medicare/Home Health Care, section I.B.5.*

These services are covered by Medicare if they are ordered by a physician pursuant to or from a plan of care and if such services are reasonable and necessary for the diagnosis and treatment of the beneficiary's illness.

Irrevocable Trust
See *Trust, Medicaid eligibility rules.*

Issue Age/Medigap
See *Medicare supplemental insurance, section II.*

(continued on next page)

J

Joint Assets/Medicaid

When an asset is held by an individual in common with another person via a joint tenancy, tenancy in common, a joint ownership or a similar arrangement, the asset is considered, for purposes of Medicaid transfer penalty rules to be transferred by the individual when any action is taken by either the individual or joint owner(s) that reduces or eliminates the individual's ownership or control of the asset.

Merely placing another person's name on the account of an asset as a joint owner ordinarily will not constitute a transfer of assets. However, actual withdrawal of funds from the account by the other person will constitute a transfer of assets.

If either the Medicaid applicant/recipient or the other joint owner can establish that funds withdrawn were in fact the sole property of the other person, and thus do not belong to the applicant/recipient, then withdrawal of those funds ordinarily will not result in the imposition of a Medicaid transfer penalty.

Joint Survivor Annuity
See *Annuity*.

Joint Tenants with Rights of Survivorship

Personal property or real property may be owned by two (2) or more owners. The basic conditions of such ownership are: (i) the owners must agree on all matters while living; (ii) one owner can terminate the joint ownership arrangement and demand his/her portion or, failing agreement between the parties, force a sale by partition proceedings and obtain the proportionate value of his/her interest; and (iii) if joint ownership continues until one owner dies, ownership of that person's interest automatically passes to the other co-owner(s).

All entries preceded by an asterisk (*) are culled or copied from the official U.S. government Medicare handbook (*Medicare & You 2011*).

K

Kennelly Widow or Widower/Medicaid

A widow or widower between ages 60 and 65 who lost his/her SSI as a result of being entitled to early widow's benefits under the Social Security survivors program. Without special protection, these individuals could lose all health care coverage because loss of SSI results in loss of automatic entitlement to Medicaid and because they are not entitled to Medicare until they turn age 65. To ensure that these individuals continue receiving Medicaid, the law considers them as if they still receive SSI. Coverage under this program provides important interim benefits for people not yet entitled to Medicare.

Keogh Plan

A retirement plan authorized by the Federal government for the self-employed and partnerships.

*Kidney Dialysis/Medicare

For people with End-Stage Renal Disease (ESRD). Medicare covers dialysis either in a facility or at home when your doctor orders it. You pay 20% of the Medicare-approved amount per session, and the Part B deductible applies.

Kidney Dialysis and Transplants/Medicare

Medicare Part B helps pay for kidney dialysis and kidney transplants.

*Kidney Disease Education Services/Medicare

Medicare may cover up to six sessions of kidney disease education services if you have Stage IV chronic kidney disease, and your doctor refers you for the service. You pay 20% of the Medicare-approved amount, and the Part B deductible applies.

All entries preceded by an asterisk (*) are culled or copied from the official U.S. government Medicare handbook (*Medicare & You 2011*).

*Kidney Transplant/Medicare

Immunosuppressive drugs are covered if Medicare paid for the transplant, or an employer or union group health plan was required to pay before Medicare paid for the transplant. You must have been entitled to Part A at the time of the transplant, and you must be entitled to Part B at the time you get immunosuppressive drugs. You pay 20% of the Medicare-approved amount, and the Part B deductible applies.

Medicare drug plans (Part D) may cover immunosuppressive drugs, even if Medicare or an employer or union group health plan didn't pay for the transplant.

(continued on next page)

L

Laboratory tests/Medicare

See *Clinical laboratory test/Medicare; Diagnostic tests/Medicare.*

Laboratory Tests, Hospital/Medicare

When a person is a hospital inpatient, laboratory tests included in the hospital bill are covered under Medicare Part A.

*Late Enrollment Penalty/Medicare Part A

If you aren't eligible for premium-free Part A, and you don't buy it when you're first eligible, your monthly premium may go up 10%. You will have to pay the higher premium for twice the number of years you could have had Part A, but didn't sign up. For example, if you were eligible for Part A for 2 years but didn't sign up, you will have to pay the higher premium for 4 years. Usually, you don't have to pay a penalty if you meet certain conditions that allow you to sign up for Part A during a Special Enrollment Period.

Late Enrollment Penalty/Medicare Part A

If a Medicare-eligible person files an application for Medicare Part A after the initial open enrollment period, no Part A penalty will be imposed, except such late filing by a voluntary enrollee.

Should a voluntary enrollee file an application after the initial enrollment period, a Part A penalty will be imposed. It is a ten- (10%) percent increase based on the monthly Part A premium price for every month of late enrollment up to twice the number of months for which the beneficiary has failed to file.

All entries preceded by an asterisk (*) are culled or copied from the official U.S. government **Medicare** handbook (*Medicare & You 2011*).

Late Enrollment Penalty/Medicare Part B

If an individual does not enroll for Medicare Part B when first eligible, he/she will be required to pay a late enrollment penalty. It is a ten- (10%) percent increase of the monthly Part B premium for each twelve- (12) month period such individual could have signed up for Part B but does not.

A late enrollment penalty will not be imposed if an individual meets certain conditions that allow him/her to sign up for Part B during a special enrollment period. A late Medicare Part A and/or Part B penalty is not application to an individual who enrolls during a special enrollment period. It relates to working individuals age 65 or over who are covered by an employer group health plan whether it is their own or that of a spouse. These persons have the option to enroll in Medicare after age 65. The enrollment period begins on the first day of the month in which the person is no longer enrolled in an employer group health plan and ends seven (7) months later. Part A or B enrollment will not result in any late enrollment penalty

Late Enrollment Penalty/Medicare Part D Drug Coverage

A beneficiary who does not enroll in a Part D plan within sixty-three (63) days of his/her initial enrollment period, and who does not have other creditable prescription drug coverage (as described below), must pay a late penalty if he/she subsequently enrolls in a Part D plan. The penalty is assessed at one (1) percent of the national average premium for each month of delayed enrollment, for the remainder of the time in which the beneficiary is enrolled in a Part D plan. Thus, a beneficiary who first becomes eligible for Part D at age 65, but who delays enrolling until age 70 may be assessed a sixty- (60) percent penalty on his/her premium (5 years x 12 months x 1%). Since the penalty is based on a percentage of the average premium each year, the dollar value of the penalty changes as the national average premium changes.

Late enrollment penalties will not be imposed if a beneficiary maintains creditable coverage," that is other coverage, equivalent to Medicare basic drug benefit (e.g., VA coverage, Medigap coverage, and most employer (or union) sponsor retiree plans). Should a beneficiary's existing drug coverage end or change and thus cease to be "creditable," he/she has up to sixty-three (63) days to enroll in a Medicare drug plan.

Laundry/Medicare

See also *Home care services.*

Laundry services generally are not covered by Medicare, except when and to the limited extent prescribed by the doctor, specifically for the patient's personal laundry.

Legacy

Personal property bequeathed to a person by a will.

Leisure Community

See *Independent living retirement community.*

Lesser of Cost or Charge Principle/Medicare

Under this principle, with certain exceptions noted below, Medicare pays certain providers the lesser of reasonable costs, or the customary charges for services furnished to Medicare beneficiaries. Reasonable costs are those actually incurred and that are necessary for the efficient delivery of services. Customary charges are the regular rates that providers charge both Medicare beneficiaries and other paying patients for the services furnished to them.

The principle does not apply to the following:

Providers

Comprehensive outpatient rehabilitation facilities;

Public providers that furnish services free of charge or at a nominal charge which is defined as a charge equal to sixty (60%) percent or less of a service's reasonable cost; and

Any provider that requests fair compensation which is the reasonable costs of covered services and that can demonstrate that a significant portion of its patients are low income and that its charges are less than costs because its customary practice is to charge patients on the basis of their ability pay.

Services

Part A inpatient hospital services that are paid for by Medicare under the prospective payment system, or that are subject to the ceiling on the rate of increase limits in operating costs set forth in CMS regulations;

Facility services related to ambulatory surgical procedures performed in outpatient hospital departments;

Services furnished by a critical access hospital;

Hospital outpatient radiology services;

Other diagnostic procedures performed by a hospital on an outpatient basis; and

Skilled nursing facility services paid for by Medicare under the prospective payment system.

Durable Medical Equipment

Such equipment provided by a home health agency is paid at eighty (80%) percent of the lesser of the actual charge for the item or the payment amount recognized under the DME fee schedule.

Level Premium/LTCI
See *Long-term care insurance.*

Licensed Facility

A facility is licensed if it has met certain minimum legal standard set by a state or local government agency.

Licensed Home Care Agency

These are private agencies from which a patient can obtain a nurse, home health aide or other personnel. They are licensed but not certified for Medicare, so that the services they render therefore are not covered by Medicare. If the facilities are licensed, it means the facilities have met certain minimum legal standards set by a local state or government agency.

Licensed Practical Nurse (LPN)

A nurse who has completed a practical nursing program and is licensed by a state to provide routine patient care under the direction of a registered nurse or a physician.

Licensed Vocational Nurse

A licensed practical nurse who is permitted by license to practice in California or Texas.

Liens/Medicaid

State Medicaid programs are authorized, but not required, to place liens on property of Medicaid recipients in two (2) limited circumstances:

> For benefits incorrectly paid, pursuant to a judgment for a court; and

> On real property of a permanently institutionalized individual when the state has determined, after an opportunity for a hearing, that the individual cannot be reasonably expected to return home. The term permanently institutionalized is not defined in the statute.

The lien on real property will dissolve if and when the Medicaid recipient is discharged from the institution and returns home. No liens can be placed on a life estate of a Medicaid recipient.

Liens cannot be imposed on homesteads if any of the following persons are lawfully residing in the institutionalized individual's home:

> His/her spouse; his/her child who is under age 21, blind or disabled; or,

> A sibling as long as he/she has an equity interest in the home and has resided there for at least one year prior to the institutionalized individual's entry into a nursing facility.

Life Care Community
See *Continuing care retirement community (CCRC)*.

Life Estate/Medicaid

A life estate is established when an individual transfers ownership of property to another individual or entity but retains for the rest of his/her life certain rights to that property. For purposes of determining Medicaid eligibility, a life estate is not considered a countable resource. Medicaid law forbids requiring an applicant to liquidate or sublease a life estate.

In the case of Medicaid transfer penalty rules, the transfer of property to a life estate is considered to be for less than fair market value whenever the value of the property transferred is greater than the value of the life estate. The transfer penalty is equal to the amount by which the value of the asset transferred exceeds the value of the life estate.

*Lifetime Reserve Days/Medicare

In Original Medicare, these are additional days that Medicare will pay for when you're in a hospital for more than 90 days. You have a total of 60 reserve days that can be used during your lifetime. For each lifetime reserve day, Medicare pays all covered costs except for a daily coinsurance.

Lifetime Reserve Days/Medicare
See also *Reserve period/Medicare.*

If a patient is hospitalized for longer than ninety (90) days during a spell of illness, Medicare will pay for up to sixty (60) additional days of care. Each of those sixty (60) days is called a reserve day and can be used only once during a beneficiary's lifetime. For each lifetime reserve day, Medicare will pay all covered costs except daily coinsurance ($578 per day in 2012).

*Limited Income/Medicare

If you have limited income and resources, you might qualify for help to pay for some health care and prescription drug costs.

The U.S. Virgin Islands, Guam, American Samoa, the Commonwealth of Puerto Rico, and the Commonwealth of Northern Mariana Islands provide their residents help with Medicare drug costs. This help isn't the same as Extra Help.

Limits to Physician's Charges/Medicare
See also *Approved charge/Medicare; Fee schedule charge/Medicare; Balance billing/Medicare.*

A physician's charges are subject to limits set by Medicare and by certain states. The limits are of three (3) different categories:

> When a physician has accepted assignment, payment of the amount of the Medicare-approved charge is complete payment for services rendered.

242

When a physician has not accepted assignment and does not perform a procedure (see paragraph below), the doctor's charge for evaluating and managing the patient's condition is limited to one-hundred fifteen (115%) percent of the Medicare-approved charges. Some states entirely bar the one-hundred fifteen- (115%) percent limiting charge permitted by Medicare and in effect mandate assignment. Some other states set a limiting charge lower than one-hundred fifteen (115%) percent.

If a physician does not accept assignment, charges for procedures performed in a hospital, outpatient department and doctor's office are limited to one-hundred fifteen (115%) percent of the Medicare-approved charge. Such procedures include surgery, anesthesiology, pathology, radiology, x-rays and most diagnostic tests.

The limiting charge does not apply to supplies or equipment.

Living Benefits
See *Accelerated benefits.*

*Living Will/Medicare

A living will is another way to make sure your voice is heard. It states which medical treatment you would accept or refuse if your life is threatened. Dialysis for kidney failure, a breathing machine if you can't breathe on your own, CPR (cardiopulmonary resuscitation) if your heart and breathing stop, or tube feeding if you can no longer eat are examples of medical treatment you can choose to accept or refuse.

Living Will
See also *Advance directive; Durable power of attorney for health care.*

A written, signed, dated and witnessed document, or provision in a document, expressing in advance the signer's wishes regarding the use or non-use of extreme life supporting measures, if the signer is ever terminally ill and incompetent to express his/her wishes. Many states have enacted statutes that enable a person to execute a living will.

Lock-in/Managed Care

This feature of a managed care system limits, or locks in, a beneficiary, such as an HMO member, to receiving covered services only from one or more of a limited group of providers.

Long-distance Caregiver

An individual who provides or organizes care for an elderly person who lives some distance away from the caregiver.

*Long-term Care/Medicare

Long-term care includes medical and non-medical care for people who have a chronic illness or disability. Non-medical care includes non-skilled personal care assistance, such as help with everyday activities like dressing, bathing, and using the bathroom. At least 70% of people over 65 will need long-term care services at some point. Medicare and most health insurance plans, including Medigap (Medicare Supplement Insurance) policies don't pay for this type of care, also called "custodial care." Medicare only pays for medically-necessary skilled nursing facility care or home health care if you meet certain conditions. Long-term care can be provided at home, in the community, in assisted living, or in a nursing home.

Long-term Care Insurance is a type of private insurance policy that can help pay for many types of long-term care, including both skilled and non-skilled (custodial) care. Long-term Care Insurance can vary widely. Some policies may cover only nursing home care. Others may include coverage for a range of services like adult day care, assisted living, medical equipment, and informal home care.

Your current or former employer or union may offer long-term care insurance. Current and retired Federal employees, active and retired members of the uniformed services, and their qualified relatives can apply for coverage under the Federal Long-term Care Insurance Program.

Resources and payments for long-term care include:

Personal Resources – You can use your savings to pay for long-term care. Some insurance companies let you use your life insurance policy to pay for long-term care. Ask your insurance agent how this works.

244

Other Private Options – *Besides long-term care insurance and personal resources, you may choose to pay for long-term care through a trust or annuity. What option is best for you depends on your age, your health status, your risk of needing long-term care, and your personal financial situation. Visit www.longtermcare.gov for more information about your options.*

Medicaid –Medicaid is a joint Federal and state program that pays for certain health services for people with limited income and resources. If you qualify, you may be able to get help to pay for nursing home care or other health care costs.

Home and Community-based Services Programs – *If you're already eligible for Medicaid (or, in some states, would be eligible for Medicaid coverage in a nursing home), you or your family members may be able to get help with the costs of services that help you stay in your home instead of moving to a nursing home. Examples include homemaker services, personal care, and respite care.*

Programs of All-inclusive Care for the Elderly (PACE) – *PACE is a Medicare and Medicaid program offered in many states that allows people who otherwise need a nursing home-level of care to remain in the community.*

Long-term Care (LTC)

There is no single recognized definition for this term broadly covering the provision of services to people who are limited in their ability to function independently over a relatively long period of time. The long-term care assistance provided to such persons, among other things, consists of help in performing basic activities of daily living and may also include services such as housework, laundry, grocery shopping, giving medication and transportation. Long-term care also embraces skilled therapeutic care for the treatment and management of chronic conditions. Long-term care can be provided in home and community-based settings as well as in institutions such as nursing homes and assisted living facilities. The major sources of funding long-term care are the private funds of older people and their families; government programs such as Medicaid and those authorized by the Older Americans Act; long-term care insurance; and assistance from not-for-profit local community agencies. Because Medicare is designed to cover acute care, its support of long-term care is limited.

(continued on next page)

LONG-TERM CARE INSURANCE

INTRODUCTION

In order to help people protect against the high cost of long-term care either in a nursing home or at home, the insurance industry in the 1980s began to offer long-term care insurance (LTCI). Since Medicare, Medicare supplemental insurance, and private health insurance are not intended to cover chronic conditions or long-term care, especially custodial care, LTCI policies were created to fill this gap.

I.   GENERAL.

LTCI policies are usually indemnity insurance that pay a daily cash amount to the policyholder, unlike service benefits paid directly to the care provider. Also unlike other health insurance, most LTCI policies are individual policies. Employers play a limited but growing role in sponsoring group LTCI available to employees, their spouses, and sometimes parents and other family members. Employees usually pay the full premium for policies. Some associations also offer their members group LTCI. Group policies do not necessarily provide less expensive premiums or better benefits than individual policies.

The Health Insurance Portability and Accountability Act of 1996 mandates that LTCI policies must contain certain provisions in order for the, policies to qualify for special tax benefits (see *section II*).

II.   COVERAGE.

Depending on the policy, LTCI covers a range of long-term care services, both skilled and personal (custodial) care, ranging from home care to assisted living to nursing home care. Most claims made under LTCI policies are for custodial care in nursing homes which is expressly excluded from Medicare coverage. Many choices involved in the purchase of an LTCI policy, such as amount of daily benefit and inflation protection, are complex and costly. Health insurance counseling received before purchasing such a policy may be very helpful and cost-saving. Many communities offer counseling programs partially supported with government funds or conducted by private organizations.

LTCI policies generally exclude coverage for the following: alcohol and drug abuse; Medicare/Medicaid reimbursable expenses; services performed by family members; services outside the United States; and assistance with instrumental activities of daily living such as preparing food, bill paying, and transportation. To be qualified for tax benefits, policies cannot exclude coverage by type of illness, treatment or medical condition or accident, with the exception of pre-existing conditions (see paragraph G below).

The period of coverage which purchasers can select may be one to two (2) years, three (3) years, four (4) to six (6) years, ten (10) years, or lifetime. The longer the period of coverage, the higher the premium.

Virtually all policies currently issued are guaranteed renewable and must be so if they are to qualify for tax benefits. This provision precludes an insurance company from canceling a policy so long as the insured pays the required premiums in a timely fashion.

III.   TYPES OF POLICIES.

The two (2) main types of individual LTCI policies are called classic and integrated policies. Both types of policies are presently available. Depending on individual circumstances, one or the other may be more suitable. Medical underwriting requirements for the two types of policies can vary. Therefore, an individual may have a better chance of being accepted under one type rather than the other.

> **Classic**. This older type of policy is usually for nursing home care with a rider attached for home health care. Some classic policies mention an alternative form of care as a coverage possibility. Usually this means that the company may consider payment at its discretion for care in an assisted living facility, as long as it is cheaper than nursing home care.
>
> In some policies, coverage for assisted living is specifically spelled out as included. Tax-qualified policies must cover adult day care.

Integrated. Under this newer type of policy, also called a pool of funds policy, a beneficiary purchases a pool of funds for flexible use. For example, an individual selects a three- (3) year LTCI policy with benefits of $200 per day, totaling $219,000. This total is determined by multiplying the daily benefit selected, (i.e., $200) times the number of days in the three- (3) year period (i.e., 1,095 days). Once the condition of the beneficiary meets the qualifying criteria for coverage, he/she may use this pool of funds as best suits his/her care needs, including care at home, in a nursing home, adult day care center, and/or assisted living facility. In addition to assistance with activities of daily living, some policies will cover other services such as cooking, laundry, and general housekeeping.

IV. TRIGGERS.

Among the many important aspects of LTCI policies, most crucial are the so-called "triggers," that is, prerequisite events which trigger coverage. Triggers include medical necessity, cognitive impairment, and limitations on activities of daily living (ADL).

Policies vary as to which ADLs are identified as trigger events, how many ADLs must be impaired before coverage starts, and especially in the definitions of ADLs. One policy, for example, may define bathing, one of the common ADLs, to include sponge baths outside a bathtub, while another policy might define it to mean washing in a shower or bathtub. Differences in definitions can mean the difference between having coverage or not.

Policy differences in the definition of "necessary assistance" with ADLs are also critical. Assistance may be defined as total reliance on another person or as supervisory assistance. Total reliance is a stricter requirement than supervisory assistance.

To be tax-qualified, policies must contain a trigger for five (5) or six (6) ADLs. To receive coverage, the insured must be unable to perform at least two (2) ADLs without substantial assistance from another individual. A doctor must certify that the ADL loss will last at least ninety (90) days. Activities of daily living are those usually performed for oneself in the course of a normal day and are usually considered to be: mobility (e.g., transfer from or to a bed or chair); dressing; bathing; self-feeding; and toileting.

Depending on the policy, the three (3) triggers of medical necessity, cognitive impairment or ADL limitations can operate separately or can be linked in different combinations. The best policies treat the triggers as single, independent events, each qualifying the beneficiary for coverage. When this is not the case, a policy linking an ADL trigger with cognitive impairment, for example, usually will not cover Alzheimer's patients who are not necessarily limited in their ADLs. Since 1997, new policies qualifying for tax benefits must have a separate, independent trigger for cognitive impairment. The insured must require substantial supervision to protect his/her health and safety due to severe cognitive impairment.

The medical necessity trigger means that a physician must certify that admission to a nursing home or the need for home care is due to illness or injury, or is medically necessary. Policies with this trigger specifically state that the insured does not need prior institutionalization or skilled level of care before being eligible for coverage.

Older LTCI policies required prior hospitalization or a step-down as a condition of coverage. According to the step-down requirement, nursing home care, for example, would have to be obtained before home benefits would be paid. Tax-qualified policies issued are forbidden to have a prior hospitalization requirement.

V. PREMIUMS.

Several major variables affect the cost of premiums, including the daily benefit amount, the length of the benefit period, the length of the deductible or elimination period, the age at which a person buys a policy, and any special coverage features such as inflation and non-forfeiture protection.

> **Level Premium.** All companies offer a level premium which means that an individual policyholder will continue to pay the premium charged to someone at the entry age when the policyholder first purchased the policy. In other words, a person who was age 65 years when he/she bought the LTCI policy will continue to pay the premium charged all 65-year-olds, regardless of the insured person's current age. Premiums cannot change unless a company receives approval from a state insurance commission to increase the rate for an entire class of policyholders. A company may not increase the premium for an individual policyholder.

Waiver of Premium. After an insured has received long-term care services for a designated period of time, most LTCI policies waive payment of premiums. Some policies count the elimination or waiting period in the waiver time period; others start counting after the elimination or waiting period. Most policies with this provision waive premiums after ninety (90) to one-hundred eighty (180) days. Tax-qualified policies must have a waiver of premium provision.

VI. BENEFITS.

Depending on the policy, LTCI provides a predetermined amount of money per day, subject to an aggregate total, for services ranging from home care to nursing home care. Policies provide benefits based upon a dollar limitation, the number of days of covered care, or a number of visits by service providers. An insured might be inclined to select and obtain a dollar limitation on benefits as more useful because the physician's care plan for the insured may call for more than one visit a day or for daily care.

VII. INFLATION PROTECTION.

Because LTCI insurance benefits may be used at some future date when long-term care costs will likely be higher than when a policy is first purchased, many companies offer, for a higher premium, three (3) different ways for insured individuals to protect against inflation. One inflation protection is an automatic percentage increase in the daily benefit amount compounded annually. The higher the percentage of inflation rate selected by the policyholder, the higher the premium. A second way of protecting against inflation is a provision to have the daily benefit amount increase annually at a simple percentage rate. A third method of inflation protection is the option to purchase additional insurance based upon the consumer price index.

Current standards for LTCI policies issued by the National Association of Insurance Commissioners provide for a five- (5%) percent compounded inflation protection. This standard is not mandatory upon companies. Some states require an insurance commission to sell LTCI policies, within their borders, with inflation protection included. All new policies qualifying for Federal tax benefits must offer customers the option to purchase inflation protection.

VIII. ELIMINATION OR WAITING PERIOD.

Much like a deductible with other insurance policies, LTCI policies impose an elimination or waiting period before paying benefits. Once an insured becomes eligible to receive benefits, he/she must wait a pre-selected period of time until the first benefit is paid. Consumers can elect an elimination period usually ranging between twenty (20) days and one (1) year. The longer the period, the smaller the premium.

IX. HOME CARE.

The home care services covered by LTCI policies vary. Most cover skilled, intermediate, and custodial care. Some policies limit coverage to services provided by skilled providers such as registered nurses and therapists. Other policies also include personal care provided by home care aides. Many policies cover a maximum of fourteen (14) days respite care and also adult day care. Most home care policies require that the insured use caregivers supplied through a licensed health care agency rather than allowing caregivers to be hired privately.

Many LTCI policies have a lower maximum benefit for home care than for institutional confinement. For example, the selected home care benefit may be limited to fifty (50%) percent of the maximum for a skilled nursing facility benefit. Or the duration of home care benefits may be limited to two (2) years, whereas the maximum period of coverage for care as an inpatient in a skilled musing facility may be four (4) years. An optimum insurance policy provides at least the same level of reimbursement and duration of benefits for home care as for institutional confinement.

X. OTHER FEATURES.

> **Non-forfeiture Clause**. Some companies offer, for a higher premium, a non-forfeiture benefit in case the insured lets a policy lapse. This provision provides that payments made on lapsed policies must be applied to purchase a fully paid reduced benefit or must be refunded in whole or in part. Without a non-forfeiture provision, premiums already paid on lapsed policies are lost. A policy lapses when the policyholder affirmatively decides to cancel it, can no longer afford the premiums, or simply forgets to pay the premiums for so long that the period of reinstatement expires. Tax-qualified policies must offer an option to purchase non-forfeiture coverage.

Unintentional Lapse. Tax-qualified policies cannot be cancelled because of a policyholder's failure to pay a premium until thirty (30) days after written notification to the policyholder or a designated third party. In the event a policyholder suffers from a cognitive impairment or loss of functional capacity and the policy lapses, it can be reinstated if requested within five (5) months after termination and if past premiums due are paid.

Pre-existing Conditions. Most older LTCI policies contain a provision disqualifying a prospective insured from obtaining coverage of a pre-existing condition either permanently or for a specified length of time. To be tax-qualified, new policies must define pre-existing condition period to be the six- (6) month period prior to the effective date of coverage; further, a policy cannot deny coverage for a pre-existing condition after six (6) months following the effective date of coverage. Currently, major carriers issue policies that immediately cover a pre-existing condition so long as it is disclosed on the application form.

Post-claims Underwriting. To be qualified for tax benefits, policies may not practice post-claims underwriting whereby a policy is automatically issued without investigation of insurability but retroactively determines whether a person is covered after a claim is filed.

Upgrading. Most LTCI policies cannot be automatically upgraded. Some companies offer the right of an insured to upgrade without additional underwriting medical examinations. Absent some type of right to upgrade, should a better policy later become available, the policyholder will have to apply anew for a policy, undergo a second underwriting medical examination, and pay a higher premium based upon his/her greater age or worsened condition in order to obtain the improved coverage.

XI. TAX STATUS.

Under the Health Insurance Portability and Accountability Act of 1996 (Act), LTCI policies are treated as accident and health insurance contracts with several favorable tax consequences. To be eligible for these tax advantages, that is to be considered tax-qualified, LTCI policies must meet certain standards. Policies issued prior to 1996 that have met existing state standards are considered qualified policies even though they may not meet the Federal requirements.

A. <u>Conditions for an LTCI Policy to be tax-qualified. An LTCI policy must satisfy a number of conditions to qualify for Federal tax advantages (see *Long-term care insurance, tax status*)</u>:

    1. A person must require services that are needed by a chronically ill individual. Such an individual is defined as someone unable to perform at least two (2) of five (5) or six (6) activities of daily living without substantial assistance from another individual or who has an equivalent level of disability that a physician projects that will last at least ninety (90) days. A chronically ill individual must require substantial supervision to protect him/her from threats to health and safety due to severe cognitive impairments.

        The LTCI contract may only provide for qualified long-term care services. The Health Insurance Portability and Accountability Act defines a qualified LTCI contract as a guaranteed-renewable long-term care insurance policy, or as a rider to a life insurance contract, under which the only insurance protection provided is coverage of qualified long-term care services. The Act defines qualified long-term services as diagnostic, preventive, therapeutic, curing, treating, mitigating and rehabilitative services and as maintenance or personal care services which are required by a chronically ill individual and provided pursuant to a plan of care prescribed by a licensed health care provider. "Maintenance or personal care services" means any care the primary purpose of which is to provide needed assistance with any of the disabilities as a result of which the individual is chronically ill, including severe cognitive impairment.

    2. The LTCI contract may not pay or reimburse expenses reimbursable by Medicare, except for coinsurance or deductible amounts.

3. The LTCI contract may not provide for a cash surrender value or other money that can be paid, pledged or borrowed.

4. The LTCI contact must contain a separate insurance coverage trigger, independent of ADLs, for cognitively impaired individuals.

5. The LTCI contract must contain certain consumer protection provisions set forth in the Long-term Care Insurance Model Act and Model Regulations developed by the National Association of Insurance Commissioners. These provisions relate to such policy features as an inflation protection option, guaranteed renewability, and adult day care coverage.

B. <u>Tax Advantages</u>.

According to the Act, there are four (4) tax advantages associated with qualified LTCI policies:

1. Subject to limitations in amount (set forth below), a taxpayer may treat LTCI premiums as un-reimbursed medical expenses and as such deduct them from Federal taxable income to the extent such expenses exceed seven and one-half (7.5%) percent of the taxpayer's adjusted gross income. The limits on deductions of annual premium dollars vary with the age of the insured and are indexed for inflation. For 2012, the limits are set forth below:

<u>Age</u>	<u>Deduction Limits (2012 tax year)</u>
40 and under	$350
41-50	$660
51-60	$1,310
61-70	$3,500
over 70	$4,370

In addition to Federal tax benefits for qualified LTCI insurance plans, some states offer their own tax incentives to encourage purchase of LTCI.

2. Employers may deduct premiums they pay for policies offered through employee benefit programs.

3. Benefits received by taxpayers under an LTCI contract are excludable from gross income for purposes of Federal income tax. However, benefits based on a fixed sum per day of disability are taxable beyond a cap ($310 per day in 2012). The dollar cap is indexed for inflation according to the medical care cost component of the consumer price index. Per-diem policies must integrate long-term care riders to life insurance policies to meet the cap. If benefit payments exceed the dollar cap, then the excess payments are excludable only to the extent of the individual's un-reimbursed costs for qualified long-term care services.

4. Employer-provided long-term care benefits are tax-free to the employee. They are not excludable by an employee, however, if provided through a cafeteria plan of benefits. Expenses for long-term care services cannot be reimbursed under a flexible spending account.

XII. STATE LONG-TERM CARE INSURANCE PARTNERSHIP PROGRAMS.

A.   Originally Limited to Certain States.

Several states following pilot projects funded by grants from the Robert Wood Johnson Foundation have enacted long-term care insurance (LTCI) programs integrating the purchase by an individual of LTCI with his/her eligibility for Medicaid. California, Connecticut, Indiana, Iowa and New York approved such plans in 1993. Federal law (COBRA 1993) previously banned extension of this type of program to other states (see below *Programs extended to all states*).

According to this plan linking LTCI with Medicaid eligibility rules, if and when private insurance benefits are exhausted, the assets of policyholders are not counted in whole (New York) or in part (the other specified states) in determining their Medicaid eligibility. However, all of their income will be counted. Under the New York plan, a person who purchases a LTCI policy may establish his/her eligibility for Medicaid when the insurance benefits run out and thereby shelter an unlimited amount of assets from recovery by Medicaid. In the four other states, a purchase of a LTCI policy will shelter assets on a dollar-for-dollar basis. The individual purchaser is able to retain an amount of assets free from Medicaid recovery equal to the amount of LTCI purchased.

B.   Programs Extended to All States.

The Deficit Reduction Act of 2005 (DRA) provides that states now may amend their Medicaid plans to include qualified long-term care partnership programs that disregard assets or resources equal to the amount of insurance benefit payments made to or on behalf of a beneficiary under a LTCI policy if the statutorily specified requirements are met regarding the insured and the policy. Under DRA, the programs in California, Connecticut, Indiana, Iowa and New York are grandfathered into the new provisions so long as the Secretary of HHS determines that each state's consumer protection standards are no less stringent than the standards applicable as of December 31, 2005. Other states that wish to offer the program may amend their Medicaid statutes to provide for the program.

C.   Requirements of a Qualified State Long-term Care Insurance Policy.

In order to qualify as a qualified state long-term care insurance partnership policy, the policy must satisfy seven (7) requirements:

1.   The insured must be a resident of the state at the time coverage first becomes effective;

2.   The policy must be a qualified LTCI policy as defined in Internal Revenue Code Section 702B(b);

3.   The policy must meet nine (9) specified sections of the Long-Term Care Insurance Model Act and nineteen (19) specified sections of the Model Regulations of the National Association of Insurance Commissioners;

4.   The policy must provide for compound annual inflation protection for persons under age 61 as of the purchase date and must also provide some level of inflation protection for persons between the ages of 61 and 75. From age 76 on, inflation protection is optional;

5.   The state Medicaid agency must provide information and technical assistance to the state insurance department to make sure that agents selling LTCI receive training and demonstrate understanding of the LTCI partnership policies and how they relate to other private and public coverage of long-term care;

6.   The insurer must provide regular reports to the Secretary of HHS regarding the performance of the program; and

7.   The state may not impose requirements on partnership policies that are not imposed on all LTCI policies.

(continued on next page)

Long-term Care Insurance, Tax Status
See also *Long-Term Care Insurance, section II.K.*

Under the Health Insurance Portability and Accountability Act of 1996, LTCI policies effective January 1, 1997 are treated as accident and health insurance contracts with several favorable tax consequences. To be eligible for these tax advantages, that is to be considered tax-qualified, LTCI policies sold after January 1, 1997 must meet certain standards. Policies issued prior to this date that have met existing state standards are considered qualified policies even though they may not meet the Federal requirements.

One standard provides that before coverage begins a person must require services that are needed by a chronically ill individual who is defined as a person unable to perform at least two (2) of five (5) or six (6) activities of daily living – eating, bathing, dressing transferring (e.g., from bed to a chair), toileting and continence – "without substantial assistance from another individual" or who has an equivalent level of disability. A physician must project that this disability will last at least ninety (90) days.

Another standard relates to individuals "requiring substantial supervision to protect [them] from threats to health and safety due to severe cognitive impairments." Such persons are deemed to be chronically ill.

To be tax-qualified, a LTCI contract must only provide for qualified long-term care services. Qualified policies must also contain a separate trigger, independent of ADLs, for cognitively impaired individuals.

Tax-qualified policies are also required to contain certain consumer protection provisions set forth in the Long-term Care Insurance Model Act and Model Regulations developed by National Association of Insurance Commissions. These provisions relate to such policy features as inflation protection option, guaranteed renewability and adult day care coverage. (For more details see *Long-term care insurance, section II. J.*)

There are four (4) tax advantages associated with qualified LTCI policies. First, subject to limitation in amount, a taxpayer may treat LTCI premiums as unreimbursed medical expenses and as such deduct them from taxable income to the extent such expenses exceed seven and one-half (7.5%) percent of the taxpayer's gross income. The limits on deductions of annual premium dollars vary with the age of the insured and are indexed for inflation.

For the 2012 tax year, the limits are set forth below.

Age	Deduction Limits (2012)
40 and under	$350
41-50	$660
51-60	$1,310
61-70	$3,500
Over 70	$4,370

Second, employers may deduct premiums they pay for policies offered through employee-benefit programs.

Third, benefits received by taxpayers under a LTCI contract are excludable from gross income, subject to a cap of $310 (2012) per day. The dollar cap will be indexed for inflation according to the medical care cost component of the consumer price index. Per diem policies, unless issued prior to July 31, 1996, must integrate long-term care riders to life insurance policies to meet the cap. If benefit payments exceed the dollar cap, then the excess payments are excludable only to the extent of the individual's unreimbursed costs for long-term care services.

Fourth, employer-provided long-term care benefits are also excludable from an employee's income. They are not excludable by an employer, however, if provided through a cafeteria plan benefits. Expenses for long-term care services cannot be reimbursed under a flexible spending account.

Long-term Hospital

A hospital that treats patients, though not acutely ill, who require an intensity of medical and skilled nursing services not available in nursing homes.

Look-back Period/Medicaid
See *Transfer penalty (civil)/Medicaid.*

Low-income Beneficiaries/Medicare Part D Drug Coverage

These beneficiaries are each a subsidy-eligible individual as defined below and according to income or status: (i) a full-subsidy-eligible individual, (ii) individuals treated (deemed) as full-subsidy eligibles, or (iii) individuals who are partial-subsidy individuals as defined below. A subsidy-eligible individual is a Part D-eligible individual who (i) is enrolled in or seeking to enroll in a Part D plan;

(ii) has an income below one-hundred fifty (150%) percent of the Federal poverty level; and (iii) has resources at or below the thresholds set forth below.

There are two groups of subsidy eligible individuals. The first group is composed of persons who either:

> are enrolled in a prescription drug plan;
>
> have incomes below one-hundred thirty-five (135%) percent of Federal poverty level;
>
> have resources in 2012 below $8,440 for an individual and $13,410 for a couple (increased in future years by the percentage increase in the consumer price index (CPI); or
>
> are full-benefit dual eligibles without regard to income and resources and without regard as to whether they meet other eligibility standards.

The second group of subsidy-eligible individuals is persons meeting the same requirements as above, except that the income level is above one-hundred thirty-five (135%) percent but below one-hundred fifty (150%) percent of the Federal poverty level and an alternative resources standard is used. The alternative standard in 2012 is $13,070 for an individual and $26,120 for a couple (increased in future years by the percentage increase in the CPI).

A full-subsidy eligible individual is an individual with full Medicaid status (full-benefit dual eligible), or an individual with (i) income below one-hundred thirty-five (135%) percent of the Federal poverty level and (ii) resources of less than $8,440 (single person) or less than $13,410 (married couple).

Individuals treated (deemed) as full-subsidy eligible individuals are those who are recipients of Supplemental Security Income without Medicaid or individuals enrolled in one of the following Medicare savings programs (also called buy-in programs):

> Qualified Medicare beneficiary (QMB);
>
> Specified low-income Medicare beneficiary (SLMB); or
>
> Qualified individual (QI) under a state's plan.

Partial-subsidy eligible individuals (non-deemed) are individuals who (i) have incomes above one-hundred thirty-five (135%) percent but less than one-hundred fifty (150%) percent of the Federal poverty level and (ii) have resources that in 2012 do not exceed $13,070 if single, or $26,120 if married.

Low-income Beneficiary/Medicare
See *Specified low-income Medicare beneficiary (SLMB)/Medicare, Medicaid.*

Low-income Qualified Individuals

An individual is selected by the state as a qualified individual. The individual must meet the qualified Medicare beneficiary criteria except that his/her income level is at least one-hundred twenty (120%) percent but less than one-hundred thirty-five (135%) percent of the Federal poverty level for a family of the size involved. The state is required to pay the full amount of Medicare Part B provision of such qualified individual, but only for premiums payable during period January 1998 through December 2002. However, the individual cannot be otherwise eligible for medical assistance under the approved state Medicaid plan.

*Low-income Subsidy (LIS) (Extra Help)/Medicare Part D Drugs
See also *Low-income beneficiaries/Medicare Part D Drug Coverage*, which gives 2012 figures.

A Medicare program to help people with limited income and resources pay Medicare prescription drug program costs, such as premiums, deductibles, and coinsurance.

You may qualify for Extra Help, also called the low-income subsidy (LIS), from Medicare to pay prescription drug costs if your yearly income and resources are below the following limits in 2010:

Single person –income less than $16,245 and resources less than $12,510

Married person living with a spouse and no other dependents – Income less than $21,855 and resources less than $25,010

These amounts may change in 2011. You may qualify even if you have a higher income (like if you still work, or if you live in Alaska or Hawaii, or have dependents living with you). Resources include money in a checking or savings account, stocks, and bonds. Resources don't include your home, car, household items, burial plot, up to $1,500 for burial expenses (per person), or life insurance policies.

If you qualify for Extra Help and join a Medicare drug plan, you will get the following:

Help paying your Medicare drug plans monthly premium, any yearly deductible, coinsurance, and copayments

No coverage gap

No late enrollment penalty

*You **automatically** qualify for Extra Help if you have Medicare and meet one of these conditions:*

You have full Medicaid coverage

You get help from your state Medicaid program paying your Part B premiums (in a Medicare Savings Program).

You get Supplemental Security Income (SSI) benefits.

To let you know you automatically qualify for Extra Help, Medicare will mail you a purple letter that you should keep for your records. You don't need to apply for Extra Help if you get this letter.

If you aren't already in a Medicare drug plan, you must join one to get this Extra Help.

If you don't join a Medicare drug plan, Medicare may enroll you in one. If Medicare enrolls you in a plan, Medicare will send you a yellow or green letter letting you know when your coverage begins.

Different plans cover different drugs. Check to see if the plan you are enrolled in covers the drugs you use and if you can go to the pharmacies you want. Compare with other plans and in your area.

If you're getting Extra Help, you can switch to another Medicare drug plan any time. Your coverage will be effective the first day of the next month.

If you have Medicaid and live in certain institutions (like a nursing home), you pay nothing for your covered prescription drugs.

If you don't want to join a Medicare drug plan (for example, because you want only your employer or union coverage), call the plan listed in your letter, or call 1-800-MEDICARE (1-800-633-4227). TTY users should call 1-877-486-2048. Tell them you don't want to be in a Medicare drug plan (you want to "opt out"). If you continue to qualify for Extra Help or if your employer or union coverage is creditable prescription drug coverage, you won't pay a penalty if you join later.

If you have employer or union coverage and you join a Medicare drug plan, you may lose your employer or union drug, and possibly health coverage even if you qualify for Extra Help. Your dependents may also lose their coverage. Call your employer's benefits administrator for more information before you join.

If you didn't automatically qualify for Extra Help, you can apply:

> *Visit www.socialsecurity.gov to apply online.*

> *Call Social Security at 1-800-772-1213 to apply by phone or to get a paper application. TTY users should call 1-800-325-0778.*

> *Visit your State Medical Assistance (Medicaid) office. Call 1-800-MEDICARE (1-800-633-4227), and say "Medicaid" to get the telephone number, or visit www.medicare.gov. TTY users should call 1-877-486-2048.*

> *You can apply for Extra Help at any time. With your consent, Social Security will forward information to your state to start an application for a Medicare Savings Program.*

> *Drug costs in 2011 for most people who qualify will be no more than $2.50 for each generic drug and $6.30 for each brand-name drug. Look on the Extra Help letters you get, or contact your plan to find out your exact costs.*

Low-Income Subsidy/Medicare Part D Drug Coverage

See also *Extra help subsidy/Medicare Part D Drug Coverage; Low-income beneficiaries/Medicare Part D Drug Coverage.*

The subsidy is financial assistance by the Federal government that lowers the premiums and copayments for beneficiaries (without SSI, or who are not dual eligible) with income below one-hundred fifty (150%) percent of the Federal poverty level and limited assets. The assistance is referred to as extra help.

Lump-Sum Death Benefit/Social Security

If a worker was fully or currently insured, the following survivors are eligible for a lump-sum death benefit of $255:

> The worker's surviving spouse if he/she was living with the worker at the time of the worker's death;

> The worker's surviving spouse even if he/she did not live with the worker but is eligible to receive benefits on the worker's account; and

A surviving child who is eligible for benefits based on the worker's account.

Lump-Sum Pension Distribution

See also *Forward averaging.*

A distribution of a participant's entire balance in a private pension plan in a manner that qualifies for forward averaging.

(continued on next page)

M

Magnetic Resonance Imaging (MRI Scan)

An MRI (or magnetic resonance imaging) scan is a radiology technique that uses magnetism, radio waves, and a computer to produce images of body structures. The MRI scanner is a tube surrounded by a giant circular magnet. The patient is placed on a moveable bed that is inserted into the magnet. The magnet creates a strong magnetic field that aligns the protons of hydrogen atoms, which are then exposed to a beam of radio waves. This spins the various protons of the body, and they produce a faint signal that is detected by the receiver portion of the MRI scanner. The receiver information is processed by a computer, and an image is produced.

The image and resolution produced by an MRI are quite detailed and can detect tiny changes of structures within the body. For some procedures, contrast agents, such gadolinium, are used to increase the accuracy of the images. An MRI scan can be used as an extremely accurate method of disease detection throughout the body. In the head, trauma to the brain can be seen as bleeding or swelling. Other abnormalities often found include brain aneurysms, stroke, tumors of the brain, as well as tumors or inflammation of the spine.

Neurosurgeons use an MRI scan not only in defining brain anatomy but in evaluating the integrity of the spinal cord after trauma. It is also used when considering problems associated with the vertebrae or intervertebral discs of the spine. An MRI scan can evaluate the structure of the heart and aorta, where it can detect aneurysms or tears.

It provides valuable information on glands and organs within the abdomen, and accurate information about the structure of the joints, soft tissues, and bones of the body. Often, surgery can be deferred or more accurately directed after knowing the results of an MRI scan.

'All entries preceded by an asterisk (*) are culled or copied from the official U.S. government **Medicare** handbook (*Medicare & You 2011*).

*Mammogram/Medicare

A type of x-ray to check women for breast cancer. Medicare covers screening mammograms once every 12 months for women 40 and older. Medicare covers one baseline mammogram for women between 35-39. Starting January 1, 2011, you pay nothing for the test if the doctor accepts assignment.

Mammography/Medicare

Part B covers x-ray screenings for the detection of breast cancer. Women age 40 or older can use the benefit every twelve (12) months. For women age 35-39, Medicare will help to pay for a baseline mammogram. The Part B annual deductible is waived for screening mammogram; the twenty- (20%) percent coinsurance amount is also waived if the doctor accepts assignment.

(continued on next page)

MANAGED CARE

INTRODUCTION

A managed care plan refers to an arrangement between individual participants and a managed care organization which provides a network of medical services to the participants on a capitated (i.e., pre-paid, fixed, periodic fee) basis. The organization is both an insurer and provider. Managed care is rapidly becoming a predominant form of delivering health care services and insuring people in the United States. More and more older people are moving into managed care.

A managed care organization utilizes a network of doctors, hospitals and other care providers and has the following primary features:

> the rendering of medical services by the network of doctors under a contract with or employed by the managed care organization;

> a relationship between a plan participant, sometimes called an enrollee;

> a primary care physician, commonly referred to as a gatekeeper, who is a medical member of the network and authorizes, arranges or coordinates medical services, and refers treatment by a specialist, for the participant; and the payment to the organization, by the participant, directly or through a group such as an employer or association, of a prepaid periodic fee, commonly referred to as a capitated fee, which usually covers all charges to a participant for an agreed upon range of the managed care organization's services regardless of how frequently utilized.

In the type of managed care plan known as the closed panel model, the participants are required to use physicians from a specific list of participating providers. When the plan does not require the primary care physician's prior

269

approval of treatment by a specialist from among the list of providers, this type of plan is known as an open panel model.

The several types of managed care organizations are set forth below. However, the distinction between the original (traditional) HMO and the various other plans types has become blurred.

1. **Traditional HMOs.**

These organizations are described in the entry *Health Maintenance Organization.*

2. **Other Managed Care Organizations.**

Other types of structured managed care organizations, which are variants of the HMO, have emerged and are expanding, including, among others: exclusive provider organization (EPO); point of service organization (POS); preferred provider organization (PPO); and, social health maintenance organization (SHMO). Each of these types of managed care organizations is described under its respective entry in the *Dictionary[+]*.

3. **Integrated Health Systems.**

Several health care systems, different from but related to HMOs, integrate the delivery of services from primary care to acute hospital services by combining physicians and hospitals such as management service organizations and physician/hospital organizations, or by linking provider organizations such as hospitals and nursing homes.

(a) Management Services Organization (MSO)

An MSO links one or more medical groups and physicians together with a hospital that is usually a wholly owned, for-profit subsidiary of a hospital/physician joint venture. Through utilization of an MSO, many individual physicians or small physicians groups are able to access managed care plans.

The MSO functions as the business manager providing the clinic premises, building services, furniture, fixtures and equipment, administrative and non-physician staff, accounting, billing, and collections and financial management.

The medical group operates as the clinic manager with responsibility for employing physicians, professional supervision and training, physician compensation and professional evaluation of clinic operations. The medical group pays the MSO a management fee for its services. The physicians remain autonomous, continuing the ownership of the group practice.

(b)   Physician Hospital Organization (PHO)

Basically, a PHO is formed when a hospital acquires or has a contractual relationship with a group of physicians. The hospital most commonly controls administrative matters, and physicians manage the clinical aspects of the business. The PHO negotiates and manages capitation contracts for the physicians and hospitals.

PHOs can differ in ownership structure. A hospital that acquires a medical group may become the owner of the PHO entities. The hospital elects its board of directors which controls the organization's operation. Physician participation in administration is generally confined to naming a medical advisory committee which addresses clinical issues such as utilization review.

In an alternate type of structure, the relationship between the physicians and hospital is contractual. Both the hospital and physicians hold ownership interest in the PHO, and the PHO manages the daily operation of the
organization and acts as a single entity.

4.   **Medicare Managed Care.**

Medicare managed care plans have been permitted by statute for more than a decade (see *Medicare health maintenance organization (HMO)*).

Historically, the only type of private health plans available to Medicare beneficiaries enrolled in Medicare Parts A and B were Medicare HMOs, which Medicare qualified under either a full risk or a cost-basis contract. With the passage of the Balanced Budget Act of 1997, the original Medicare HMO was replaced by an array of Medicare Advantage (previously Medicare+Choice) plans.

5.   **Medicaid Managed Care.**

Traditionally, Medicaid services have been provided under fee-for-service arrangements. In recent years, however, states have begun shifting Medicaid recipients into managed care plans. Use of these plans by states varies considerably.

Medicaid managed care arrangements include HMOs, prepaid health plans, health insuring organizations, and primary care case management which are described elsewhere in the *Dictionary*[+].

The Balanced Budget Act of 1997 authorized states to require Medicaid recipients to enroll in a managed care entity which includes managed care organizations and a primary care case management arrangement. (See *Medicaid mandatory managed care.*)

(continued on next page)

Mandated Benefits/LTCI

Benefits that state regulators require to be included in all policies licensed for sale within a state. The existence of mandated benefits makes policies more uniform, thus facilitating comparisons, and protects consumers from purchasing policies that are so restrictively written that it is unlikely that anyone will collect benefits. However, mandated benefits can make policies more expensive. In general, there is no standardization of LTCI policies, as there is with Medigap policies.

Mandated Benefits/Medicaid
See *Medicaid, section III.A.*

Mandatory Supplemental Benefits/Medicare Advantage

These benefits are services not covered by Medicare; an enrollee must purchase them as part of a Medicare Advantage plan. The enrollee directly pays for these services through premiums or cost sharing.

Marital Deduction

The marital deduction is an unlimited deduction that permits a married decedent to avoid completely the payment of any Federal estate taxes on all property passing from the decedent to the surviving spouse.

Every property, other than a "terminable interest" in property, may pass to a surviving spouse and qualify for a marital deduction. The transfer of property may be made in a variety of ways in addition to a will – for example, passing property under a joint tenancy of a husband and wife with rights of survivorship, or the payment of life insurance proceeds outright to a surviving spouse or to a trust that qualifies for a marital deduction.

An interest in property is terminable if the gift of that interest terminates upon the lapse of time or the occurrence of an event. Illustrations of such terminable interests are a life estate, annuity and lease term of years, all of which terminate upon a lapse of time and hence do not qualify as a marital deduction. A notable exception to the terminable interest property rule is a transfer of a qualified terminable interest property.

Marital Property

Commonly refers to property which is accumulated by a married couple during marriage, except gifts or inheritances.

Maximum Allowable Charge/Medicare
See *Balance billing/Medicare.*

Meals on Wheels

This program provides a hot, nutritious home-delivered meal once and sometimes twice a day, five (5) days a week to persons who are unable to cook for themselves. There is usually a sliding fee (or no fee) for meals determined by an individual's ability to pay. Often referred to as meals on wheels, this service is covered by Medicaid waivers in certain states, by area agencies on aging under the Older Americans Act and by social services block grants.

Means-tested Program

A government program such as SSI and Medicaid where eligibility is not general but is limited to those whose income and/or assets (i.e., means) fall below specified levels.

(continued on next page)

MEDICAID

INTRODUCTION

Medicaid (Title XIX of the Social Security Act) is a welfare program of medical assistance. Financed jointly by the state and Federal governments, the program is administered primarily by the states. The Federal government sets the guidelines for Medicaid. Each state designs its own particular program within the limits of Federal law and regulations.

At the Federal level, the Department of Health and Human Services (DHHS), through the Centers of Medicare and Medicaid Services (CMS), issues regulations and guidelines and monitors state compliance with Federal laws and rules. DHHS publishes the State Medicaid Assistance Manual for use by the states in administering the program. At the state level, a state agency is responsible for issuing rules and regulations and guidelines for Medicaid eligibility. Local agencies are responsible for day-to-day administration of the Medicaid program.

The Medicaid program enables a Medicaid recipient to receive medical services. The bill of the Medicaid individual for medical services received is sent to the state Medicaid agency for payment. Each Medicaid recipient gets a plastic identification card, which must be presented when services are received. Medicaid pays doctors, hospitals, nursing homes and other providers directly, provided they have agreed to accept Medicaid clients and agree to accept Medicaid payment as payment in full.

Individuals age 65 and over, blind or disabled persons, low-income pregnant women and certain low-income families with children may qualify for this assistance. Medicaid recipients must be American citizens or fall within specified categories of permanent resident aliens.

Medicaid is a means-tested program. Unlike Medicare (which is available regardless of financial need to most persons age 65 or older and to certain disabled individuals), Medicaid is available only to individuals with limited income and resources. All the states plus Puerto Rico, the Virgin Islands, Guam and the District of Columbia participate in Medicaid; Arizona has a limited program.

Within the Medicaid program, there are several sub-programs known as buy-in programs, or medical programs, which assist low-income Medicaid beneficiaries to pay some or all of the premiums, copayments and deductibles associated with the Medicaid program: namely, the qualified Medicare beneficiary program, specified low-income Medicare beneficiary, and qualified individuals. These individuals may buy-in to these sub-programs without applying for full Medicare coverage. The payments are made by state Medicaid agencies.

In general, states serve two groups of persons through their Medicaid programs. First, they must serve the categorically needy, defined to include aged (65 and older), blind, and disabled persons eligible for benefits under the Supplemental Security Income (SSI) program. Second, states are permitted, but not required, to serve the medically needy, which refers to those persons in need of medical assistance whose income levels disqualify them from the SSI programs.

Congress created the SSI program in 1972, to take effect January 1, 1974. The SSI eligibility criteria were broader than some of the prior state-established criteria. Congress added §209(b) to the Supplemental Security Income Act, 42 U.S.C. § 1396a(f), to encourage continued participation by states with stricter criteria. States choosing the § 209(b) option are not required to provide Medicaid to persons who would not have been eligible under the state medical assistance plan in effect on January 1, 1972, prior to the enactment of SSI. States electing the 209(b) option are required (with few exceptions) to operate a program for the medical needy, and to adopt an income spend-down provision. The 209(b) states are: Connecticut, Hawaii, Illinois, Indiana, Minnesota, Missouri, Nebraska, New Hampshire, North Carolina, North Dakota, Ohio, Oklahoma, Utah and Virginia.

When a medically needy applicant's income or resources exceed the applicable state's Medicaid eligibility limits, the spend-down rule may apply. Under this rule, the applicant may be able to spend down excess income or resources, by applying them to outstanding medical bills, to become eligible for Medicaid. Income spend-down is the process whereby an applicant's income is reduced for the purpose of determining Medicaid eligibility by the amount of incurred but unpaid medical expenses. Resource spend-down is the process that allows Medicaid applicants to offset their resources by incurred but unpaid medical bills.

The Balanced Budget Act of 1997 amended the Social Security Act so that states may require individuals eligible for Medicaid medical assistance to enroll in a managed care entity (see *Medicaid mandatory managed care, section VIII*).

On February 8, 2006, President Bush signed into law the Deficit Reduction Act of 2005 (DRA). This law placed severe new restrictions on the ability of the elderly to transfer assets before qualifying for Medicaid coverage of nursing home care.

I. APPLICATION FOR MEDICAID ASSISTANCE.

An individual eligible for Medicaid may apply for assistance by following the application process described below:

A written application on a state-prescribed Medicaid application form is submitted by the applicant to the state agency designated to handle Medicaid applications. This agency is commonly a department of social services, or public welfare. In certain states, application can be made at a Social Security office.

A personal interview is necessary. The state agency will accommodate a disabled individual by sending a worker to his/her home.

The state agency will require extensive documentation to establish eligibility, (e.g., age 65 or over, citizenship, and income and resources at or below the levels established by the state).

The state agency will make a determination on the applicant's Medicaid eligibility and provide the applicant with a written notice of acceptance or denial. Medicaid reimbursement is generally retroactive to the third month preceding the month of application, if the applicant met eligibility requirements during that period.

Medicaid is usually for an authorized period such as one year. At the end of the authorized period, the Medicaid recipient is required to submit a state Medicaid form seeking recertification for continued eligibility. The request is required to notify the state of any changes, which may affect his/her eligibility.

Applications for personal care require completing further documentation prescribed by the state agency (see section V).

II.   ELIGIBILITY FOR MEDICAID ASSISTANCE.[*]

Medicaid eligibility for services depends upon the following four eligibility factors:

Certain status standards (see A);

Whether the Medicaid-eligible person resides in an SSI state or a section 209(b) state (see B);

Income and resource standards (see C); and,

Several categories of eligibility (see D). The types of services provided by Medicaid differ among three groups of Medicaid eligibles: categorically needy, medically needy, and optionally categorically needy.

A.   Status Test

The status test is one of the four (4) eligibility factors.

Any elderly, disabled or blind person who is a United States citizen or among a limited category of qualified aliens (permanent resident alien status) is eligible to apply for Medicaid. The individual must be age 65 or older or meet the SSI definition of blindness or disability, or a state's more restrictive definition of blindness or disability if the person is in a 209(b) state (see paragraph B below).

According to the Personal Responsibility and Work Opportunity Act of 1996, aliens lawfully residing in the United States and receiving SSI on August 22, 1996 may continue to receive Medicaid medical assistance as if they were citizens. Likewise, aliens who lawfully resided in the United States on August 22, 1996 and who met the statutory definition of blind or disabled are also entitled to receive such benefits. Legal immigrants arriving in the country after August 22, 1996 generally are barred (banned) from Medicaid medical assistance during the first five (5) years after their entry into the United States. However, five (5) categories of these immigrants are excepted from this ban:

---

[*] This section duplicates and repeats matter contained in the Overview "Eligibility for Medicaid Services." The author believes that direct access to the subject will be convenient and helpful to the reader.

honorably discharged U.S. military veterans and active duty personnel, their spouses and unmarried dependents;

individuals who singly or collectively with their spouse have worked forty (40) qualified quarters of Social Security coverage;

current and future refugees;

individuals granted political asylum; and,

individuals granted status as Cuban, Haitian or Amerasian entrants.

All five (5) categories of the legal immigrants specified above are eligible for Medicaid medical assistance for seven (7) years after their entry into this country.

B. Residence in SSI States and Section 209(b) States – Spend-down Process

This is one of the four (4) eligibility factors.

1. **SSI States**

Medicaid eligibility, to a significant extent, is tied to eligibility for benefits under the SSI program. An SSI state is one that determines eligibility for Medicaid by using SSI financial and citizenship criteria. In SSI states, persons who receive SSI benefits due to age, blindness or disability are automatically eligible for Medicaid and are mandatorily considered categorically eligible. Like the SSI program, Medicaid, is a strict categorical program and is in effect in thirty-seven (37) states (known as SSI states).

In SSI states, the three (3) categorical status standards for Medicaid coverage of individuals (other than children) are age (65 or older), blindness or disability. Medicaid does not provide a definition of blindness or disability. The SSI states have adopted the definition of those words as set forth in the SSI program and are governed by these SSI definitions.

2. **209(b) States (Spend-down Process).**

As in SSI states, the three (3) status standards for Medicaid coverage of individuals (other than children) residing in 209(b) states are: age (65 or older), blindness or disability. The definitions of blindness and disability in 209(b) states are different and may be more restrictive than the definitions in SSI states. While the age standard (65 or older) is the same, section 209(b) permits states which so desire the option to use income standards (levels) that are more restrictive than those provided in SSI states. Fourteen (14) states exercise the option (known as the 209(b) option after the section of the public law under which it was enacted): Connecticut, Hawaii, Illinois, Indiana, Minnesota, Missouri, Nebraska, New Hampshire, North Carolina, North Dakota, Ohio, Oklahoma, Utah and Virginia. The right to spend down (described below) applies to each of these states. Spend down occurs in either of two particular areas of Medicaid eligibility. First, individuals in 209(b) states whose income is higher than the state's prescribed financial levels have the right of spend down so as to become eligible for Medicaid as discussed below. Second, persons eligible under a state's medically needy program may spend down to the state's prescribed financial levels, and thereby become eligible for Medicaid; the categorically needy and optional categorically needy groups have no right to spend down.

Section 209(b) states must allow people with incomes above their more restrictive standard to become eligible for Medicaid if they spend down their excess income on incurred medical bills. More specifically, in 209(b) states, an individual who does not satisfy the income and resources standards prescribed by that state may spend down his/her income on incurred medical expenses in order to reduce one's income to a state's prescribed standard for purposes of becoming eligible for Medicaid. Some states also permit a resource spend down, applying the same principle. The spend-down process is described below.

Four 209(b) states have either partial (Oklahoma), or no (Indiana, Ohio and Missouri) medically needy programs. However, this is not of great significance since 209(b) states are required to have a spend-down program regardless of whether they have a medically needy program so that elderly people can get Medicaid if their medical bills are sufficiently high. There is a technical statutory difference. States with a medically needy program require that individuals be permitted to spend down not only income but also resources; however, 209(b) states, while required to permit income spend-down, may permit (but are not required to allow) applicants to spend down resources. The statutory language covering 209(b) states provides for a spend-down. However, the medically needy states have no statutory spend-down language, though the statutory language covering these states has been interpreted as spend-down provisions.

2.1   Description of the Spend-down Process

If a state has a medically needy program, or is a 209(b) state, it must apply all incurred medical expenses to reduce a Medicaid applicant's income when determining Medicaid eligibility. If he/she still does not meet the state's medically needy income level (MNIL) – or in a 209(b) state, the lower income standard that the state uses – Medicaid will advise the individual of the amount by which the individual continues to be over income. This amount is called the spend-down amount. SSI states (and generally 209(b) states) must deduct from "over-income" any amounts that would be deducted in determining SSI eligibility. Examples of such deductions, or disregards, are: (i) first $20 earned or unearned income per household; (ii) unearned income disregard of $65 per month, plus half the remainder; and, (iii) infrequent or irregular income.

Incurred medical expenses (including health insurance premiums and other cost-sharing, deductibles and coinsurance charges, as well as other medical and remedial expenses recognized under state law), whether or not they are covered by the state's Medicaid plan, will be considered by the state both in its eligibility determination, and subsequently in determining when the spend-down is met. Medical expenses need only be incurred, not paid. Therefore, medical bills need not actually have been paid so long as they were incurred and the individual is currently liable for the expenses. Any legitimate medical expenses, whether or not covered by the state's Medicaid plan, may be deducted. Thus, there may be deducted: Medicare and other health care premiums, deductibles and coinsurance incurred by the individual and family; necessary medical and remedial expenses including prescriptions, over-the-counter drugs, eyeglasses, transportation, most dental expenses, etc.

The prospective period during which an applicant must spend down his/her over-income or over-resource is called the budget period. It usually varies up to six (6) months for persons living at home and one (1) month for institutionalized persons. To be Medicaid eligible, an individual must incur medical expenses equal to or greater than his/her income for a prescribed period up to six (6) months (the individual must repeat this spend-down every six (6) months). Once the individual has incurred medical expenses that reduce his/her income to the MNIL or the 209(b) standard, he/she is entitled to have Medicaid pay for covered care and services for the duration of the budget period. The individual will be considered eligible under this program if the medical expenses incurred equal or exceed the difference between the individual's available net income and resources, and the medically needy income and resource eligibility limits prescribed by the state.

C.   Income and Resource Test.

This test is one of the four (4) eligibility factors and revolves around the following rules and criteria, applicable to the following subjects:

> Countable Income (section 1 below)
>
> Countable Resources (section 2 below)
>
> Trust Income and Resource Rules (section 3 below)
>
> Deeming of Income and Resources of Spouses (section 4 below)

1.   Countable Income.

The general term income means any payment from any source of any kind (money, goods or services). Payment made on a one-time basis and on a recurring basis is considered income. It includes earned income such as salary, unearned income, and in-kind income (see (a), (b) and (c) below).

Individuals must have countable income below state-prescribed standards that the state in which the Medicaid applicant resides establishes for Medicaid eligibility. To be counted (i.e., included) in determining income of a Medicaid applicant, the income must be available to the individual; that is, within his/her possession or control or obtainable with reasonable effort. Medicaid applicants and recipients are required to take all necessary steps to obtain any annuities, pensions, retirement, disability benefits and other income to which they are entitled, unless they can show good cause for not doing so.

Countable income includes:

> one-half (½) of earned income (see (a) below) each month after deducting applicable disregards;
>
> unearned income (see (b) below), after deducting the applicable disregards; and
>
> certain in-kind income (see (c) below).

Not all of the income available to a recipient is counted in determining his/her financial eligibility for Medicaid assistance. SSI states must deduct (disregard) from income any amounts that would be deducted in determining financial eligibility under SSI. Some 209(b) states use the SSI methodology as well. These deductions are known as SSI disregards, and include:

> The first $20 per month of unearned income. Only one $20 disregard is permitted per couple.

> A certified blind or certified disabled child living with parents is entitled to a separate $20 disregard from his/her total unearned income.

> If a person's unearned income is under $20, the balance will be deducted from earned income.

> The first $65 of earned income.

> One-half of the remaining earned income.

> Infrequently or irregularly received income up to $20 of unearned income per month, and $10 of earned income per month.

The three types of countable income are described below:

> (a) **Earned Income**. This is income received as a result of working, including, but not limited to, wages, salaries, tips, commissions, and bonuses. It also includes income from self-employment or a small business. Some of the allowable business expenses that may be deducted to arrive at net income from self-employment or a small business include: rental of quarters and equipment; salaries and fringe benefits of employees; and cost of goods for resale.

> (b) **Unearned Income**. This is income that is not received as compensation for work performed. It includes, but is not limited to: Social Security retirement or disability payments; inheritances and spouse's right to the new elective share; pensions, annuities, dividends, interest; insurance compensation; income from roomers, boarders and lodgers; and other sources classified as unearned income for the purpose of determining SSI eligibility.

Unearned income also includes income from rental property. This type of income, after allowable business expenses are deducted, is considered available unearned income. The following business expenses illustrate examples of expenses that should be deducted to arrive at net income from this source:

Property, school, water and sewer taxes;

The cost of utilities if they are included in the rent; and

Interest payments on mortgages for the property (but not payments on the principal of the mortgage).

(c) **In-kind Income.** This is income received in goods or services rather than in money. Generally, contributions of goods and services from a third party to support a Medicaid recipient are not counted as income provided the third party's contribution(s) go directly to the vendor or service provider. Payment for a recipient's food, shelter and medical bills are examples of in-kind support, which a third party can pay to a vendor or service provider for a Medicaid recipient, and is not countable income. Contributions from a legally responsible person (e.g., a parent) to a Medicaid recipient of food, shelter or clothing in certain states may constitute countable income, not however to exceed one-third (⅓) of such contributions. Contributions other than food, shelter or clothing are not countable income. New York does not include Medicaid in-kind payments of any sort as countable income.

2. **Countable Resources**

(a) Countable resources comprise property of all kinds, real or personal, tangible or intangible, including: (i) cash on hand, stocks and bonds, certificates of deposit, mutual fund shares, bank accounts (including joint accounts), pension funds, retirement funds, and insurance; (ii) real property (other than a homestead); and (iii) deemed property whether in a spouse's sole name or the joint name of both spouses.

Countable resources also include:

Entrance Fee for a Continuing Care Retirement Community. The entrance fee for a continuing care retirement community (CCRC) is considered an available resource to the individual residing in the CCRC to the extent that: (i) the individual is able to use the entrance fee; (ii) the contract allows the entrance fee to be used to pay for the individual's care if her income or other resources are insufficient; and (iii) the individual is eligible for a refund of the remainder of the entrance fee on the individual's death or termination of the contract and departure from the CCRC, and the fee does not grant an ownership interest in the CCRC.

If a nursing facility is part of a CCRC, pursuant to the CCRC admission agreement, residents may be required to spend their resources (that are declared for purposes of admission) on their care before applying for Medicaid.

Home Value in Excess of Certain Amounts. The family home is no longer an unqualifiedly exempt asset. Home equity in excess of $500,000 (an amount a state may elect to increase to $750,000) is treated as an available resource. The $500,000 amount (or other amount set by the state) is increased every year, starting in 2011, based on the Consumer Price Index and rounded to the nearest $1,000. The foregoing provision of this subparagraph, does not apply if the individual's spouse or child (under age 21 or disabled) resides in the home. The individual may use a home equity loan or reverse mortgage to reduce the equity. These provisions may be waived by the state in cases of demonstrated hardship.

(b)   Exempt resources are not counted as available resources to a Medicaid applicant or recipient in determining financial eligibility if they are any one of the following exempt (i.e., excluded) resources:

> Home (including the land), subject to a home valued in excess of certain amounts (see preceding paragraph)
>
> Household goods
>
> Personal effects
>
> Automobile
>
> Value of any burial place
>
> A separately identifiable $1,500 burial fund set aside per individual

Life insurance policies with a face value of $1,500 or less regardless of cash surrender value.

3. **Trust Income and Resources Eligibility Rules**

   (a) **Established Trust**

For purposes of determining Medicaid eligibility, special trust rules apply to established trusts. A trust is considered to be an established trust only if: (i) assets of the grantor constitute the principal of the trust; and (ii) the trust is established, other than by will, by an individual spouse or by an entity such as a court or legal guardian acting on behalf of the individual/spouse.

The trust rules may apply differently depending upon whether an established trust is a revocable living trust or an irrevocable living trust. These two trusts are defined below.

Revocable living (*inter vivos*) trust. This is a trust created by a grantor during his/her lifetime and may be amended or revoked by the grantor at any time or at the end of a designated period.

The trust may be funded at the time of the trust's creation by the transfer of assets to it, or unfunded until the occurrence of some event.

Irrevocable living (*inter vivos*) trust. This trust is created by a grantor during his/her lifetime for the purpose of irrevocably transferring assets to another beneficiary. The grantor loses all control over the trust assets (principal) and may not amend or revoke the trust.

In the case of a revocable living trust, the entire principal is considered to be an available resource. All of the payments from the trust to or for the benefit of the grantor are considered available income.

Only if and to the extent payments from the trust can be made to or for the benefit of the grantor, the portion of the principal (or the income on the principal) from which payment to the individual can be made is considered available resources of the individual. All payments from any portion of the principal or income of the irrevocable trust, which are made from, to or for the benefit of the grantor, are considered available income of such individual.

(b)　Supplemental Needs Trust

This type of trust, also known as a special needs trust, is an irrevocable trust, funded by assets of a third party (and therefore is not an established trust), created for a disabled beneficiary, and intended to supplement government benefits. The beneficiary has no power to control distributions.

Generally, for Medicaid eligibility purposes, payments from a supplemental needs trust are governed by SSI income principles. If payments are made for food, clothing or shelter, or if payments are made directly to the beneficiary, the amounts are counted as income to the beneficiary for purposes of eligibility and will disqualify the beneficiary's Medicaid eligibility status. The more common arrangement with supplemental needs trusts, which will not disqualify the beneficiary's Medicaid eligibility, is for the trustee to make direct payments to vendors of services or goods that are not food, clothing or shelter; such payments are not considered income to the beneficiary.

(c)　Third-Party Grantor Trust

This trust is set up by a third party for the benefit of either spouse and is considered to produce available income (and resources) for the Medicaid recipient only to the extent that funds are actually transferred to the beneficiary. The trustee's power to pay a larger amount will not cause the larger amount to be deemed as available to the beneficiary.

(d)　Trigger Trust

This trust is designed to divert from a Medicaid applicant income (or principal) that would otherwise be paid to such Medicaid applicant upon entry into a hospital or nursing home, and thereby remove payment as a disqualification for Medicaid eligibility. Standards may vary from state to state as to the validity of a trigger trust. The state of New York has, by statutory enactment, declared void any *inter vivos* trust which suspends, or diverts the payment of income (or principal) in the event the creator's spouse applies for Medicaid assistance, hospital, nursing or long-term care.

(e)　Medicaid Qualifying Trust

The Medicaid qualifying trust, contrary to its name, actually disqualifies an individual for Medicaid eligibility. Under this trust an individual or his/her spouse may be the beneficiary of all or part of the payments of principal and/or income from the trust; the trustee has discretion as to the amounts to be distributed. Even if not actually distributed, the law will consider the maximum amounts of payments which the trustee may distribute to the grantor or his/her spouse; this may disqualify the grantor and his/her spouse from Medicaid eligibility.

(f)   Exempt Trusts

Certain categories of established trusts set forth below are by statute expressly considered exempt from Medicaid income and resource eligibility rules. One trust (income-only trust) is exempt (and the assets of the trust are not considered available) by virtue of an administrative ruling.

Trust for Disabled Person under Age 65. This trust contains that person's assets and is established for his/her benefit by his/her parent, grandparent, legal guardian or a court. This trust is exempt from the Medicaid eligibility rules if it provides that the state will receive all amounts remaining in the trust upon the death of the disabled person up to the amount of Medicaid assistance provided to this person by the state.

Miller Trust. Composed of an individual's pension and/or Social Security income, this trust is exempt from Medicaid eligibility rules if the following conditions are met:

The trust is composed only of the individual's pension, Social Security or other income payable to the individual, including accumulated trust income. Neither the income transferred to this type of trust nor the right to recover the income is counted in determining the individual's eligibility for Medicaid.

The state will receive all amounts remaining in the trust upon the person's death up to the amount of Medicaid assistance provided to this person by the state.

The individual resides in a state that does not have a medically needy program for nursing facility services and that uses a special income limit for eligibility for certain long-term care services.

Such a state is called an income cap state or a three-hundred-(300%) percent state (see *section D.3*).

Should any principal be transferred to a Miller trust, this will disqualify the trust from its exempt status. A transfer to the trust of the ownership rights to a stream of income (e.g., Social Security benefits) constitutes a transfer of a resource and will also cause the trust to lose its exempt status.

Pooled Trust. Established for a disabled individual, regardless of age, this trust contains the assets of that individual. If it meets the following conditions, a pooled trust is exempt from Medicaid eligibility rules:

The trust is established and managed by a non-profit association.

Each trust beneficiary has a separate account, but the trust pools these accounts for investment and management of the funds.

These accounts are established solely for the disabled individual's benefit by the individual, the individual's parent, grandparent, legal guardian or a court.

Any amounts remaining in the trust after the beneficiary's death and not retained by it are paid over to the state up to an amount equal to the total amount of Medicaid services provided to the beneficiary.

Income-only Trust. This is an irrevocable trust established by an individual which provides that income only from the trust shall be paid to the grantor for life, but excludes distribution of the trust principal to the grantor. CMS has interpreted the trust Medicaid eligibility rules to preclude the counting of such trust's principal as available to the grantor since it cannot under any circumstances be distributed to, or for the benefit of, the grantor or his/her spouse.

Undue Hardship. The state Medicaid agency must establish procedures, in accordance with standards specified by the Secretary of HHS, whereby the state waives the application of the trust eligibility rules in cases where the individual establishes that these rules will cause undue hardship if applied to him or her.

4.   **Income and Resource Eligibility Rules for Couples**

(a)   **Deeming of Income and Resources of Spouses**

Medicaid rules impose upon married couples the financial responsibility to provide for one another. (This legal duty is severed only when the income or resources of one spouse are made unavailable to the other spouse.) The available income and non-exempt income resources of the Medicaid applicant's spouse, and the available income and non-exempt resources of the other spouse are pooled together and counted as available to the other spouse in calculating the applicant's financial eligibility for Medicaid. This is known as the rule of deeming. This rule is one of the significant determinants of a person's Medicaid financial eligibility. It applies only to a married couple living together in the community.

Deeming ceases upon the occurrence of events set forth below:

When a Couple Stops Living Together Other Than for Reason of Institutionalization (e.g., divorce). The couple's income and resources are counted as available to each other, for the month the couple ceases living together, and for the ensuing six- (6) month period.

Thereafter, deeming ceases, and each of the previously married spouses is treated as a single individual.

When a Married Couple Stops Living Together upon Institutionalization of One of Them. When one spouse is institutionalized (i.e., likely to be in a medical institution or nursing home for at least thirty (30) days) and applies for Medicaid, that individual (applicant spouse) is known as an institutionalized spouse. The person married to the institutionalized spouse who remains in the community is known as the community spouse.

Deeming will also cease when one spouse (applicant) (i) resides in the community, (ii) needs Medicaid community services and home care services, all of which are non-waivered services, and

(iii) the non-applicant spouse submits a written letter to Medicaid (spousal refusal letter) that he/she is unable or unwilling to contribute financial support to the applicant spouse. The applicant will be considered as a single individual, and Medicaid will base its eligibility determination for the non-waivered services solely on the income and resources of the applicant.

(b)   **Protection of Community Spouse Against Impoverishment**

Medicaid restricts the amount of income and assets a Medicaid applicant is allowed to retain after institutionalization. Otherwise, this could lead to the impoverishment of the community spouse.

Consequently, states are required to permit an institutionalized individual (or at states' option, an individual who is a recipient of waivered home health benefits), who is married and receives Medicaid assistance, to contribute to his/her spouse, remaining in the community in order to bring that community spouse's income, up to a minimum monthly income allowance and resources up to a minimum resource allowance. In addition, the community spouse is assured a family allowance (for family dependents living with the community spouse) and an excess shelter allowance.

Medicaid will make an assessment of resources of a couple at the request of either the community spouse or the applicant and may do so at any time of the institutionalization of the applicant. The colloquial term "snapshot rule" refers to the act of assessing such resources, for the purposes of Medicaid eligibility, at the beginning of a period of institutionalization of one member of the couple. A snapshot of the couple's resources is taken when one begins a nursing home stay expected to last a period of thirty (30) days or more (continuous period of institutionalization), regardless of whether an application is made at that time. The non-exempt resources of the couple are pooled as of the snapshot day.

Following the assessment, Medicaid will determine the eligibility amount for the community spouse minimum monthly income allowance, excess shelter allowance, and family allowance based on the following factors:

States are required to adopt the community spouse minimum monthly income allowance (basic allowance) for the community spouse which is equal to 150% of the then Federal poverty level for a two- (2) person family (even though the community spouse is only one person). This amounts to a minimum monthly income allowance of $1,838 (2012). The allowance is adjusted annually for inflation. The community spouse maximum monthly income allowance is $2,841 (2012). States are required to calculate and provide an excess shelter allowance where the costs (e.g., rent, mortgage, taxes, maintenance charges on a condo, insurance and utilities) of maintaining the principal residence exceeds thirty (30%) percent of the applicable percentage of the poverty level. The excess shelter allowance will be added to the basic allowance.

In addition, states are required to provide a family allowance (see 4(e) below).

There is a cap of $2,841 (2012) as adjusted for inflation, on the total of the basic allowance and the excess shelter allowance.

In lieu of the allowance computed with the above two components (the basic allowance and the excess shelter allowance), a state may elect a flat monthly maintenance allowance. (California and New York have, for example, made this election.) This allowance is subject to a cap of $2,841 (2012) indexed for inflation.

If the community spouse resource allowance is insufficient to generate the statutory minimum monthly income allowance, then the community spouse may resort to a fair hearing to increase his/her resource allowance to make up the income deficiency. However, the community spouse may not resort to the fair hearing process to increase his/her resource allowance unless prior thereto the institutionalized spouse has first made available to the community spouse, out of his/her income, an amount sufficient to make up the deficiency. (This is referred to as the income-first rule.)

In addition, the amount allowed for the community spouse whether consisting of the basic allowance plus excess shelter allowance, or the flat monthly maintenance allowance, is subject to increase by an award of a higher figure at a fair hearing based upon "exceptional circumstances resulting in significant financial duress requiring the provision of additional income."

(c)   Maximum and Minimum Community Spouse Resource Allowance – Spousal Share

Medicaid, in determining the eligibility of an institutionalized person with a spouse in the community, provides that the community spouse must be allowed to retain resources (spousal share) equal to one-half of the couple's assessed total countable resources, but not less than the minimum community spouse resource allowance and not more than the maximum community spouse resource allowance permitted under Federal law. The maximum community spouse resource allowance under Federal law is $113,640 (2012); and the minimum community spouse resource allowance is $22,728 (2012). Each figure is subject to adjustment for inflation. A state may establish a dollar amount which is both the minimum and maximum amount.

The spousal share is determined by the spouse as of the beginning of the most recent continuous period of institutionalization of the institutionalized spouse. Continuous period of institutionalization means at least thirty (30) consecutive days of institutional care in a medical institution and/or nursing facility, or receipt of home and community-based waiver services, or a combination of institutional and home and community-based waiver services. Absence from a medical institution/facility or discontinuance of home and community-based waiver services or the Program of All-inclusive Care for the Elderly (PACE) services for thirty (30) consecutive days is the criteria used to determine if a continuous period of institutionalization has been broken.

When the first month of the most recent continuous period of institutionalization is prior to the month for which Medicaid coverage is sought, use of the spousal share figure will require social services districts to complete two assessments of a couple's resources. The first assessment will determine the total countable resources of the couple for purposes of establishing the spousal share. This assessment must be based on the resources of the couple as of the beginning of the most recent continuous period of institutionalization. The second assessment will determine the total countable resources of the couple for the month Medicaid coverage is sought. The spousal share amount, as determined by the first assessment, is used in the second assessment to determine the community spouse resource allowance and the Medicaid eligibility of the institutionalized spouse.

When the community spouse's spousal share is less than the minimum community spouse resources allowance, the institutionalized spouse is required to transfer to the community spouse an amount sufficient to increase the latter's resources up to the spousal share. This transfer to the sole name of the community spouse should be made within ninety (90) days of the initial eligibility determination in order to protect the spousal allowance from further consideration as an available resource. Resources not shifted by the deadline will be considered available resources for the institutionalized spouse.

(d)   **Spousal Refusal**

As noted above, the minimum community spouse resource allowance is $22,728 (2012), and the maximum community spouse resource allowance is $113,640 (2012). If the spousal share (i.e., one-half of the combined countable resources of both spouses) exceeds $22,728 (2012), the community spouse is allowed to retain resources in an amount equal to the spousal share but not to exceed $113,640 (2012). If, in fact, the community spouse has resources in excess of the spousal share, the excess is considered to be available to the institutionalized spouse, and the community spouse is required to contribute the excess amount to the cost of care of the institutionalized spouse. If the community spouse should fail or refuse to contribute these excess resources, the refusal is termed spousal refusal. In case of a spousal refusal, the resources of the community spouse will no longer be considered available to the institutionalized spouse, and the latter can still receive Medicaid:

> if the institutionalized spouse assigns to his/her state rights to support from the community spouse;
>
> if the institutionalized spouse lacks the ability to execute an assignment due to physical or mental impairment, but the state has the right to bring a support proceeding against the community spouse; or,
>
> if denial of eligibility would work an undue hardship.

(e)   **Permitted Deductions**

The Medicaid statute requires that all of the income of the institutionalized spouse, after permitted deductions, be applied to the cost of institutional care. These permitted deductions are set forth below:

The community spouse's minimum monthly income allowance. Personal needs allowance, an amount of at least $30 per month) (see *(f) below*).

Family allowance for each family member (who is residing with the community spouse and who has over fifty (50%) percent of his/her maintenance needs met by the community spouse and/or the institutionalized spouse), – an amount equal to at least one-third of the amount by which the minimum monthly needs allowance (not including the excess shelter allowance) exceeds the amount of the monthly income of a family member.

Amounts for incurred expenses for medical or remedial care for the institutionalized spouse.

States may deduct an amount for the maintenance of the home of the institutionalized spouse for six (6) months or less if a physician certifies that the individual is likely to return home within that period.

(f)   **Personal Needs Allowance (PNA)**

This is an amount of money required to be set aside for an institutionalized individual receiving nursing facility services in order to pay for personal needs such as clothing, reading material, stationery, and snacks not required to be provided by the facility, and activities not required to be provided by the facility. At a minimum, the allowance must be $30 per month. States can (and twenty-six (26) states have elected to) increase the personal needs allowance above the minimum.

The PNA also applies (except as to amount) to an institutionalized spouse living in the community who is receiving either a waiver service or participating in the Program of All-inclusive Care for the Elderly (PACE). The PNA amount for persons who meet the definition of an institutionalized spouse residing in the community (and who are receiving community waiver services or are participating in the PACE program) is higher than the $30 PNA that institutionalized residents are allowed to retain. The PNA amount for these waiver recipients PACE participants is $350 (2010).

D.   CATEGORIES OF ELIGIBILITY

This is one of the four eligibility factors.

There are three (3) significant categories of SSI and Medicaid eligibles: categorically needy, optional categorically needy, and medically needy. (Also, there are miscellaneous categories of eligibility set forth in (d) below.)

1.   Categorically Needy

All states must provide Medicaid coverage to persons who are in the categorically needy group. An individual, otherwise Medicaid eligible, who satisfies the SSI financial eligibility standards of a state's Medicaid program, historically is considered to be Medicaid eligible as categorically needy. More specifically, the classification describes individuals who satisfy the categorical requirements of being age 65 or over or are blind or disabled, and in addition satisfy a state's Medicaid financial eligibility requirements of having assets or income below state-determined levels.

In most states an individual who receives SSI is automatically considered to be within this group. A person who is categorically needy is not allowed to spend down.

2.   Medically Needy

The medically needy group is optional to states. Thirty-seven (37) states and the District of Columbia have this category. It is for persons who meet the non-financial status requirements (age, disability) for categorical assistance, but whose income and/or resources are over the categorical needy levels. Unlike the categorically needy or optional categorically needy, a medically needy person has the right to reduce his/her income to below state-prescribed levels through the deduction of incurred medical expenses, a process commonly referred to as spending down.

Medically needy programs will not necessarily provide to a "spendowner" all requisite medical assistance. A state with a medically needy program may elect to provide nursing home facilities or not. In those states whose programs do provide nursing home facilities to the medically needy, the expenses that may be deducted from countable income and resources are both the medical and nursing home expenses of an individual. In those states whose programs do not provide nursing home facilities, individuals cannot spend down to become nursing home eligible – i.e., there is no spend down for the incurred or paid medical expenses in order to obtain eligibility for nursing home care.

3. Optional Categorically Needy

Some states, referred to income cap states, do not have a medically needy program serving nursing facility residents. In these states individuals are not allowed to spend down to the SSI income level to become eligible for Medicaid-covered nursing home care. Income cap states avail themselves of an optional Medicaid program termed the optional categorically needy program under which individuals are provided limited nursing facility coverage. Under the program individuals qualify for Medicaid nursing home coverage if their countable income does not exceed a cap of a prescribed percentage, usually three-hundred (300%) percent, of the SSI benefit for one person; the three-hundred- (300%) percent cap is an absolute dollar cap. It is categorically fixed and severe: one dollar of excess income above the cap will disqualify the individual. An individual is not permitted to spend down for medical expenses, nor can he/she forego collection of a pension, Social Security benefits or interest income in order to fall within the income cap. The income cap states are Alabama, Alaska, Colorado, Delaware, Idaho, Mississippi, Nevada, New Mexico, Ohio, South Dakota and Wyoming.

A possible method for reducing the income of an individual seeking to qualify under the optional categorically needy program, also commonly referred to as the three-hundred- (300%) percent program, is to obtain from a state court a qualified domestic relations order which allocates pension payments to the community spouse. The community spouse as the payee arguably is the beneficiary of the pension, and payments to him/her would constitute his/her income under the name-on-the-check rule, not income of the institutionalized spouse who was the original pensioner.

Another method of qualifying for the optional categorically needy program is available under the provisions of Consolidated Omnibus Budget Reconciliation Act (COBRA) of 1993. With this law Congress allowed individuals in income cap states to become eligible for Medicaid nursing home assistance by putting their income (e.g., pension, Social Security benefits) into a so-called Miller trust. During the Medicaid recipient's lifetime, all but a small portion of the money in the trust must go toward paying the nursing home bill. If any money remains in the trust after the recipient's death, it must be paid to the state, up to the amount of Medicaid assistance that was rendered.

4. Miscellaneous Classifications of Eligibility

Federal laws mandate eligibility must be extended to individuals who are within certain other special classifications. Certain of these classifications (see below) have been created to correct for some statutory entitlement or benefit increase which caused persons in that group, who were Medicaid eligible, to lose their Medicaid eligibility.

Individuals Covered by the Pickle Amendment. The Social Security Act was amended to deal with the inadvertent consequences of the automatic cost-of-living increase granted by Congress. These increases caused some people to lose Medicaid coverage because the increased income brought them over the SSI level. At the urging of Representative Pickle, Congress passed a provision designed to alleviate this unintentional problem caused by the cost-of-living increases.

The Pickle amendment mandates that cost-of-living increases are not to be considered in determining Medicaid eligibility. Any individual who would be eligible for Medicaid as categorically needy but for the cost of living is eligible for Medicaid.

COBRA Widows (Widowers). The Social Security Act was amended to provide disabled widows or widowers with increased disability benefits. As a result of these increases, many within this group lost their Medicaid coverage because the increased income brought them over the SSI level.

The Consolidation Omnibus Budget Reconciliation Act of 1985 extended protection of these individuals by allowing entitlement to Medicaid benefits for the categorically needy, which they otherwise would have had, but for the increase of their disability benefits.

Kennelly Widows (Widowers). This group consists of elderly widows and widowers who lost their SSI as a result of their entitlement to "early" widows' benefits. These widows, age 60 or over, but not yet 65 and, therefore, not yet eligible for Medicaid benefits, are by statute, considered to be Medicaid eligible as categorically needy, as if they did not receive these additional benefits.

Low-income Medicare Beneficiaries. Medicaid will pay certain Medicare benefits (deductibles, copayments, coinsurance, and/or premiums) for low-income Medicare beneficiaries, as set forth below:

Qualified Medicare Beneficiary (QMB). Federal law requires state Medicaid programs to "buy in" Medicare coverage for certain low-income Medicare beneficiaries. The buy-in consists of payment of deductibles and coinsurance costs under Medicare Part A and Part B, payment of premiums under Part B, and payment of premiums under Part A for those not entitled to Part A by virtue of receiving Social Security benefits. These beneficiaries are known as qualified Medicare beneficiaries.

QMBs must:

meet federally prescribed income and resource standards. Individuals must have incomes below one-hundred (100%) percent of the Federal poverty level, and their non-exempt resources cannot exceed twice the SSI resource standard ($4,000 for an individual and $6,000 for a family of two).

be entitled to Part A hospitalization. If they otherwise would be eligible for QMB benefits but are not automatically eligible to Medicare Part A, the state must pay their Part A premiums to make them eligible for Part A.

A subset of QMBs is known as dual eligibles. They are individuals whose income is below one-hundred (100%) percent of the Federal poverty level and have low assets and are eligible for full coverage under both Medicare and Medicaid. They are exempt from mandatory enrollment in Medicaid managed care. Virtually all individuals receiving Medicaid or age 65 and over are entitled to Medicare Part B at least. State Medicaid programs pay the Medicare Part B premiums for dual eligibles, and they should also pay Medicare Part A premiums for those not entitled to Part A by virtue of receiving Social Security retirement benefits. All dual eligibles are QMBs, but not all QMBs are dually eligible. They are entitled to the full spectrum of both Medicaid and Medicare benefits.

Specified Low-income Medicare Beneficiary (SLMB). An individual entitled to Medicare Part A benefits whose income is between one-hundred (100%) percent and one-hundred twenty (120%) percent of Federal poverty guidelines and whose non-exempt resources are $4,000 or less ($6,000 in the case of a couple) is eligible to have Medicaid pay his/her Medicare Part B premium. This individual is referred to as a SLMB within the qualified Medicare beneficiary program. The SLMB program is managed by the state agency that provides medical assistance under Medicaid.

Low-income Qualified Individual (QI). An individual is selected by the state as a qualified individual (QI). QIs meet the QMB criteria, except that their income level is at least one-hundred twenty (120%) percent but less than one-hundred thirty-five (135%) percent of the Federal poverty level for a family of the size involved and their non-exempt resources are $4,000 or less ($6,000 in the case of a couple). The state is required to pay the full amount of the Medicare Part B premiums of a QI (but only for premiums payable during a statutorily prescribed period). However, the individual cannot be otherwise eligible for medical assistance under the approved state Medicaid plan.

Qualified Disabled and Working Individuals. State Medicaid programs must pay only Medicare Part A premiums, but not other Medicaid services, for individuals whose income is below two-hundred (200%) percent of the Federal poverty level; who are entitled to Medicare on the basis of disability; who are in a trial work period and are entitled to continue Medicare coverage while they are in that work period; whose non-exempt resources do not exceed twice SSI resource levels ($4,000 for individuals plus $1,500 for burial expenses, and $6,000 plus $3,000 for burial expenses in the case of couples); and who are not otherwise eligible for Medicaid.

III.   SERVICES COVERED BY MEDICAID.

(See also *section IV.*)

Medicaid will pay for a wide range of medical and related assistance consisting of specific services (list of Medicaid services) plus "any other medical care, and any other type of remedial care recognized under state law" that may be specified by the Secretary of HHS.

The services which are available depend on the state where one resides and the category (e.g., medically needy) of an individual's eligibility. Certain of these services (mandated services) are required to be provided by all states; other services (optional services) are optional to the states.

A.   Mandated Services.

Federal law requires that all states provide the categorically needy and optional categorically needy recipient at least the following mandated services:

> inpatient hospital services;
>
> outpatient hospital services;
>
> laboratory and x-ray services;
>
> nursing facility services for people over age 21;
>
> early and periodic screening, diagnosis and treatment for people under age 21;
>
> family planning services and supplies for individuals of child-bearing age;
>
> physicians' services and some dental services;
>
> midwife services;
>
> home health care services; and,
>
> psychiatric care on an inpatient and outpatient basis.

Of the foregoing services, nursing facility services and home health care services are most commonly associated with Medicaid long-term care. Nursing facility services are provided in institutional settings to individuals requiring skilled nursing or rehabilitative care or other health-related services above the level of room and board.

1. Home Health Care Services

Medicaid must provide home health care services to the categorically needy and optional categorically needy recipients who are entitled to nursing facility placement, and to medically needy individuals living in a state that has opted to provide skilled nursing services. These services include:

> nursing services provided on a part-time or intermittent basis from a home health agency;
>
> home health aide services, provided by a certified home health agency;
>
> medical supplies and equipment; and
>
> physical and occupational therapy, speech-language pathology and audiology services, provided by a home health agency.

The first three items are required components of home health care services under a state Medicaid plan. (The therapy and other services listed in the last item are optional to the state under a Medicaid state plan.) Providing private daily nursing, optional to states, is not characterized by CMS as a home health service.

2. Conditions to Obtaining Home Health Care Services

Unlike Medicare, Medicaid does not necessarily require that patients be homebound, or that they need skilled nursing services or therapy, as a condition to obtaining home health care. A Medicaid beneficiary must satisfy the following conditions to obtain home health care:

> The individual must be eligible for Medicaid coverage of nursing facility services under the state plan.
>
> Home health services must be provided in the recipient's home, which does not include hospitals, skilled nursing facilities or intermediate care facilities.
>
> The services must be prescribed by the client's physician and provided by a certified home health agency.
>
> The services must be provided under a written plan, reviewed every sixty (60) days by a physician.

While Medicaid statutorily does not have part-time or intermittent nurse limitations or definitions, as does Medicare, Medicaid regulations adopt the Medicare statutory limitations and definitions on nursing. These nursing services are available on a part-time or intermittent basis. This restriction does not appear to apply to home health aide services.

State law may impose practical limits on the number of hours of home health care.

A person who requires home care costing nearly as much as, or more than, Medicaid nursing facility care may be required to be institutionalized, to participate in a long-term care program (such as the Lombardi program in New York), or to be provided other more cost-effective services. Refusal to do so may result in denial of Medicaid benefits.

The eligibility of a recipient who receives home health services does not depend upon his/her need for or discharge from institutional care.

B. Optional Services

1. Medically Oriented Services

The following medically oriented services are optionally available to the states:

medical or remedial care recognized under state law, furnished by licensed practitioners (e.g., chiropractor, optometrists, podiatrists);

private duty nursing services;

clinic services;

dental services;

physical therapy and related services;

prescribed drugs, dentures, prosthetic devices, and prescribed eyeglasses;

other diagnostic screening preventive, and rehabilitation services;

inpatient hospital, skilled nursing facility (SNF), and intermediate care facility (ICF) services for individuals age 65 or over in an institution for tuberculosis or mental diseases;

ICF services;

inpatient psychiatric facility services for persons under age 21;

hospice care;

case management services;

respiratory care services;

services furnished by a certified pediatric nurse practitioner or certified family nurse practitioner;

home and community care for functionally disabled elderly individuals; and,

community-supported living arrangement services.

2. Non-Medically Oriented Services.

States have the option of providing a variety of non-medically oriented services: personal care and other services under a Medicaid waiver program.

(a) Personal Care (see also *section V*). Personal care provided by Medicaid comprises some or total assistance with personal hygiene, dressing, feeding, nutritional and environment support functions and health related tasks. Personal care services do not necessarily have to be in support of a skilled service.

The following basic requirements must be met:

The services must be according to a physician's written plan of care (or at the state's option, in accordance with a service plan approved by the state) and may not be provided by a family member.

Under existing CMS regulations, the services need not be supervised by a registered nurse.

The services must be provided at home, or at a state's option in another location. Accompaniment to work, school or for shopping or other appointments is permissible, however. Medicaid coverage of personal care is not available to an individual who is an inpatient at a hospital facility, nursing facility, intermediate care facility for the mentally retarded or an institution for mental diseases.

The services must be medically necessary as determined by the physician.

The client's health and safety must be able to be maintained in the home.

Personal care services include:

basic personal care and grooming, including bathing, hair care, and assistance with clothing;

assisting with bladder and bowel requirements, including helping the patient to the bathroom or with a bed pan;

assisting with medications that are ordinarily self-administered;

assisting with food, nutrition, and diet, including preparing meals, if incidental to a medical need; and,

performing household services if related to a medical need and essential to the patient's health and comfort at home.

The personal care services must be essential to the maintenance of the recipient's health. Essential household and chore services may be considered an integral but subordinate part of personal services. The word "integral" means services directly related to the patient's medical condition or services reflected in the physician's plan of treatment and furnished in conjunction with direct patient care. Household and chore services are subordinate so long as they count for no more than one-third of the total time expended by the personal care worker.

(b)   Medicaid Waivered Services. Federal law requires states to provide certain prescribed services for Medicaid-eligible persons. States may provide additional services, or, in some instances, may redesign their whole Medicaid program under a Federal waiver of certain provisions of the Medicaid

Act, including provisions requiring that recipients have free choice of provider, that services be offered statewide, that they be offered to all individuals within the eligibility category and that they be comparable to those offered to other individuals.

Under waiver programs, states can serve very small numbers of individuals, offering them a discrete package of services, or they can require whole portions of their Medicaid population to participate in managed care programs.

Through the process of obtaining from CMS a waiver of requirements that would otherwise be imposed by Federal law, states may provide Medicaid services beyond those required by Federal Medicaid regulations. The waiver programs most relevant to older and disabled individuals are those that provide services to:

individuals at risk of institutionalization in a nursing home or intermediate care facility for the mentally retarded; and

individuals age 65 or older at risk of institutionalization.

In the absence of a Federal waiver, a state Medicaid program can pay only for extremely limited home care. Waivers for home and community-based long-term care services have proven to be particularly helpful to older and disabled individuals. CMS periodically publishes a Medicaid waiver fact sheet that summarizes the waivers for home and community-based services for each state. Some of the waivered services relevant to long-term care include:

Adult day care services	Moving assistance
Case management	Nutritional/education services
Emergency response systems	Respite care
Foster care	Respiratory therapy
Home-delivered meals	Shift nursing
Home maintenance tasks	Social transportation
House improvement	

The Deficit Reduction Act of 2005 (Act) has amended the Social Security Act to expand, effective January 1, 2007, access to home and community-based services for the elderly and the disabled. These services are included as an optional benefit to those individuals, in addition to home and community-based services offered under waiver under existing sections of the Social Security Act.

Under the Act the Secretary of HHS is required to grant a waiver to provide that a state plan shall include as "medical assistance" payment for part or all of the cost of home or community-based services (other than room and board) which are provided pursuant to a written plan of care to individuals 65 years of age or older with respect to whom there has been a determination that but for the provision of such services the individuals would be likely to require the level of care provided in a skilled nursing facility or intermediate care facility, the cost of which could be reimbursed under the state plan. Such medical assistance will include (to the extent consistent with written plans of care) case management services, homemaker/home health aide services, personal care services, adult day health services, habilitation services, respite care, and such other services requested by the state as the Secretary of HHS may approve and for day treatment or other partial hospitalization services, psychosocial rehabilitation services, and clinic services (whether or not furnished in a facility) for individuals with chronic mental illness. The term "habilitation services" means services designed to assist individuals in acquiring, retaining, and improving the self-help, socialization, and adaptive skills necessary to reside successfully in home and community-based settings.

A state may provide for the provision of medical assistance for home and community-based services for individuals eligible for medical assistance under a state plan whose income does not exceed one-hundred fifty (150%) percent of the poverty line, without determining that but for the provision of such services the individuals would require the level of care provided in a hospital or a nursing facility or intermediate care facility for the mentally retarded.

In addition, under the Act a state may allow an eligible individual or the individual's representative to receive self-directed services (as defined by the new amended provision of the Social Security Act) which are planned and purchased under the direction and control of such individual or the individual's authorized representative.

IV. SALIENT CHARACTERISTICS RELATING TO MEDICAID SERVICES.

Salient factors relating to Medicaid services are set forth below:

States must cover services in sufficient amount, duration and scope to reasonably achieve their purpose. Limitations cannot be based on diagnosis, type of illness or condition.

Services provided to the categorically needy cannot be less in amount, duration and scope than those provided to the medically needy. Services must be provided statewide.

Recipients are entitled to a free choice of provider, unless the recipient is enrolled in a Medicaid managed care plan.

Providers must take Medicaid payment as payment in full, including nominal copayments, for services rendered.

Reimbursement must be sufficient to enlist enough providers to ensure that services are available to the extent they are available to the general public.

Reimbursement to institutions must be adequate to meet the costs of an efficiently and economically operated facility.

Hospitals serving a disproportionate share of low-income individuals are entitled to enhanced reimbursement, so-called disproportionate share payments.

V. APPLICATION FOR PERSONAL CARE.

Applications for personal care generally follow the procedures set forth below:

The applications based upon a physician's order will be processed by Medicaid offices, designated by the state, to review such applications.

A physician's order form will customarily provide required information including the client's medical condition and his/her need for assistance with personal care tasks. The physician or the patient must forward the completed signed form to the appropriate state office together with a Medicaid application if the patient is not yet receiving Medicaid.

Upon receipt of the physician's order, the state Medicaid agency will require a nursing assessment by a registered nurse. The nursing assessment must contain an evaluation of the functions and tasks required by the patient, the degree of assistance required for each function, and, together with the patient, the development of a plan of care. The nurse's assessment will recommend services for a designated number of days per week, and hours per day of personal care services.

Upon receipt of a personal care application, the state Medicaid agency will make a social assessment of the need for personal care services. An assigned case manager will visit the patient and then complete a social assessment form.

When personal care services will be required for more than sixty (60) continuous days, then additional assessments will be made: an assessment of other services and efficiencies to ensure that the most cost-effective services are being used in every plan of care; and a fiscal assessment.

The home health agency which is to deliver the services customarily will perform these assessments, subject to approval by a state Medicaid agency.

VI.   COPAYMENTS AND DEDUCTIBLES.

In some instances, states are permitted to charge Medicaid recipients cost-sharing, such as copayments (also called coinsurance) and deductibles, but only nominal amounts. A copayment is a percentage of the cost of a Medicaid service. A deductible is a fixed sum that a Medicaid recipient may be required to pay for services before Medicaid will pay the rest of the cost of services. These charges can be required of both medically needy and categorically needy recipients; however, states may not impose copayments for certain specified services.

VII.   APPEAL RIGHTS.

Medicaid applicants and recipients are entitled to a notice and a full evidentiary hearing to challenge any agency action to terminate, suspend or reduce Medicaid eligibility or services. If an individual is already eligible, he/she is entitled to continued assistance until the hearing.

Medicaid claimants have the right to appeal adverse decisions made by the Medicaid program. These decisions involve, among other matters, eligibility requirements; the denial, suspension or reduction of benefits; and the number of hours of homecare services. Claimants have a right to written notice about their claims and the reason for a decision. Generally, the state or local Medicaid agency must mail the notice at least ten (10) days before benefits are reduced and discontinued. This period may be shortened to five (5) days in a fraud matter. Toappeal a decision, a claimant should follow the process and procedures outlined below.

Request for a Fair Hearing.

To request a fair hearing review of a claim, a Medicaid applicant or recipient is entitled to a reasonable time, not to exceed ninety (90) days, from the mailing of the notice of the adverse decision. If a Medicaid recipient (not a new applicant) requests a fair hearing within ten (10) days of the mailing of the notice of the adverse decision, he/she has a right to receive continuing Medicaid benefits, known as aid continuing, until a decision has been reached after a fair hearing. The right to aid continuing applies to those already receiving Medicaid benefits, not to new applicants.

Fair Hearing.

A hearing officer who has not participated in the local Medicaid agency's initial adverse decision conducts a fair hearing. The hearing officer's decision is mailed to the Medicaid claimant four (4) to six (6) weeks following the hearing.

De Novo Hearing.

Within fifteen (15) days of the mailing of the fair hearing decision, a claimant may appeal to the state Medicaid agency for a new hearing, commonly called a *de novo* hearing. If a claimant does not specifically request a *de novo* hearing but merely a general request for a new hearing, the state agency will review only the record of the local hearing, as contrasted to a hearing that includes new and independent evidence. Following the hearing, the claimant will receive a written notice of the decision within ninety (90) days from the date of the request for a hearing.

Judicial Review by a State Court.

A claimant may appeal an adverse fair hearing decision to a state court.

In addition to the formal procedures, a claimant may seek an informal review by calling or meeting with a caseworker at the Medicaid agency. The request for this type of conference review is not a fair hearing request and does not replace such a request nor extend the time limitation for seeking a hearing or a continuation of benefits. A request for an informal review customarily is and should be made together with a request of a fair hearing.

VIII.   TRANSFER PENALTY (CIVIL)

A.   General.

The following is an overview of the salient aspects of the Medicaid transfer penalty.

Medicaid imposes a civil penalty on certain transfers of assets (see *section B* below). This penalty consists of a period of ineligibility (see *section C* below).

The civil penalty is imposed when a person transfers any asset for less than fair market value (called uncompensated value of transferred assets), and applies for Medicaid assistance to pay for certain long-term care services during a period called the look-back period (see *section D* below).

Historically the look-back period was thirty-six (36) months for all transfers, except transfers into a trust were subject to a sixty- (60) month look-back period. The thirty-six- (36) month period has been extended to sixty (60) months; the extension was phased in (applying to all transfers) as follows:

Phase-in Period	Extension of Period
1993 until Jan. 30, 2009	36 months
February 1, 2009	36 + 1 = 37 months
March 1, 2009	36 + 2 = 38 months
Every month through February 1, 2011	Period extended by one month
February 1, 2010	36 + 13 = 49 months
February 1, 2011	60 months

The penalty consists of the imposition of the period of ineligibility for Medicaid assistance covering only certain designated services as defined in section E below.

The transfer penalty must be applied in cases of individuals seeking nursing home care, or its equivalent, and waivered home care services. It affects Medicaid non-waivered home care services, only if a state so elects (see *section D.2* below).

Certain asset transfers are considered to be exempt transfers and are not subject to the transfer penalty (see *section F* below).

The well-known term "Medicaid planning" is the process of a Medicaid applicant (or prospective Medicaid applicant) planning to transfer non-exempt assets for less than fair market value, out of reach of the Medicaid authorities, and without running afoul of the civil transfer penalty. The subject of the civil transfer penalty requires an understanding of a number of terms including: look-back period; period of ineligibility; designated services; institutionalized person; and, non-institutionalized person.

States will waive transfer penalties if their application would cause undue hardship.

B.   Assets.

The term "assets," as used in the context of Medicaid transfer of assets penalty rule, includes:

1.   **The income and resources of an individual or the individual's spouse** which either have been placed in a trust (see *section G* below) or have been transferred to someone else for less than fair market value.

2.   **An annuity**, unless it:

falls under IRC § 408(b) or (q); or

is purchased with the proceeds from a trust or account under IRC § 408(a)(c) or (p), a simplified employee pension, or a Roth IRA; or

is irrevocable and non-assignable, "actuarially sound" (using actuarial publications of the office of the SSA Chief Actuary), and provides payments in equal amounts during the annuity term. There can be no deferred annuity or annuity with balloon payments which pay interest, plus a relatively small amount of principal monies rather than being actuarially sound, with equal monthly payments.

The Deficit Reduction Act of 2005 (DRA) treats the purchase of an annuity as the transfer of an asset for less than fair market value unless the annuity meets the following specific requirements:

The state is either the remainder beneficiary in the first position for at least the full amount of medical assistance received by the Medicaid recipient; or

The state is listed as the beneficiary in the second position after the community spouse or disabled or minor child; and the state is named in the first position if either the spouse or the child's representative disposes of the remainder for less than fair market value.

Though annuities which meet the requirements set forth in the first part of this section will not constitute transfers of an asset for less than fair market value, they will be subject to estate recovery upon the death of the Medicaid recipient unless there is a surviving spouse or disabled or minor child or unless the annuity is sheltered because of the Medicaid recipient's participation in the Robert Wood Johnson Program.

Under the DRA, state Medicaid applications, including recertification applications, must include a description of any interest the applicant or community spouse has in an annuity or a similar financial instrument, even though the annuity is considered actuarially sound. The recertification application must include a statement that the state, by providing Medicaid, becomes the remainder beneficiary under the annuity or instrument. The state notifies the issuer of the annuity of the state's right as the preferred remainder beneficiary. The issuer may notify persons with other remainder interests of the state's interest. The state must consider that information in determining the individual's eligibility for Medicaid or the amount of the state's obligation for Medicaid.

3. **Funds used to purchase a mortgage, or for a loan or promissory note** unless the repayment term is actuarially sound, provides for payments in equal amounts during the term of the loan without deferrals or balloon payments, and prohibits the cancellation of the balance on the lender's death. For those mortgages, loans or notes that do not satisfy these requirements, the value of the mortgage, loan or a note is the outstanding balance on the date of the individual's Medicaid application.

4. **Income or resources which an individual is entitled to but does not receive** because of his/her own actions, such as a disclaimer, waiver of pension income, waiver of his inheritance, or because of the action of an entity or another person with legal authority to act in place of the individual, such as a court guardian, or attorney-in-fact. (Medicaid eligibility rules treat income and resources separately from each other.)

5.   **Funds used to purchase a life estate in another's home** unless the buyer resides in the home for at least one (1) year after the purchase.

C.   Period Of Ineligibility.

The period of ineligibility is the period stated as a number of months that an individual who has made a transfer of assets for less than fair market value within the look-back period (defined in section D below) remains ineligible for certain Medicaid services.

For an institutionalized person, the period of ineligibility equals, and for a non-institutionalized person is not greater than, the number of months calculated by dividing: (i) the total uncompensated value of all assets an individual disposed of during the look-back period by (ii) a patient's average cost of nursing facility care per month.

The period of ineligibility begins:

in the case of transfer of assets made before the date of enactment (the "enactment date") of the Deficit Reduction Act of 2005 (DRA), the commencement date is the first day of the first month during or after the assets have been transferred for less than fair market value and which does not occur during any other period of ineligibility; or

in the case of transfer of assets made on or after the enactment date of the DRA, the commencement date is (i) the first day of the month during or after which assets have been transferred for less than fair market value or (ii) the date on which the individual is eligible for medical assistance under the date plan and would otherwise be receiving institutional level care (e.g., nursing home facility services), but for the application of the penalty period, whichever is later and which does not occur during any other period of ineligibility.

D.   Look-back Period.

The term look-back period refers to a number of months prior to the Medicaid application for which the Medicaid agency will ask the applicant to account for any transfers of assets, including transfers for less than fair market value. Federal law applies a sixty- (60) month look-back period. States must use the federally designated look-back period.

The commencement date of the look-back period in the case of an institutionalized person is the date the individual is deemed both an institutionalized person and an applicant for state Medicaid assistance. In the case of a non-institutionalized person, the commencement date is the date that the individual applies for state Medicaid aid, or, if later, the date that the individual disposes of assets for less than fair market value.

When multiple transfers are made during the look-back period, they are treated as follows:

> For multiple transfers during the look-back period when assets have been transferred in amounts or in frequency that would make the calculated periods overlap, the transfers must be added together and then divided by the average monthly payment for nursing facilities within a state, or, at the option of the state, within a designated region of the state. The total amount transferred will be treated as if it was all transferred over on the first day of the month following the month in which the first transfer is made; or

> When multiple transfers are made in such a way that the penalties for each do not overlap, each transfer is treated as a separate event, with its own penalty period.

E. TRANSFER PENALTY NOT APPLICABLE TO ALL MEDICAID SERVICES

The transfer penalty rule does not apply to all Medicaid services, only to the following designated services: (i) nursing home services, (ii) waivered services (under a Federal waiver that a state requested of the Federal government), and (iii) at the option of a state, home health care. Thus, in New York State, for example, the transfer penalty rule does not apply to home health services. In New York, a Medicaid applicant who is not institutionalized and who is eligible for home health care is entitled to obtain non-waivered services (such as nurses and home health aides) and may make transfers of his/her assets, irrespective of the amount of the transfers, without any concern for the transfer penalty rules which do not apply to the non-waivered services.

The designated services affected by the transfer penalty rules differ in the case of institutionalized and non-institutionalized person:

1. **For institutionalized individuals** designated services include the following:

>Nursing home services;

>A level of care in any institution equivalent to that of nursing facility services such as skilled nursing or custodial care in a hospital while awaiting transfer to a nursing home; and

>Home or community-based care authorized under the waiver program (waivered services).

2. **For all non-institutionalized persons**, only in the case where the state has elected to apply the transfer penalty rules to such persons, will the following designated services be covered and affected by the transfer penalty rules:

>Home health care;

>Any other type of remedial care recognized under state law specified by the Secretary of HHS; or

>Community-supported living arrangements related to services to assist disabled individuals, as statutorily defined, in activities of daily living to permit them to live in their own home, apartment, family home or rental unit furnished in a community-supported living setting. Services include personal assistance, training, twenty-four- (24) hour emergency response system.

F. TRANSFERS EXEMPT FROM PENALTY RULES

A number of transfers are exempt from the civil penalty rule:

>Transfers made outside the statutory look-back period, that is, more than sixty (60) months prior to Medicaid application. Since such transfers are made outside the statutory look-back period, they do not result in any imposition of a period of ineligibility.

>Transfers by homebound individuals applying for or receiving non-waivered Medicaid services in states which have opted not to

apply Medicaid transfer penalties to non-waivered services. A transfer will not make such individuals ineligible for receipt of the non-waivered services. That is, such a transfer will not result, under civil transfer penalty rules, in a denial of reimbursement from Medicaid for non-waivered services.

Transfers for fair market value or where the individual intended to receive fair market value.

Transfers exclusively for a purpose other than qualifying for Medicaid eligibility.

Transfers to child under age 21 or to a child of any age who is blind or disabled as defined by SSI, or to a trust established for that child's benefit.

Transfers to or from an individual's spouse or to a third party for the sole benefit of the individual's spouse, as well as transfers from the individual spouse to the other spouse for the sole benefit of the spouse.

Transfers of an individual's home, if transferred to:

> the individual's spouse;

> the individual's child who is under age 21, or who is blind or disabled;

> the sibling of an individual who had an equity in the home and resided in it for one year prior to the individual's institutionalization;

> an individual's child (other than a child who is under age 21, blind or disabled) who resided in the home at least two (2) years prior to the individual's institutionalization and who provided services to the individual that delayed institutionalization.

Transfers to a trust for a disabled person under age 65 of that person's assets, established for his/her benefit by the person's parent, grandparent, legal guardian or court. Upon the death of the disabled person, any funds remaining in the trust must be used to repay the state for the person's Medicaid assistance. (see *Section G* below) – these trusts are called "pay-back trusts."

Transfers where the transferred assets have been returned.

and,

Transfers where the state determines that a penalty would result in undue hardship. The facility where the institutionalized individual resides may file an undue hardship waiver for her and with her consent or the consent of her personal representative. While the undue hardship waiver application is pending, if the application meets criteria specified by Secretary of HHS, the state may pay the facility for thirty (30) days of care in order to hold the bed for the resident.

G. TRUST TRANSFER PENALTY RULES

As itemized and set forth below, the transfer penalty rules impose a penalty upon certain, but not all, transfers of assets into and from certain kinds of trusts. The transfer penalty rules apply to, and impose a penalty on, transfers to and from an irrevocable trust, pooled trust and income-only trust. The rules do not apply to (i) revocable trusts, (ii) trusts for the disabled under age 65, or (iii) Miller trusts, each of which is considered an exempt trust as discussed below.

Revocable Trust. The principal of this trust is not subject to the transfer of assets rules. This is also true for the establishment of a revocable trust. Moreover, payments from the trust are subject to transfer rules and penalties only to the extent payments are made to or for the benefit of someone other than the individual applying for or receiving Medicaid.

Irrevocable Trust. Transfers of assets into an irrevocable trust are penalized if the assets cannot be paid to the individual Medicaid applicant. Any portion of the assets which could be paid to or used for the benefit of the individual creating the trust is outside the purview of the penalty rules. Payments from this trust are penalized if they are not paid to or for the benefit of the individual whose assets established the trust but are paid to or for the other individuals' benefit.

Trusts for the Disabled. Transfer rules expressly exempt from coverage transfers to trusts established for a disabled child and to a trust established for disabled individuals under age 65. Any funds remaining in the trust must be used to repay the state for the person's Medicaid assistance.

Miller Trust. The transfer of income into this trust will not be penalized if and to the extent that the trust instrument provides that such income will be used to pay for medical care provided to the individual. The transfer of any income not used (e.g., income which exceeds the amount paid for these medical services) will be penalized.

Pooled Trust. This trust is not exempt from the transfer of assets rules. However, a transfer to a pooled trust is exempt if the transfer is made by a disabled person under age 65 at the time the trust is established.

Income-only Trust. The value of the trust principal will be treated, for transfer penalty purposes, as a transfer of assets for less than fair market value, and therefore is subject to transfer penalty.

IX.   TRANSFER PENALTY (CRIMINAL).

The Balanced Budget Act of 1997 (Act) makes it a Federal crime for an individual for a fee to knowingly and willfully counsel or assist another individual to dispose of the latter's assets so that such individual can become eligible for Medicaid. More specifically, the Act provides: "whoever for a fee knowingly and willfully counsels or assists an individual to dispose of assets (including by any transfer in trust) in order for an individual to become eligible for medical assistance under a state plan under Title XIX if disposing of the assets results in the imposition of a period of ineligibility for such assistance shall be guilty of a misdemeanor and upon conviction thereof fined not more than one year or both." This provision is directed solely to the individual who counsels and advises, and not to the person who is so advised. The constitutionality of the above provisions of the Act has been successfully challenged in lower Federal courts. The office of U.S. Attorney General (then, Honorable Janet Reno) has stated that the Department of Justice will not take any steps to enforce the Act's provision. (A future Attorney General could determine to enforce the Act.)

Only transfers that result in the imposition of a period of ineligibility for Medicaid assistance are made criminal; those specifically protected by existing law from penalty are not.

Although clarification is still required, it appears likely that certain other transfers would not be considered by the Act to be criminal transfers:

Transfers made outside the statutory look-back period that is more than sixty (60) months prior to application for Medicaid. Since such transfers are made outside the statutory look-back period, they do not result in any imposition of a period of ineligibility.

Transfers for which a period of ineligibility, less than the look-back period, has run out by the time of application for Medicaid assistance. The new law is less clear about these transfers. The only assured protection from criminal prosecution is to avoid applying for benefits during the look-back period.

Transfers by homebound individuals applying for or receiving non-waivered Medicaid services in states which have opted not to apply Medicaid transfer penalties to non-waivered services. A transfer will not make such individuals ineligible for receipt of the non-waivered services. That is, such a transfer will not result under civil transfer penalty rules, in a denial of reimbursement from Medicaid for non-waivered services. The absence of the imposition of a period of ineligibility suggests such transfer should not be subject to criminal penalties.

As mentioned, the penalty provisions of the Act state that the crime covered by it is a misdemeanor punishable by a fine up to $10,000 or one year in prison, or both. According to the felony portion of the Act, "any person(s) furnishing...items or services...under a program [is] guilty of a felony and upon conviction thereof are fined not more than $25,000 or imprisoned for not more than five (5) years, and/or both." This appears to apply only to the providers of services for Medicare or Medicaid recipients and not to the recipients or persons advising them.

X. RECOVERY BY MEDICAID.

A. Liens On Real Property Of Medicaid Recipient.

State Medicaid programs are authorized, but not required, to place liens on property of Medicaid recipients in two limited circumstances:

> For benefits incorrectly paid, pursuant to a judgment from a court; and

> On real property for a permanently institutionalized individual when the state has determined, after an opportunity for a hearing, that the individual cannot be reasonably expected to return home.

Liens cannot be imposed on homesteads if any of the following persons are lawfully residing in the institutionalized individual's home:

> His/her spouse; his/her child who is under age 21, blind or disabled or;

> A sibling as long as he/she has an equity interest in the home and has resided there for at least one year prior to the institutionalized individual's entry into a nursing facility.

No liens can be placed on a life estate of a Medicaid recipient. Medicaid does not consider a life estate as a countable resource.

B.   Medicaid Recovery From Community Spouse.

When a community spouse has excess resources over and above the community spouse's resource allowance and the community spouse refuses (spousal refusal) to turn over his/her resources available to meet the Medicaid recipient's needs, states may and are likely to seek recovery of costs expended on the Medicaid recipient's care.

(continued on next page)

MEDICAID MANDATORY MANAGED CARE

INTRODUCTION

The Balanced Budget Act of 1997 amended the Social Security Act with the addition of Section 1932, titled Provisions Relating to Managed Care. This authorizes states to require individuals eligible for Medicaid medical assistance, subject to some exceptions noted below, to enroll in a managed care entity. Managed care entity refers to either a Medicaid managed care organization, or primary care case manager. These latter two terms are defined in section VIII below. In a managed care entity, a primary care physician coordinates and approves an array of services in addition to providing primary care services. Usually, physicians are paid case management fees in addition to their regular fee-for-service payments for the primary care services they provide.

The salient topics of Medicaid mandatory managed care are discussed below.

I. EXEMPTIONS FROM MANDATORY ENROLLMENT.

Children under age 19 with special needs (e.g., children receiving foster care) and dual eligible individuals are exempt from mandatory enrollment but may voluntarily enroll.

II. FREEDOM OF CHOICE.

A state must give individuals a choice of at least two managed care entities or primary care case managers. In rural areas, eligible individuals must be permitted to: receive such assistance through no fewer than two (2) physicians or case managers to the extent that they are available to provide such assistance in the area; and obtain Medicaid medical assistance from any other provider under appropriate circumstances as set forth by CMS regulations.

III.   GUARANTEED ELIGIBILITY.

Individuals enrolled with a Medicaid managed care organization or a primary care case manager are guaranteed Medicaid eligibility for six (6) months from the date of enrollment.

IV.   TERMINATION AND CHANGE OF ENROLLMENT.

An individual must be permitted to terminate or change enrollment at any time for cause and may do so without cause during the ninety- (90) day period beginning on the day he/she receives notice of enrollment and at least once annually thereafter.   States must establish notice of termination requirements as well as a method for determining enrollment priorities in the event a managed care organization does not have the capacity to enroll all individuals seeking enrollment.

The state must establish a default enrollment process for enrolling any person who does not choose a managed care organization during a state's specified enrollment period.   This process must provide for enrollment in a managed care organization that maintains existing provider-individual relationships or has contracted with providers that have traditionally served Medicaid recipients.

V.   PROVISION OF INFORMATION.

Each state or managed care organization must provide all enrollment notices and other information in easily understood form.   Upon request, each Medicaid managed care organization must make available to enrollees and potential enrollees information concerning providers, enrollees' responsibilities and rights, grievance and appeals procedures, and information on covered items and services.

A state requiring enrollment in a managed care organization must annually provide Medicaid recipients a list identifying available managed care organizations, their benefits, cost sharing, service area, quality and performance.

VI.   EMERGENCY SERVICES.

Each Medicaid managed care organization or primary care case manager must provide coverage for emergency services without regard to prior authorization or the emergency care provider's contractual relationship with the organization or manager. Emergency services are inpatient and outpatient medical services that are rendered by a provider qualified to furnish them and that are needed to evaluate or stabilize an emergency medical condition.

An emergency medical condition manifests itself by acute symptoms of sufficient severity, including severe pain, such that a lay person can reasonably expect the absence of immediate medical attention to seriously jeopardize the health of an individual, or in the case of a pregnant woman, the health of the woman or her unborn child; or result in serious impairment to bodily functions or serious dysfunction of any bodily organ or part.

VII. ENROLLEE-PROVIDER COMMUNICATIONS.

A Medicaid managed care organization may not prohibit or otherwise restrict a health professional from advising the enrollee who is a patient of that professional about the enrollee's health status or the medical care and treatment of his/her condition(s), regardless of whether benefits for such care or treatment are provided under the organization's contract.

VIII. DEFINITIONS.

A. Medicaid Managed Care Organization.

The entities considered a Medicaid managed care organization are:

a health maintenance organization;

an eligible organization with a contract under Section 1876 of the Social Security Act;

a Medicare Advantage organization with a contract under Part C of Title XVIII of Medicare;

a provider-sponsored organization; or

any other public or private organization that meets the requirements of Section 1902(w) of the Social Security Act.

B. Primary Care Case Management.

One type of arrangement under which Medicaid provides managed care is called primary care case management (PCCM). Under PCCM arrangements, a primary care physician coordinates and approves an array of services in addition to providing primary care services. In most PCCM systems, physicians are paid case management fees in addition to their regular fee-for-service payments for the primary care services they provide. In a few PCCM systems, physicians are placed at financial risk for some services, usually ambulatory care. They may determine the level of their Medicaid caseloads, up to a state-specified limit.

Medicaid Planning

The well-known term Medicaid planning is the process of a Medicaid applicant (or prospective Medicaid applicant) planning to transfer non-exempt assets for less than fair market value, out of reach of the Medicaid authorities, and without running afoul of the civil transfer penalty.

Medicaid-qualifying Trust

A trust under which an individual or his/her spouse may be the beneficiary of all or part of the payments of principal and/or income from the trust; the trustee has discretion as to the amounts to be distributed. Even if not actually distributed, the law considers the maximum amounts of payments which the trustee may distribute to the grantor or his/her spouse as available income to the grantor or his/her spouse. This may disqualify the grantor and his/her spouse from Medicaid eligibility. The term applies to trusts established before August 1993, the effective date of the Omnibus Budget Reconciliation Act of 1993.

Medicaid Waivers
(See also *2176 waivers/Medicaid; Section 1115 demonstration waivers/Medicaid; Section 1915 program waivers/Medicaid;* and *Waivered services/Medicaid.*)

Federal law requires states to provide certain prescribed services for Medicaid-eligible persons. States may provide additional services, or, in some instances, may redesign their whole Medicaid program under a Federal waiver of certain provisions of the Medicaid Act, including provisions requiring that recipients have free choice of provider, that services be offered statewide, that they be offered to all individuals within the eligibility category and that they be comparable to those offered to other individuals. Thus, under waiver programs, states can serve very small numbers of individuals, offering them a discrete package of services, or they can require whole portions of their Medicaid population to participate in managed care programs.

The waiver process allows states to apply to CMS for permission to provide home care to persons who would otherwise be institutionalized. Home care services provided under waivers include home-delivered meals, home maintenance tasks and respite care. In addition, specified personal care services may be provided through a personal care option granted to states.

Medical Benefit Notice/Medicare

In the case of services covered by Medicare Part A, the fiscal intermediary will make payment directly to the provider (e.g., hospital), and then forward to the patient a medical benefit notice which explains the action taken by the intermediary.

Medical Expense Exclusion

If an individual pays for another person's medical expenses, these payments are excluded from (that is, not subject to) gift tax, provided the payment is made directly to the facility or person providing the service.

Medical Expense Tax Deduction

Expenses paid by a taxpayer for medical care for himself/herself, his/her spouse and dependents constitute itemized deductions for Federal income tax purposes. This deduction is available for all unreimbursed medical expenses, in excess of seven and one-half (7.5%) percent of adjusted gross income.

The term "medical care" as defined in the Internal Revenue Code includes expenses paid for:

> The diagnosis, cure, mitigation, treatment or prevention of disease;
>
> The purpose of affecting any structure or function of the body;
>
> Transportation primarily for and essential to medical care;
>
> Insurance covering medical care; and
>
> Qualified long-term care services (defined in the *Dictionary*[+] under a separate entry).

Under the Internal Revenue Code, a dependent in general includes a parent and/or child of the taxpayer, as long as the taxpayer provides over one-half of the dependent's support.

Medical Hospital Social Worker

A social worker, with a master's or higher degree in social work, who suggests resources such as home health agencies and nursing homes and generally assists patients and their families. Discharge planning in hospitals is an important area of practice for medical social workers.

Medical Necessity Exclusion/Medicare

See also *Exclusions/Medicare; Reasonable and necessary/Medicare.*

Medicare applies a general exclusion from coverage of services if they are not reasonable and necessary for the treatment of illness or injury. This is commonly referred to as the medical necessity exclusion. Medical necessity determinations are made by a wide array of agencies including Medicare carriers and intermediaries, and hospitals, either directly or through their utilization review committee.

Medical Necessity Trigger/LTCI

To collect benefits under a LTCI policy with a medical necessity trigger, a person must obtain certification from a doctor that institutional or home care is required to treat that person's health condition(s). Depending on the policy, certification may have to be repeated at intervals, and the insurance company's own doctor or utilization review staff may be given some power to review the medical necessity or continued medical necessity of the insured person's treatment. Some newer policies do not require a medical necessity trigger.

*Medical Nutrition Therapy/Medicare

Medicare may cover medical nutrition therapy and certain related services if you have diabetes or kidney disease, or you have had a kidney transplant in the last 36 months, and your doctor refers you for the service. Starting January 1, 2011, you pay nothing for these services if the doctor accepts assignment

*Medical Savings Account (MSA) Plans/Medicare

A plan that combines a high deductible health plan with a bank account. Medicare deposits money into the account (usually less than the deductible). You can use the money to pay for your health care services during the year.

Medical Savings Account (MSA)

See also *Medicare Advantage/Medical Savings Account.*

In the private sector a medical savings account operates in the following manner. An employer enables an employee to obtain and pay for a high-deductible catastrophic health insurance policy by paying a fixed premium for the policy to the insurance company. The insured employee might share this cost. The difference between what the employer would customarily pay for traditional health coverage, and the premium for catastrophic health insurance coverage, is placed into the employee's medical savings account (MSA) solely to pay for the qualified medical expenses of the employee, his/her spouse, and dependents.

In 1996, Congress enacted the Health Insurance Portability and Accountability Act of 1996 (HIPAA), established a four-year experimental MSA program (HIPAA MSA), effective January 1, 1997 (and has since extended the program periodically), allowing a maximum of 750,000 individuals in businesses with fifty (50) or fewer employees as well as self-employed and uninsured individuals who are covered by a high-deductible health plan, and no other plan except for certain permitted insurance, to create an MSA limited to making distributions for qualified medical expenses. These expenses are defined as amounts paid by an MSA account holder for his/her medical care or that of his/her spouse and/or dependents, but only to the extent such amounts are not compensated by insurance other than long-term care insurance, continuation insurance (COBRA) coverage, or coverage while the individual is receiving unemployment. The salient features of the MSA program are below:

Tax Treatment

HIPAA MSA account holders and their MSAs receive the following tax treatment:

> An individual covered under a high-deductible health plan – defined as a plan with a minimum annual deductible of $2,050 (2011) and a maximum deductible of $3,050 (2011) – can deduct from his/her adjusted gross income for Federal income tax purposes a defined percentage of the annual deductible paid into that individual's MSA. The defined percentage is up to sixty-five (65%) percent of the deductible or seventy-five (75%) percent for plans with a spouse or dependents.

> Interest on MSA balances accumulates tax free.

> Withdrawals from the MSA for qualified medical expenses of the account holder, his/her spouse or dependents are allowed as a tax deduction.

Penalties are imposed on withdrawals from the MSA, except for qualified medical expenses or unless made after age 65, death or disability.

Eligibility for Tax Benefits

To be eligible for the tax benefits, the person for whom the medical expenses are incurred under a high-deductible health plan must have no other health plan in effect except for the following specified types of insurance coverage:

Liabilities incurred under workers' compensation law;

Tort liabilities;

Liabilities relating to ownership or use of property or such other similar liabilities as the Secretary of HHS may specify by regulation;

Insurance for a specified disease or illness; and

Insurance paying a fixed amount per day (or other period) of hospitalization.

Medicare is not one of the allowable insurance coverages. Therefore, Medicare beneficiaries are not eligible to participate in the HIPAA MSA project.

Note: Congress, in 2003, enacted the Medicare Prescription Drug Improvement and Modernization Act, establishing the Health Savings Account as a substitute for the private MSA.

For the benefit of Medicare beneficiaries, the Balanced Budget Act of 1997 created the Medicare Advantage MSA plan (originally called Medicare+ Choice). The plan employs the traditional MSA feature of a high-deductible catastrophic health policy, a public sector variant of the private MSA (discussed above).

Medical Savings Program/Medicare/Medicaid
See *Buy-in programs/Medicare/Medicaid.*

Medical Social Services/Medicare

See also *Dependent home health care services/Medicare.*

Medical social services are one of the five (5) Medicare dependent home health care services which Medicare covers under certain conditions. Medical social services represent counseling services necessary to resolve social or emotional problems. When these problems are, or are expected to be, an impediment to the effective treatment of a beneficiary's medical condition or his/her rate of recovery, Medicare will cover them. An example might be a family member engaging in abusive or neglectful behavior toward the beneficiary. Services must be provided by or under the supervision of a qualified medical social worker. The service also includes assessment of financial resources. Medical social services must be ordered by a physician, be under the direction of a physician and included in a plan of care.

Medical Supplies/Medicare

See *Dependent home health care services/Medicare.*

One of the five (5) Medicare dependent home health care services, medical supplies are covered by Medicare if they are essential to the home health care treatment of a beneficiary. There are two (2) types of supplies:

Routine. These supplies are customarily used during the course of most home care visits by home health agency staff and are not designated for a specific patient (for example, swabs, thermometers and masks). The cost for such supplies is included in the cost per visit of the home health care service.

Non-routine. These supplies must be specifically ordered by a physician for use in treating a specific patient. The charge for these supplies is separate from the per visit cost of a home health agency. Included in non-routine supplies are catheters, syringes and sterile dressings.

Drugs and biologicals are not considered medical supplies and are not covered by Medicare for outpatient or home care treatment.

*Medically Necessary/Medicare

Services or supplies that are needed for the diagnosis or treatment of your medical condition and meet accepted standards of medical practice.

Medically Necessary/Medicaid

The basic standard of measure of whether a particular service must be provided to a particular individual. Generally speaking, Medicaid programs must provide, within the scope of the services they offer, all medically necessary services to eligible individuals.

Medically Necessary/Medicare

See *Reasonable and necessary/Medicare*.

Medically Needy/Medicaid

See also *Medicaid, section II.D.2; Income cap states/Medicaid*.

The medically needy group is one of the three categories of Medicaid eligibility. The medically needy program is optional to states. Medically needy individuals may have too much income, or in some instances the resources qualify under the other two categories of eligibility: mandatory or optionally needy. This option permits them to spend down to the income and, in some instances, resource limits prescribed by a state for Medicaid eligibility by deducting from their income incurred medical expenses.

The following states and the District of Columbia have medically needy programs: California, Connecticut, Georgia, Hawaii, Illinois, Kansas, Kentucky, Maine, Maryland, Massachusetts, Michigan, Minnesota, Montana, Nebraska, New Hampshire, New Jersey, New York, North Carolina, North Dakota, Pennsylvania, Rhode Island, Tennessee, Utah, Vermont, Virginia, Washington, West Virginia and Wisconsin. A second group of states – Arizona, Arkansas, Florida, Iowa, Louisiana (subject to the availability of state funds for those above the income cap), Oklahoma and Oregon plus Texas which does not cover the elderly – have medically needy programs but do not permit nursing home expenses to be counted in calculating the spend-down expenses.

Medically Oriented Home Care

Medically oriented home care, usually referred to as "home health care," is often needed following an acute medical episode (for example, a heart attack) and is provided under doctor's orders, according to a doctor's plan of care. Home health care is skilled care that includes the following:

Part-time skilled nursing care;

Physical and occupational therapy and speech language pathology; or

Hospice care for the terminally ill.

*Medicare (CMS Handbook)

Medicare Benefits (Part A and B) Obtained Automatically by Some Eligibles

In most cases, if you're already getting benefits from Social Security or the Railroad Retirement Board (RRB), you will automatically get Part A and Part B starting the first day of the month you turn 65. If your birthday is on the first day of the month, Part A and Part B will start on the first day of the prior month.

If you're under 65 and disabled, you automatically get Part A and Part B after you get disability benefits from Social Security or certain disability benefits from the RRB for 24 months.

You will get your red, white and blue Medicare card in the mail 3 months before your 65th birthday or your 25th month of disability. If you don't want Part B, follow the instructions that come with the card, and send the card back. If you keep the card, you keep Part B and will pay Part B premiums.

If you live in Puerto Rico and you get benefits from Social Security or the RRB, you will automatically get Part A. If you want Part B, you will need to sign up for it. Contact your local Social Security office or RRB for more information.

If you have ALS (Amyotrophic Lateral Sclerosis, also called Lou Gehrig's disease), you automatically get Part A and Part B the month your disability benefits begin.

Maximum Medicare Benefit (Part A, Part B) Only Obtained by Application

If you aren't getting Social Security or RRB benefits (for instance, because you're still working) and you want Part A and Part B, you will need to sign up (even if you're eligible to get Part A premium-free). If you're not eligible for premium-free

Part A, you can buy Part A and Part B. You should contact Social Security 3 months before you turn 65. If you worked for a railroad, contact the RRB to sign up.

If you have End-Stage Renal Disease (ESRD), you should visit your local Social Security office, or call Social Security at 1-800-772-1213 to sign up for Part A and Part B. TTY users should call 1-800-325-0778.

Medicare Enrollment Periods

You can sign up when you're first eligible for Part B. (For example, if you're eligible for Part B when you turn 65, this is a 7-month period that begins 3 months before the month you turn 65, includes the month you turn 65, and ends 3 months after the month you turn 65.)

If you enroll in Part B during the first three months of your Initial Enrollment Period, your coverage start date will depend on your birthday:

If your birthday isn't on the first day of the month, your Part B coverage starts the first day of your birthday month.

If your birthday is on the first day of the month, your coverage will start the first day of the prior month.

If you enroll in Part B the month you turn 65 or during the last 3 months of your Initial Enrollment Period, your Part B start date will be delayed. For example, Mrs. Simpson turns 65 in July. When her coverage starts depends on the month she enrolls.

General Enrollment Period

If you didn't sign up for Part A and/or Part B (for which you pay monthly premiums) when you were first eligible, you can sign up between January 1 – March 31 each year. Your coverage will begin July 1. You may have to pay a higher premium for late enrollment.

Special Enrollment Period

If you didn't sign up for Part A and/or Part B (for which you pay monthly premiums) when you were first eligible because you're covered under a group health plan based on current employment, you can sign up for Part A and/or Part B as follows:

Any time that you or your spouse (or family member if you're disabled) are working, and you're covered by a group health plan through the employer or union based on that work.

During the 8-month period that begins the month after the employment ends or the group health plan coverage ends, whichever happens first.

5-Star Special Enrollment Period

Medicare uses information from member satisfaction surveys, plans, and health care providers to give overall performance star ratings to plans. A plan can get a rating between one to five stars. A 5-star rating is considered excellent. These ratings help you compare plans based on quality and performance.

You can switch to a 5-star Medicare Advantage Plan at any time during the year. The overall plan star ratings are available at www.medicare.gov/find-a-plan. You can only join a 5-star Medicare Advantage Plan if one is available in your area. You can only use this special enrollment period to switch to a 5-star plan one time each year. You can't use this period to join a Medicare cost plan.

Medicare, Part A Premium

You usually don't pay a monthly premium for Part A coverage if you or your spouse paid Medicare taxes while working.

If you aren't eligible for premium-free Part A, you may be able to buy Part A if you meet one of the following conditions:

You're 65 or older, and you're entitled to (or enrolling in) Part B and meet the citizenship and residency requirements.

You're under 65, disabled, and your premium-free Part A coverage ended because you returned to work. (If you're under 65 and disabled, you can continue to get premium-free Part A for up to 8.5 years after you return to work.)

Medicare Part B Premium

You pay the Part B premium each month. Most people will pay the standard premium amount. However, if your modified adjusted gross income as reported on your IRS tax, return from 2 years ago (the most recent tax return information provided to Social Security by the IRS) is above a certain amount, you may pay more.

Your modified adjusted gross income is your adjusted gross income plus your tax exempt interest income. Each year, Social Security will notify you if you have to pay more than the standard premium. Whether you pay the standard premium or a higher premium can change each year depending on your income.

What Does Part A (Hospital Insurance) Cover?

Part A helps cover the following:

> *Inpatient care in hospitals*
>
> *Inpatient care in a skilled nursing facility (not custodial or long-term care)*
>
> *Hospice care services*
>
> *Home health care services*
>
> *Inpatient care in a Religious Nonmedical Health Care Institution*

Medicare Part A Covered Services

> *Blood*
>
> *Home Health Services*
>
> *Hospice Care*
>
> *Hospital Stays (Inpatient)*
>
> *Religious Nonmedical Health Care Institution (Inpatient Care)*
>
> *Skilled Nursing Facility Care*

Medicare Part B (Medical Insurance) Service Coverage

Part B helps cover medically-necessary services like doctors' services and tests, outpatient care, home health services, durable medical equipment, and other medical services. Part B also covers some preventive services. Look at your Medicare card to find out if you have Part B.

Below is a list of common Part B-covered services. Medicare may cover some services and tests more often than the timeframes listed if needed to diagnose a condition:

> *Abdominal Aortic Aneurysm Screening*

336

Ambulance Services

Ambulatory Surgical Centers

Blood

Bone Mass Measurement (Bone Density)

Cardiac Rehabilitation

Cardiovascular Screenings

Chiropractic Services (limited)

Clinical Laboratory Services

Clinical Research Studies

Colorectal Cancer Screenings

Defibrillator (Implantable Automatic)

Diabetes Screenings

Diabetes Self-Management Training

Diabetes Supplies

Doctor Services

Durable Medical Equipment (like walkers)

EKG Screening

Emergency Department Services

Eyeglasses (limited)

Federally Qualified Health Center Services

Flu Shots

Foot Exams and Treatment

Glaucoma Tests

Hearing and Balance Exams

Hepatitis B Shots

HIV Screening

Home Health Services

Kidney Dialysis Services and Supplies

Kidney Disease Education Services

Mammograms (screening)

Medical Nutrition Therapy Services

Mental Health Care (outpatient)

Non-doctor Services

Occupational Therapy

Outpatient Medical and Surgical Services and Supplies

Pap Test and Pelvic Exams (includes clinical breast exam)

Physical Exams

Physical Therapy

Pneumococcal Shot

Prescription Drugs (limited)

Prostate Cancer Screenings

Prosthetic/Orthotic Items

Pulmonary Rehabilitation

Rural Health Clinic Services

Second Surgical Opinions

Smoking Cessation (counseling to stop smoking)

Speech-Language Pathology Services

Surgical Dressing Services

Telehealth

Tests (other than lab tests)

Transplants and Immunosuppressive Drugs

Travel (health care needed when traveling outside the United States)

Urgently-Needed care

Payment for Part B-Covered Services

The charts [in the Medicare and You handbook] give general information about what you pay if you have Original Medicare and see doctors or providers who accept assignment. You will pay more for doctors or providers who don't accept assignment. **If you're in a Medicare Advantage Plan (like an HMO or PPO) or have other insurance, your costs may be different.**

Under Original Medicare, if the Part B deductible applies you must pay all costs until you meet the yearly Part B deductible before Medicare begins to pay its share. Then, after your deductible is met, you typically pay 20% of the Medicare-approved amount of the service. There is no yearly limit for what you pay out-of-pocket.

Starting January 1, 2011, you will pay nothing for most preventive services if you get the services from a doctor or other health care provider who accepts assignment. For some preventive services, you will pay nothing for the service, but you may have to pay coinsurance for the office visit when you get these services.

Medicare Part C (Medicare Advantage Plans)

*A **Medicare Advantage Plan** (like an HMO or PPO) is another Medicare health plan choice you may have as part of Medicare. Medicare Advantage Plans, sometimes called "Part C" or "MA Plans" are offered by private companies approved by Medicare. If you join a Medicare Advantage Plan, the plan will provide all of your Part A (Hospital Insurance) and Part B (Medical Insurance) coverage. In all types of Medicare Advantage Plans, you're always covered for emergency and urgent care. Medicare Advantage Plans must cover all of the* *services that Original Medicare covers except hospice care. Original Medicare covers hospice care even if you're in a Medicare Advantage Plan. Medicare Advantage Plans aren't supplemental coverage.*

Medicare Advantage Plans may offer extra coverage, such as vision, hearing, dental, and or health and wellness programs. Most include Medicare prescription drug coverage (Part D). In addition to your Part B premium, you usually pay one monthly premium for the services included. Medicare pays a fixed amount for your care every month to the companies offering Medicare Advantage Plans. These companies must follow rules set by Medicare. However, each Medicare Advantage Plan can charge different out-of-pocket costs and have different rules for how you get services (like whether you need a referral to see a specialist or if you have to go to only doctors, facilities, or suppliers, that belong to the plan for non-emergency or non-urgent care). These rules can change each year.

There are different types of Medicare Advantage Plans

Other Significant Factors of Medicare Advantage Plans

As with Original Medicare, you still have Medicare rights and protections, including the right to appeal.

Check with the plan before you get a service to find out whether they will cover the service and what your costs may be.

You must follow plan rules, like getting a referral to see a specialist to avoid higher costs if your plan requires it. Check with the plan.

You can join a Medicare Advantage Plan even if you have a pre-existing condition, except for End-Stage Renal Disease.

You can only join or leave a plan at certain times during the year.

If you go to a doctor, facility, or supplier that doesn't belong to the plan, your services may not be covered, or your costs could be higher, depending on the type of Medicare Advantage Plan. In most cases, this applies to Medicare Advantage HMOs and PPOs.

If the plan decides to stop participating in Medicare, you will have to join another Medicare health plan or return to Original Medicare.

340

You usually get prescription drug coverage (Part D) through the plan. In some types of plans that don't offer drug coverage, you can join a Medicare Prescription Drug Plan. **If you're in a Medicare Advantage Plan that includes prescription drug coverage and you join a Medicare Prescription Drug Plan, you will be disenrolled from your Medicare.** *You can't have prescription drug coverage through both a Medicare Advantage Plan and a Medicare Prescription Drug Plan.*

You don't need to buy (and can't be sold) a Medigap (Medicare Supplement Insurance) policy while you're in a Medicare Advantage Plan. It won't cover your Medicare Advantage Plan deductibles, copayment, or coinsurance.

Medicare Advantage Plans can't charge you more than Original Medicare for certain services like chemotherapy, dialysis, and skilled nursing facility care.

Medicare Advantage Plans will have an annual cap on how much you pay for Part A and Part B services during the year. This annual maximum out-of-pocket can be different between Medicare Advantage Plans. You should consider this when you choose a plan.

You can generally join a Medicare Advantage Plan if you meet these conditions:

You have Part A and Part B

You live in the service area of the plan

You don't have End-Stage Renal Disease (ESRD) (permanent kidney failure requiring dialysis or a kidney transplant).

NEW-Making changes to your coverage after December 31

Between January 1 – February 14, 2011, if you're in a Medicare Advantage Plan, you can leave your plan and switch to Original Medicare. If you switch to Original Medicare during this period, you will have until February 14 to also join a Medicare Prescription Drug Plan to add drug coverage. Your coverage will begin the first day of the month after the plan gets your enrollment form. During this period, you can't do the following:

Switch from Original Medicare to a Medicare Advantage Plan.

Switch from one Medicare Advantage Plan to another.

Switch from one Medicare Prescription Drug Plan to another.

Join, switch, or drop a Medicare Medical Savings Account Plan.

In most cases, you must stay enrolled for that calendar year starting the date your coverage begins. However, in certain situations, you may be able to join, switch, or drop a Medicare Advantage Plan at other times. Some of these situations include the following:

If you move out of your plan's service area.

If you qualify for Extra Help.

If you live in an institution (like a nursing home).

Medicare Part D (Drug Coverage) – *Medicare offers prescription drug coverage to everyone with Medicare. Even if you don't take a lot of prescriptions now, you should still consider joining a Medicare drug plan. To get Medicare prescription drug coverage, you must join a plan run by an insurance company or other private company approved by Medicare. Each plan can vary in cost and drugs covered. If you decide not to join a Medicare drug plan when you're first eligible, and you don't have other creditable prescription drug coverage, you will likely pay a late enrollment penalty.*

<u>*There are two ways to get Medicare prescription drug coverage.*</u>

Medicare Prescription Drug Plans. *These plans (sometimes called "PDPs") add drug coverage to Original Medicare, some Medicare Cost Plans, some Medicare Private Fee-for-Service (PFFS) Plans, and Medicare Medical Savings Account (MSA) Plans.*

Medicare Advantage Plans *(like an HMO or PPO) or other Medicare health plans that offer Medicare prescription drug coverage. You get all of your Part A and Part B coverage, and prescription drug coverage (Part D), through these plans. Medicare Advantage Plans with prescription drug coverage are sometimes called "MA-PDPs."*

(continued on next page)

342

MEDICARE

INTRODUCTION

Medicare was established by Congress in 1965 as Title XVIII of the Social Security Act. It is a Federal health insurance program (commonly referred to as "original" or "traditional" Medicare fee for services), wholly funded by the Federal government with no state participation. Its coverage is divided into Medicare Part A (Hospital Insurance) and Medicare Part B (Supplementary Medical Insurance). Part A basically covers the costs of acute care (i.e., short-term care following an episode of illness or accident) in hospitals, limited post-hospital care in a skilled nursing facility, hospice, and limited at-home health care. Part B is voluntary supplemental medical insurance to cover the costs of physicians' and other health professionals' services, and for a variety of outpatient hospital services and limited at-home health care. No premium is required to be paid for Part A coverage by Medicare beneficiaries. There is a monthly premium for Part B coverage, which is either billed to the beneficiary quarterly or deducted from the beneficiary's Social Security check. Medicare does not focus upon chronic care (i.e., long-term care for a condition or illness) needed to treat and manage the needs of the ill or disabled elderly at home. Medicare expressly excludes coverage of custodial care (i.e., personal care to help with bathing, dressing, use of the bathroom, and eating).

The Tax Equity and Fiscal Responsibility Act of 1982 (TEFRA) authorized as an alternative to Original Medicare, the creation of Medicare privately managed care plans (known as Risk Health Maintenance Organizations (HMOs). The word *risk*, in the term risk HMOs, referred to the contractual arrangement that the private plan had with Medicare whereby the HMO offered to receive a set amount (capitated amount) from Medicare to provide Medicare-covered services (Part A and Part B) for plan enrollees (TEFRA risk enrollees), and accepted the risk that if costs for a particular beneficiary were higher than the set amount, the plan assumed the full insurance risk for those enrollees. Medicare in the mid-1980s, with the advent of TEFRA, began offering beneficiaries (entitled to Part A benefits and enrolled in Part B), the option of enrolling in these private managed-care HMOs as an alternative to Original Medicare.

The Balanced Budget Act of 1997 ("BBA") created Medicare Part C replacing Medicare Risk Contracts with contracts under a Medicare+Choice program. The program expanded the HMOs into a variety of private managed-care plan options for Medicare beneficiaries. (These plans were originally called Medicare+Choice and are currently called Medicare Advantage.)

The Medicare Prescription Drug Improvement and Modernization Act of 2003 (MMA): (i) created Medicare Part D, establishing a voluntary prescription drug benefit program to Medicare beneficiaries entitled to Part A; (ii) authorized, among other matters, changes to the Medicare+Choice program and replaced the term Medicare+Choice (phased out in 2005-2006) by the term Medicare Advantage (MA); and (iii) expanded the array of private managed plans available to Medicare enrollees, as alternatives to Original Medicare. An individual is eligible for the Medicare prescription drug program if he or she is entitled to Medicare Part A or is enrolled in Part B. These beneficiaries are able to obtain prescription drugs with either (i) a stand-alone prescription drug program available to enrollees in Original Medicare or (ii) a Medicare Advantage plan.

The salient topics of Medicare are discussed below. The following ten (10) topics which are cross-referenced in this overview are described in detail in separate Overview entries:

> Denial Notices;
>
> Durable Medical Equipment (DME);
>
> Home Health Care;
>
> Mental Health Services;
>
> Outpatient Department Hospital Services;
>
> Outpatient Prescription Drug Program (Part D);
>
> Outpatient Skilled Therapy;
>
> Preventive Disease Management Services;
>
> Private Contracts; and
>
> Prospective Payment System

I. ADMINISTRATION.

Overall responsibility for the administration of the Original Medicare program rests with the Secretary of the Department of Health and Human Services (DHHS).

The Centers for Medicare and Medicaid Services (CMS), previously known as the Health Care Financing Administration (HCFA), a division of DHHS, directly manages and administers the Original Medicare program. Its day-to-day administration of payment of Medicare Part A and B bills is operated through private companies under contract with the Secretary of DHHS. In the case of Part A services, they are called fiscal intermediaries, and in the case of Part B services (except for homebound beneficiaries whose claim administration is through fiscal intermediaries), they are called carriers. The Medicare Prescription Drug and Improvement Modernization Act of 2003 (MMA) mandates that the Secretary of DHHS replace the fiscal intermediaries and the carriers with medical administrative contractors. The implementation of this program is scheduled for 2005-2011.

Medicare independent review entities, consisting of groups of practicing physicians and other health care experts, participate (as private contractors for DHHS) in the administration of the Medicare program. These entities are called quality improvement organizations (QIO) (formerly known as peer review organizations (PRO)). The QIO's functions consist of the following: (i) responsibility for making determinations regarding the necessity and reasonableness of health care provided by Medicare; (ii) reviewing of non-coverage notices issued by hospitals to Medicare beneficiaries changing coverage of their continued stay; (iii) evaluating the efficiency and economy of the health care services provided; (iv) ensuring that such services meet professional and accepted medical quality of care standards; and (v) reviewing the professional activities of prescription drug sponsors pursuant to contracts under Medicare Part D. In addition, the QIOs review complaints by beneficiaries relating to the quality of care in settings such as inpatient hospitals, hospital outpatient departments, hospital emergency rooms, skilled nursing facilities, home health agencies, private fee-for-service plans, and ambulatory sites. QIOs make an initial determination in hospital cases, but do not issue payments; they authorize the appropriate contractor to issue payment.

CMS has established new entities called quality independent contractors (QICs) to conduct a second level of administrative reviews (called reconsideration(s)) of Part A claim denials made by fiscal intermediaries, carriers and QIOs. The QIC's participation in the claims appeal process, commencing January 1, 2006, constitutes a replacement of the fair hearing level of appeals of Part B claims.

The MMA created the role of ombudsman as the principal point of contact with CMS for Medicare beneficiaries. The ombudsman's responsibilities include: 1) responding to complaints, grievances and inquiries concerning any aspect of the Medicare program; 2) assisting beneficiaries in collecting information needed to file appeals; 3) helping beneficiaries with enrollment and disenrollment problems; 4) assisting beneficiaries with issues related to premiums; and 5) working with the aging and disability communities to improve beneficiaries' understanding of their rights and protections within the program.

II.   ELIGIBILITY AND ENROLLMENT.

Enrollment in Part A and Part B is automatic for a Medicare-eligible person who is entitled to and receiving Social Security or Railroad Retirement benefits.

Application for retirement benefits triggers enrollment without the necessity of a separate application. All other Medicare beneficiaries are required to file an application to qualify for Medicare coverage. The eligibility criteria and enrollment process of Medicare Part A and Part B are described below. (The criteria and process are also applicable to Medicare+Choice/Medicare Advantage plans.)

A.   Part A (Hospital Insurance).

1.   Eligible Persons.

— Persons age 65 and over, entitled to receive either Social Security or Railroad Retirement benefits. Also eligible are spouses or former spouses of these persons who qualify for Social Security benefits as dependents and who have attained 65 years of age.

Note: Persons who elect retirement at age 62 are not eligible for Medicare until they turn 65. Persons who elect to postpone Social Security retirement benefits and continue working after age 65 can begin receiving Medicare benefits at age 65.

Note: Employers with twenty (20) or more employees must offer employees over 65 the option of receiving the same private health insurance package that they offer other employees in lieu of, or in addition to, receiving Medicare.

— Persons under age 65 who have received Social Security or Railroad Retirement disability benefits for twenty-four (24) months. Eligibility begins on the twenty-fifth (25th) month. Medicare benefits will continue up to ninety-three (93) months after the individual has stopped receiving disability benefits because of successfully completing a nine- (9) month trial work period.

— Transitional group of persons, not eligible for Social Security or Railroad Retirement benefits, who reached age 65 before 1968 or who became age 65 and had three (3) quarters of coverage for each year between 1967 and 1974.

— Persons under age 65 with end-stage renal disease who require dialysis or a kidney transplant (if fully insured or currently insured or if the wife or dependent child of such insured person). Most of these persons are eligible for Medicare benefits after a three- (3) month waiting period. The waiting period does not apply to transplant candidates, provided their surgery takes place before the third month or to individuals who participate in a self-care training program before the beginning of the third month.

— Persons diagnosed with Amyotrophic Lateral Sclerosis who receive either Social Security or Railroad Retirement disability benefits.

— Employees of the Federal government from 1983 on, as well as state and local government employees hired after March 1986. In each case these government employees must have the required work credits (quarters of coverage) under the Social Security program and meet several other technical requirements. Dependents and survivors of these workers are also covered.

— Voluntary enrollees who: (a) attained age 65, (b) are not eligible for either Social Security or Railroad Retirement benefits, (c) are residents of the United States, and (d) are either citizens of the United States or aliens lawfully admitted for permanent residence (who have continuously resided in the

United States for not less than five (5) years immediately before the month in which application for enrollment is made). These individuals may purchase Medicare coverage by payment of a monthly premium that CMS determines annually. In order for a voluntary enrollee to receive coverage in Medicare Part A, he/she must enroll in Medicare Part B.

2.   **Automatic Enrollment.**

Enrollment is automatic for most persons age 65 or older who are entitled to and are receiving Social Security or Railroad Retirement benefits. Application by these persons for these benefits is considered to be an application for Medicare Part A and Part B (unless they indicate they do not want Part B), and automatically triggers the enrollment process without the necessity of a separate application.

Enrollment is also automatic for a person, irrespective of age, who has been a disability patient receiving benefits under the Social Security Act or Railroad Retirement Act for twenty-four (24) months. Such patient will automatically receive his/her Medicare card for Part A and Part B benefits.

Should a person be eligible for Social Security or Railroad Retirement benefits but not be receiving those benefits, then eligibility for Medicare Part A is not automatic, and he/she must file an application.

3.   **Application for Enrollment.**

All Medicare-eligible persons who are not automatically enrolled must apply for enrollment during one of three (3) enrollment periods.

4.   **Enrollment Periods.**

There are three (3) enrollment periods – initial enrollment period, general (annual) enrollment period and special enrollment period, as set forth below:

Initial enrollment period. This is a period of seven (7) months. It begins with the third month prior to the month when the prospective enrollee reaches age 65 and continues for three (3) months after the month of his/her 65th birthday. If an individual does not file during the initial enrollment period, then he/she can file during the general enrollment period.

Enrollment during the first three (3) months of the initial enrollment period will result in coverage the first day of the month the individual attains age 65. Enrollment after the first three (3) months will cause a delay in coverage. Enrollment in the month when the beneficiary reaches age 65 will result in coverage on the first day of the second month after the applicant enrolls. If the applicant enrolls during the last three (3) months of the initial enrollment period, there may be a delay in coverage of one (1) to three (3) months.

Should a voluntary enrollee file an application after the initial enrollment period, a Part A and Part B penalty surcharge will be imposed. Should other Medicare-eligible persons file an application after the initial enrollment period, no Part A penalty will be imposed.

However, such individuals, except those qualifying for the special enrollment period (see below), will be subject to a Part B penalty surcharge.

General (annual) enrollment period. This is held during the period January 1 through March 31 of each year. Coverage begins on July 1 after the application is filed.

Special enrollment period. This period relates to working individuals age 65 or over who are covered by an employer group health plan covering 20 or more employees, whether it be their own or that of a spouse. These persons have the option to enroll in Medicare after age 65. The enrollment period begins on the first day of the month in which the person or spouse is no longer working in the employer group health plan and ends eight (8) months later. Enrollment will not result in any penalty payment of late enrollment charges.

B.   Part B (Supplemental Medical Insurance).

1.   **Eligible Persons.**

Medicare Part B is a voluntary program for eligible individuals who enroll in the program and pay a premium quarterly, or by having it deducted from their monthly Social Security check. Eligibility for Part B does not depend on Part A eligibility, although all individuals over age 65 eligible for Part A are automatically entitled to Part B. An individual age 65 or over is eligible for enrollment for Part B if he/she is either entitled to hospital insurance under Part A or is a United States resident who is either an American citizen or a permanent resident alien who has resided in the United States for the five (5) years immediately before the month of application for enrollment.

2. **Automatic Enrollment.**

Persons age 65 or older who are entitled to Social Security or Railroad Retirement benefits <u>and</u> are receiving such benefits are automatically eligible for Medicare Part B. As in the case of Medicare Part A, a separate Medicare enrollment for Part B is unnecessary.

3. **Application for Enrollment.**

If a person is eligible for but not receiving Social Security or Railroad Retirement benefits, he/she must file an application for Medicare Part B benefits. As in the case of Medicare Part A coverage, the application for Medicare Part B coverage should be filed during the initial enrollment period to maximize the entitlement benefits.

Should an individual fail to file an application during the initial enrollment period, then he/she (unless entitled to enroll during the special enrollment period) will be subject to a late enrollment charge and will not be able to enroll until the next general enrollment period (January 1 – March 31). The late penalty is ten (10%) percent added to the premium for each full year of late enrollment. Beneficiaries age 65 or older who are covered by an employer group health plan through their own employment or the employment of their spouse are entitled to a special enrollment period without incurring any late enrollment charges (see *section II.A.4, special enrollment period*). If a person enrolls for Part B benefits during the general enrollment period, coverage will not begin until July of that year.

As in the case of Medicare Part A benefits, a person age 65 or over who is a U.S. citizen or a permanent resident alien residing in the United States for at least five (5) years immediately prior to application, can purchase Medicare Part B benefits by filing an application and paying monthly premiums which CMS fixes annually.

C. **Cancellation of Medicare Coverage.**

Medicare Part A coverage will cease in the following instances:

> When a beneficiary's Medicare hospital insurance (Part A) is based on a spouse's work record, coverage will end if the

beneficiary and his/her spouse are divorced during the first ten (10) years of their marriage. If the beneficiary is covered by Part A based on his/her own work record, coverage will continue as long as he/she lives.

If the beneficiary has purchased Medicare Part A by paying monthly premiums, he/she will lose it upon cancellation of Medicare Part B or non-payment of the monthly premium.

Medicare Part B coverage will cease in the following instances:

If the beneficiary fails to make required monthly premiums.

If a beneficiary cancels Part B coverage and then later decides to re-enroll, he/she will have to wait for a general enrollment period (January 1—March 31 of each year).

III.   MEDICARE HEALTH INSURANCE CARD.

Medicare-eligible persons receive a Medicare card in the mail following an application for Medicare or in certain cases automatically. The card is red, white and blue. It shows the name of the Medicare person, his/her Medicare claim number (Social Security number), entitlement to Hospital Insurance (Part A) and/or Supplemental Medical Insurance (Part B), and the effective date of each.

If the Medicare eligible should lose or damage the Medicare health insurance card, he/she can order a new card on line at *www.socialsecurity.gov* (selecting a number from the subject list) or by calling the Social Security Administration at 1-800-772-1213. Persons who are deaf, hard of hearing or have speech impairments, can call 1-800-325-0778.

IV.   SERVICES.

A.   **Part A (Hospital Insurance).**   Part A covers four categories of services:

1.   **Inpatient Hospital Care**

1.1   *Covered Services.*   With the exception of certain deductibles and copayments explained below, Medicare Part A will pay one-hundred (100%) percent of the following inpatient hospital services (except where otherwise indicated):

— Bed and board in a semi-private room (two to four beds). Medicare will pay the cost of a private room only if it is required for medical reasons. Nursing services provided by or under the supervision of licensed nursing personnel other than services of a private duty nurse or attendant.

— Services of hospital medical social workers.

— Use of regular hospital equipment, supplies and appliances, such as oxygen tents, wheelchairs, crutches, casts, surgical dressings and splints.

— Drugs and biologicals, supplies and equipment ordinarily furnished by the hospital.

— Diagnostic or therapeutic items and services ordinarily furnished by the hospital or by others, under arrangements made with the hospital.

— Operating room costs, including hospital costs for anesthesia services.

— Services, medical and surgical, of interns and residents in training under an approved teaching program.

— Blood transfusions, after the first three (3) pints.

— X-rays and other radiology services, including radiation therapy, billed by the hospital.

— Lab tests.

— Dialysis services.

— Cost of special care units such as intensive care and coronary care units.

— Rehabilitation services such as physical therapy, occupational therapy and speech-language pathology services.

— Medicare will cover rehabilitation hospitalization in a freestanding rehabilitation hospital or in a rehabilitation unit of an acute care hospital. Such coverage is dependent upon satisfying certain requirements: The care must be reasonable and necessary and not be available in a skilled nursing facility or on an outpatient basis. The hospital must be a certified Medicare facility, and a physician must certify that the patient needs inpatient hospital care for the rehabilitation.

— Psychiatric care in a hospital. *(See Medicare/ Mental Health Services)*

Medicare Part A will help to pay up to one-hundred ninety (190) days of inpatient care in a participating psychiatric hospital. Psychiatric care provided at general hospitals is not subject to the one-hundred ninety- (190) day limit. Inpatient care in a participating psychiatric hospital is subject to the same terms and conditions, deductible and copayments as those for other Medicare inpatient hospital care.

— Ambulance transportation.

1.2 *Notices to Beneficiary.* All hospitals are required by Medicare to provide beneficiaries with two notices. The first is "An Important Message from Medicare" which sets forth the patient's rights during hospitalization. The second is the "Hospital Issued Notice of Non-coverage" (see *Notice of non-coverage/Medicare*).

1.3 *Deductibles and Coinsurance Payments.* For each benefit period or spell of illness requiring hospitalization, (i) the first sixty (60) days are fully paid by Medicare subject to the requirement that the beneficiary must pay a deductible for the first day's charges ($1,156 in 2012); (ii) for days 61-90, a coinsurance payment by the beneficiary of $289 (2012) per day is required; and (iii) for days 91-150 ("lifetime reserve days"), coinsurance payment by the beneficiary of $578 (2012) per day is required. Medicare will pay for all covered costs except the daily coinsurance required. These sixty (60) reserve days can be used by the beneficiary only once during his/her lifetime. Beneficiaries must also pay a deductible of the first three (3) pints of blood used each year, unless the beneficiary or someone else donates blood to replace blood which the beneficiary used.

1.4   *Excluded Services.* The following hospital services are not covered by Medicare:

> The medical and surgical services of a physician (coverage is under Part B).
>
> Personal convenience items such as a telephone and television;
>
> Private duty nurses or attendants unless the patient's condition requires such services and the nurse or attendant is a hospital employee; and
>
> The first three (3) pints of blood.

2.   Inpatient Care in a Skilled Nursing Facility (SNF)

A skilled nursing facility is specially staffed and equipped to provide intensive nursing and rehabilitative care to patients. Care is provided by registered and other licensed nurses or licensed therapists under the supervision of a doctor. Medicare's requirement for admission to a skilled nursing facility (SNF), the benefits covered and the period of coverage are set forth below.

2.1   *Requirements for Admission.* Subject to certain limits, Medicare Part A will help pay for a patient's care in a Medicare-participating SNF if a patient meets all of the following six (6) requirements:

> The patient's condition must require daily skilled nursing or skilled rehabilitation services which, as a practical matter, can only be provided in a SNF.
>
> The patient must have been in a hospital at least three (3) days in a row (not counting the day of discharge) before admission to a participating SNF.
>
> The patient must be admitted to the facility within a short time (generally thirty (30) days) after leaving the hospital.
>
> The patient's care in the SNF must be for a condition that was treated in the hospital or for a condition that arose while receiving care in the SNF.

A physician must certify that the patient needs and receives daily skilled nursing or skilled rehabilitation services.

The Medicare fiscal intermediary must not disapprove the patient's stay.

2.2   *Notice to the Beneficiary.*   The SNF, prior to the beneficiary's admission, will assess the beneficiary and determine whether there is Medicare coverage.   Should the SNF deny Medicare to the beneficiary, it may at the beneficiary's request admit the beneficiary and submit the beneficiary's claims to the fiscal intermediary.   The SNF makes decisions generally through its utilization review committee.   It will give written notice of its decision to the beneficiary, provide the services, and bill ("no-payment billing") the fiscal intermediary only provided that the beneficiary agrees to pay if Medicare does not pay.   The SNF will not bill the beneficiary until there is a determination by the fiscal intermediary.

2.3   *Coverage.* Medicare will provide:

— Nursing care that is provided or supervised by a registered nurse (RN).

— Bed and board in a semiprivate room or a ward, unless the patient's condition requires isolation or no semiprivate rooms or wards are available.

— Speech, physical and occupational therapy.

— Medical social services.

— Drugs, biologicals, supplies, appliances, and equipment.

— Certain medical services provided by an intern or resident-in-training.

— Certain diagnostic or therapeutic services including certain other medical and health services, respiratory therapy service that is prescribed by the doctor for the purpose of assessing, diagnosing, evaluating, treating, managing and monitoring patients who have deficiencies and abnormalities of cardiopulmonary function, and ambulance transportation that would meet the general "medical necessity" requirements of the regulations.

— Other services necessary, to the health of the patient and, generally provided by SNFs.

2.4 *Exclusions.* Medicare will not provide:

A physician's services (usually covered by Part B).

A private duty nurse or attendant.

Personal care services.

Services which generally would not be included in inpatient hospital services (e.g., personal laundry service).

Services not generally provided by SNFs (e.g., an operating room).

2.5 *Period of Coverage and Coinsurance.* Patient skilled nursing care is furnished to a patient in a skilled nursing facility up to one-hundred (100) days of each benefit period or spell of illness, depending on the patient's condition. Medicare Part A will pay one-hundred (100%) percent of covered services for the first twenty (20) days. For each day from the twenty-first (21st) to the one-hundredth (100th) day, the patient must pay a coinsurance amount of $144.50 (2012) per day, with Medicare paying the balance. (See *section V B.2*)

3. Limited Home Health Care

Medicare will help pay, in part for post-institutional medically oriented home health care of a homebound-eligible beneficiary which is provided over a limited time benefit period by a skilled nurse, therapist, or speech-language pathologist obtained through a certified home health agency. The services, previously covered under Hospital Insurance (Part A) are now in the main covered by Supplemental Medical Insurance (Part B).

4. Hospice Care

Hospice care is designed for terminally ill persons and is covered by Medicare Part A. Hospice programs will care for patients in a hospice facility or whenever possible in their homes and emphasize relieving pain and managing symptoms rather than undertaking curative procedures. An individual may elect to receive hospice care rather than regular Medicare benefits for the management of his/her illness. For routine home care, Medicare coverage is available for the level of care that is reasonable and necessary. For periods of crisis, Medicare will cover continuous home care, including nursing for up to twenty-four (24) hours per day. The beneficiary need not be homebound. During a person's lifetime, Medicare pays for up to two (2) ninety- (90) day benefit periods of hospice care following by an unlimited number of sixty (60) day periods that the individual elects to receive hospice, provided the following four (4) conditions are met:

The attending physician either in the employ of the hospice, or under contract with the hospice as an independent physician or part of an independent physicians group, and the medical director of the hospice must establish and periodically review a written plan for hospice care and at the beginning of each of the successive periods mentioned above, certify that a patient is terminally ill, i.e., that the patient's life expectancy is six (6) months or less.

The patient must elect to receive care from a hospice instead of standard Medicare medical benefits for the terminal illness. A patient may elect to revert to standard

Medicare benefits, but will then be required to pay any applicable deductibles and copayments.

Care must be provided by a Medicare-certified hospice program.

The individual must be eligible for Part A benefits.

If the foregoing four (4) conditions are met, Medicare will pay for the following services:

—   Nursing services;

—   Doctor's services;

—   Drugs, including outpatient drugs for pain relief and symptom management;

—   Physical, occupational and speech-language therapy;

—   Home health aides and homemaker services;

—   Medical social services;

— Medical supplies (including drugs and biologicals) and appliances;

— Short-term inpatient care including, procedures necessary for pain control, and acute and chronic symptom management;

— Training and counseling for the patient and family members; and any other item or service which is specified in the plan mentioned above and for which payment may otherwise by paid by Medicare;

— Prescription drugs for pain relief and symptom management, for which patients can be charged five (5%) percent of the reasonable cost, but no more than five dollars ($5) per prescription; and

— Respite care, for which a patient can be charged about five dollars ($5) per day, depending on the area of the country.

[Medicare will not cover respite care except in the case of hospice benefits. Respite care may be provided in respite care facilities, or in nursing homes, or provided by respite agencies or home care agencies or is home-visited by volunteers from a community organization.]

There is no deductible for these hospice care benefits. Copayments, however, are required for two (2) benefits: (i) Prescription drugs for pain relief and symptom management for which payments can be charged five (5%) percent of the reasonable cost, but no more than $5 per prescription; and (ii) respite care for which a patient can be charged about $5 per day, depending on the area of the country.

B. Part B (Supplemental Medical Insurance).

Part B coverage is voluntary. It covers a variety of services mostly provided on an outpatient basis including: physician services for care in and outside a hospital, durable medical equipment, medical supplies, psychiatric care, chiropractor services and outpatient hospital services. In addition, with the advent of the Balanced Budget Act of 1997, Part B covers limited home health care. Part B is financed by general revenues and monthly premiums paid by beneficiaries for

Part B coverage either billed quarterly or deducted from a beneficiary's Social Security check. Details about these services are explained below.

1.   **Covered Services**

—   Services of physicians (including diagnosis, therapy, consultations and home, office and institutional calls) surgeons, pathologists, radiologists, anesthesiologists and osteopaths, and services of certain non-physician health care practitioners which are incidental to the services of a physician.

[Before any surgery, Medicare recommends an opinion from a second doctor to help clarify the patient's decision. Medicare will help pay for both a second and, if necessary, a third opinion, if the first and second opinions contradict each other.]

—   Physicians' assistants, nurse practitioners, clinical nurse specialists, certified nurse midwives, clinical psychologists, clinical social workers, physical therapists and occupational therapists.

—   Limited home health care service. (See *Medicare/ Home Health Care*)

—   Services by chiropractors with respect to treatment of subluxation (i.e., partial dislocation) of the spine by means of manual manipulation (Medicare will not pay for any other diagnostic or therapeutic services, excluding x-ray).

—   Fees of podiatrists, including the treatment of plantar warts, but not for routine foot care.

—   The cost of diagnosis and treatment of eye and ear ailments, including treatment of aphasia.

—   Plastic surgery for repair of an accidental injury, an impaired limb or a malformed part of the body.

—   Radiological or pathological services furnished by a physician to a hospital inpatient.

— The cost of blood-clotting factors and supplies necessary for the self-administration of the clotting factors, for hemophiliac patients.

— Immunosuppressive drugs used in the first three (3) years after transplantation, plus an extension of up to eight (8) additional months.

— Outpatient physical and occupational therapy and speech-language pathology service. (See *Outpatient Occupational Therapy Physical Therapy and Speech-language Pathology/Medicare*).

— Outpatient hospital services. (See *Medicare/Outpatient Hospital Services*)

— Outpatient mental health services furnished by hospital outpatient units and qualified community health services. *(See Medicare/Outpatient Mental Health Services)*

— Radiation therapy with x-ray, radium or radioactive isotopes.

— Surgical dressings, splints, casts and other devices for reduction of fractures and dislocations.

— Rental or purchase of durable medical equipment, such as iron lungs, oxygen tents, hospital beds and wheelchairs for use in the patient's home; prosthetic devices, such as artificial heart valves or synthetic arteries, designed to replace part or all of an internal organ (but not false teeth, hearing aids or eyeglasses); braces, artificial limbs, artificial eyes. (See *Medicare/Durable Medical Equipment*)

— Ambulance service to and from the hospital, nursing home and the patient's home if the patient's condition does not permit the use of other methods of transportation.

— Certain of the costs relating to diabetes: The cost of training services (including the skills of self-administrative injection drugs) in an ambulatory setting for diabetes outpatient self-management, if recommended by a physician; a blood glucose lancet monitor and, every three (3) months, one-hundred (100) lancets plus one-hundred (100) test strips. [See M*edical nutrition therapy* under kidneys below.]

— The following costs relative to kidneys:

Kidney dialysis equipment and necessary supplies.

The cost of care for kidney donors including all reasonable preparatory, operation and post-operation recovery expenses associated with the donation, without regard to the usual Medicare deductibles, coinsurance and premium payment.

The costs of all supplies and equipment, including portable equipment, necessary to perform home dialysis.

The costs of monitoring the patient's home adaptation, visits by qualified provider or facility personnel in accordance with the plan prepared and periodically reviewed by a professional team, installation and maintenance of dialysis equipment, and testing and treatment of the water.

The costs of medical nutrition therapy services for individuals who have diabetes or kidney disease (unless on dialysis) with a physician's referral. These services are covered for three (3) years after a kidney transplant.

— Transplants. Heart transplants when performed in specialized facilities by trained personnel, and liver and lung transplants.

— The cost of a flu shot each fall, and one pneumonia shot per lifetime. Neither the annual deductible nor the twenty- (20%) percent coinsurance applies to the pneumonia shot.

— The cost of hepatitis B vaccine for high- and intermediate-risk individuals when it is administered in a hospital or renal dialysis facility.

— Screen tests, as a preventative of disease. (See *Medicare/Preventative Disease*)

— The cost of an injectable drug approved for the treatment of a bone fracture related to post-menopausal osteoporosis under the following conditions: the patient's attending physician certifies the patient is unable to learn the skills needed to self-administer, or is physically or mentally incapable of self-administering the drug; and the patient meets the requirements for Medicare coverage of home health services.

— One pair of eyeglasses following cataract surgery.

— The cost of bone mass measurements for women over age 65 who are at high risk for osteoporosis, and for beneficiaries with vertebral abnormalities and certain bone defects.

— Intravenous immune globulin (IVIG) for treatment of primary immune deficiency diseases when medically necessary.

— Diagnostic x-ray tests, diagnostic laboratory tests, and other diagnostic tests are covered by Medicare Part B and are not subject to the payment of any deductible or coinsurance. The tests must be ordered by the physician who is treating the beneficiary. The tests may be provided by an independent laboratory which must accept assignment for the test.

— Psychiatric care. (See also *Medicare/Mental Health Services.*) Medicare helps pay for services received for non-hospital treatment of mental illness. This includes services from doctors, comprehensive outpatient rehabilitation facilities, physician assistants, psychologists and clinical social workers. Services for non-hospital treatment of a mental illness are subject to a special payment rule which is explained in the Overview *Medicare/Mental Health Services.* Partial hospitalization services for treatment of mental illness are not subject to this special payment rule.

— Emergency hospital care. Hospitals are required by federal law to examine all persons seeking care in the hospital emergency room to determine whether an emergency condition exists; or, if so, the hospital must provide stabilizing treatment so that when the person is transferred from the hospital, his/her condition is not likely to deteriorate.

2. Exclusions

2.1 *General.* The two largest Medicare exclusions that may affect most people are prescription drug coverage (except as mentioned above), and long-term care (especially custodial care, in a nursing home or at home). Since most long-term care needs are custodial, Medicare therefore does not cover most long-term care.

2.2 *Express Exclusions.* Medicare expressly excludes coverage of many services:

— full-time nursing care;

— routine foot care, or orthopedic shoes;

— meals delivered to the home;

— cosmetic surgery;

— homemaker chores (e.g., general housekeeping, meal preparation, shopping) unrelated to patient care;

— custodial care;

— services that would not be covered as inpatient hospital services;

— routine physical examinations, and tests directly related to such examinations (except some Pap smears, mammograms, and prostate cancer and other specified screenings);

— eye or ear examinations (optometrists) to prescribe or fit eyeglasses or hearing aids;

— immunizations, except flu vaccinations, pneumococcal pneumonia and hepatitis B vaccinations, or immunizations required because of any injury or immediate risk of infection;

— acupuncture;

— most chiropractic services;

— dental care;

— private room, TV and radio;

— private nurses;

— services payable by workers compensation, auto insurance, employer health plan or other governmental programs; and

— services provided outside the United States.

2.3 *Reasonable and Necessary Requirement Exclusion.* Medicare excludes any services that are not reasonable and necessary for the diagnosis or treatment of illness or injury, or to improve the functioning of a malformed body organ. There are no judicial decisions interpreting this term. However, the legislative history and Medicare manuals recognize that reasonable and necessary care needs to be practical and individualized. CMS in turn has established many policies applying the general exclusion provision, frequently referred to as the medical necessity exclusion. Further, Medicare coverage decisions relating to this exclusion frequently are made on a case-by-case basis by Medicare carriers and intermediaries and by providers of health services.

V. PREMIUMS, DEDUCTIBLES, AND COPAYMENTS/ COINSURANCE.

Federal law requires hospitals that participate in Medicare and have an emergency room to examine all persons seeking care in the emergency room to determine whether they have an emergency medical condition. If staff personnel determine that an emergency condition exists, they must provide stabilizing treatment, that is requisite medical treatment so that when the person is transferred from the hospital, no deterioration of the person's condition is likely to result.

A. General.

With respect to a variety of Medicare-covered services, the Medicare beneficiary is required to pay certain payments before Medicare will make any payment. These payments are designated as deductibles and copayments, or coinsurance.

B. Deductibles and Coinsurance Payments.

1. Inpatient Hospital Care

Medicare eligibles must pay:

> the first day's deductible charge of $1,156 (2012);
>
> for days 61-90, a coinsurance payment of $289 per day (2012);
>
> for days 91-150 (lifetime reserve days), a coinsurance payment of $578 per day (2012); and
>
> for costs of first three (3) pints of blood used per year.

2. Patient Skilled Nursing Home

Medicare eligibles pay nothing for the first twenty (20) days. From the twenty-first (21st) to the one-hundredth (100th) day, the patient must pay a coinsurance amount of $144.50 (2012) per day, with Medicare paying the balance.

3. Home Health Services

There are no deductibles, copayments or coinsurance under Part A. There are deductibles for durable medical equipment under Part B.

4. Annual Part B Deductible

This deductible of $140 (2012) must be paid by Medicare eligibles enrolled in Part B.

5. Part B Coinsurance

Coinsurance equal to twenty (20%) percent of Medicare's maximum approved charges for Medicare-covered services, including durable medical equipment, must be paid by Medicare eligibles. (Special rules apply to certain mental health conditions. See the Overview *Medicare/Mental Health Services.*)

The deductibles, coinsurance and copayments represent so-called "gaps" in Medicare coverage. To fill these gaps (i.e., the difference between the amount paid by Medicare and the Medicare-approved charges), Medicare eligibles may obtain private Medigap insurance policies to protect against these areas in which the Medicare program is deficient in coverage. (See *Medicare Supplemental Insurance – Medigap*)

C.   Premiums.

1.   Part A Premiums

Individuals age 65 or older, who are entitled to Social Security retirement or Railroad Retirement benefits generally are entitled to Part A benefits without payment of premiums. (Persons not entitled to Part A benefits may be able to purchase them.)

2.   Part B and Medicare Prescription Drug Premiums

There is a standard Part B premium <u>and</u> a Medicare prescription drug premium.   In both cases Medicare beneficiaries are required to pay more, as a surcharge, on premiums, depending on beneficiaries' income. The higher income-related premium applies to beneficiaries with Federal adjusted gross income over a basic amount (the standard premium) of $85,000 per individual or $170,000 for a couple.

The basic or standard Part B premium in 2012 is $99.90.   The premium in the case of prescription drugs varies according to plan. If the income is above $85,000 (singles) or $170,000 (couples), then beneficiaries will pay a Medicare Part B surcharge (see chart on next page). Social Security will use the income reported two years ago on the beneficiary's IRS income tax return to determine his/her premium (if unavailable, SSA will use income from three years ago). SSA will then take the following steps to determine the beneficiary's Part B premium.

— determine the beneficiary's adjusted gross income and tax exempt income;

— add the adjusted gross income and tax exempt income to determine what is called modified adjusted gross income (MAGI); and

— compare the beneficiary's MAGI with the income thresholds (MAGI range) set by Medicare law.

As stated above, the premium in the case of prescription drugs varies according to plan.

The 2012 standard monthly Part B premiums <u>and</u> the prescription drug monthly premiums with surcharges are set forth in the charts below:

CHART I

If a beneficiary is single and filed an individual tax return, or married and filed a joint tax return, the following chart will apply:

Modified Adjusted Gross Income (MAGI)	Part B Monthly Premium Amount	Prescription Drug Plan Monthly Premium Amount
Individuals with a MAGI of $85,000 or less Married couples with a MAGI of $170,000 or less	**2012 Standard premium = $99.90**	**Prescription Drug Plan Premium**
Individuals with a MAGI above $85,000 up to $107,000 Married couples with a MAGI above $170,000 up to $214,000	Standard premium + $40	Prescription Drug Plan Premium + $11.60
Individuals with a MAGI above $107,000 up to $160,000 Married couples with a MAGI above $214,000 up to $320,000	Standard premium + $99.90	Prescription Drug Plan Premium + $29.90
Individuals with a MAGI above $160,000 up to $214,000 Married couples with a MAGI above $320,000 up to $428,000	Standard premium + $159.80	Prescription Drug Plan Premium + $48.10
Individuals with a MAGI above $214,000 Married couples with a MAGI above $428,000	Standard premium + $219.80	Prescription Drug Plan Premium + $66.40

(continued on next page)

CHART II

If a beneficiary is married and lived with his/her spouse at some time during the taxable year, but filed a separate tax return, the following chart will apply:

Modified Adjusted Gross Income (MAGI)	Part B Monthly Premium Amount	Prescription Drug Plan Monthly Premium Amount
Individuals with a MAGI of $85,000 or less	**2012 Standard premium = $99.90**	**Prescription Drug Plan Premium**
Individuals with a MAGI above $85,000 up to $129,000	Standard premium + $159.80	Prescription Drug Plan Premium + $48.10
Individuals with a MAGI above $129,000	Standard premium + $219.80	Prescription Drug Plan Premium + $66.40

Medicare Advantage organizations are authorized to offer a reduction in the Part B premium as an additional benefit under one or more of the Medicare Advantage plans.

D.   Low-income Beneficiaries.

Medicaid will pay certain Medicare benefits (deductibles, copayments, coinsurance, and/or premiums for low-income Medicare beneficiaries, as set forth below:

1.   Qualified Medicare Beneficiary (QMB)

Federal law requires state Medicaid programs to buy-in Medicare coverage for certain low-income Medicare beneficiaries. The buy-in consists of payment of deductibles and coinsurance costs under Medicare Part A and Part B, payment of premiums under Part B, and payment of premiums under Part A for those not entitled to Part A by virtue of receiving Social Security benefits. These beneficiaries are known as Qualified Medicare Beneficiaries (QMB).

QMBs must:

> meet federally prescribed income and resource standards. Individuals must have incomes below one-hundred (100%) percent of the Federal poverty level, and their non-exempt resources cannot exceed twice the Supplemental Security

Income resource standard ($4,000 for an individual and $6,000 for a family of two).

be entitled to Part A hospitalization. If they otherwise would be eligible for QMB benefits but are not automatically eligible to Medicare Part A, the state must pay their Part A premiums to make them eligible for Part A.

[QMBs are a subset of dual eligibles. Dual eligibles are individuals whose income is below one-hundred (100%) percent of the Federal poverty level and have low assets and are eligible for full coverage under both Medicare and Medicaid. They are exempt from mandatory enrollment in Medicaid managed care. The state Medicaid program pays the Medicare Part B premiums for dual eligibles and should also pay Medicare Part A premiums for those not entitled to Part A by virtue of receiving Social Security retirement benefits. All dual eligibles are qualified Medicare beneficiaries. They are entitled to the full spectrum of both Medicaid and Medicare benefits.]

2.   **Specified Low-income Medicare Beneficiary (SLMB)**

An individual entitled to Medicare Part A benefits whose income is between one-hundred (100%) percent and one-hundred twenty (120%) percent of Federal poverty guidelines and whose non-exempt resources are $4,000 or less ($6,000 in the case of a couple) is eligible to have Medicaid pay his/her Medicare Part B premium. This individual is referred to as a SLMB. As with the QMB program, the SLMB program is managed by the state agency that provides medical assistance under Medicaid.

3.   **Low-income Qualified Individual (QI)**

An individual is selected by the state as a qualified individual (QI). A QI is an individual who meets the QMB criteria, except that his/her income level is at least one-hundred twenty (120%) percent but less than one-hundred thirty-five (135%) percent of the Federal poverty level for a family of the size involved and his/her non-exempt resources are $4,000 or less ($6,000 in the case of a couple). (There is no resource criterion in New York State and some other states.) The state is required to pay the full amount of the Medicare Part B premiums of such a qualifying individual, but only for premiums payable during a statutorily prescribed period. However, the individual cannot be otherwise eligible for medical assistance under the state-approved plan.

4. **Qualified Disabled and Working Individual (QDWI)**

State Medicaid programs must pay Medicare Part A premiums for the individuals whose income is below two-hundred (200%) percent of the Federal poverty level who are entitled to Medicare on the basis of disability; who are in a trial work period and are entitled to continue Medicare coverage while they are in that work period; whose non-exempt resources do not exceed twice SSI resource levels ($4,000 for individuals, and $6,000 in the case of couples); and who are not otherwise eligible for Medicaid. They are not entitled to other Medicaid services.

VI. BILLING AND PAYMENT FOR PART A AND PART B SERVICES AND SUPPLIES.

A. Billing.

1. For Part A Services

A request (bill) for payment is submitted to the fiscal intermediary by an institutional provider (e.g. hospital, skilled nursing facility, home health agency, hospice); it is not necessary for a patient to submit bills to Medicare in order for payment to them to be made for services. The provider in turn may bill the beneficiary for applicable coinsurance and deductibles.

2. For Part B Services

A claim (bill) for payment may be submitted to the carrier by physicians, practitioners, medical suppliers either on their own behalf for payment to them, or on behalf of the beneficiary for payment to him/her; depending upon whether the provider has entered into a participation agreement with Medicare to accept assignment by the beneficiary or not. A provider who agrees to accept assignment is known as a participating provider.

2.1 *Where provider has accepted assignment.* The beneficiary will assign, by signing an assignment statement, his/her right to payment for services and supplies rendered [rendered and supplied] to the provider, and authorize the bill for these services to be paid by Medicare to the provider. Medicare will pay eighty (80%) percent of the Medicare approved (allowed) charges to the provider, who in turn will bill the beneficiary for the remaining twenty (20%) percent, and any unmet deductible. By accepting assignment, the provider agrees to accept the amount approved by Medicare as the full charge for the services and items rendered and supplied.

2.2 *Where provider has not accepted assignment (assignment of services).* Although payment is made to the beneficiary, the provider is responsible for handling, on the beneficiary's behalf, the paper work of claims to Medicare for payment. The provider will bill and seek payment to the beneficiary on the basis of an itemized bill. This method of billing is known as balance billing. Payment will be made by Medicare to the beneficiary for eighty (80%) percent of the Medicare-approved charge. The beneficiary is responsible for paying the bill which amount may not legally exceeds one-hundred fifteen (115%) percent of the Medicare-approved charge. This approved charge is also known as the limiting charge or actual charge. Several states by statute have prohibited balance billing, and thus in effect have mandated assignment.

B.   Payment of Bills.

      1.   **In the case of services rendered under Part A and Part B by institutional providers (hospitals, skilled nursing facilities, home health agencies, hospices),** payments are made by Medicare directly to the provider. The provider in turn may then charge the beneficiary for applicable deductibles and coinsurance payments.

      2.   **In the case of services rendered under Part B by physicians, practitioners, durable equipment suppliers,** payment may be made by Medicare to the physician or other providers only if the right to payment is assigned to them by the beneficiary, and they agree to be paid according to the rules of assignment (see *section VI.A.2.1* above).

VII. MEDICARE SUMMARY NOTICE.

After the provider of Medicare-covered services, such as a hospital, skilled nursing home or home health agency, sends a claim to a fiscal intermediary or carrier, Medicare will forward to the Medicare beneficiary a Medicare summary notice (MSN) for Part A and/or Part B services. The MSN lists all the services or supplies that were billed to Medicare for a thirty- (30) day period – the amount the provider billed, and the amount paid by Medicare to the provider for unassigned claims. The MSN, among other things, in addition, lists the Medicare-approved charges for the listed services and supplies; the amount that the beneficiary must be billed by the provider for deductibles and coinsurance; appeals information and notice that the beneficiary may request an itemized statement. The MSN may or may not state the reasons to explain a denial; it may merely state that the care provided was not reasonable and necessary.

In several geographic areas, Medicare is testing a new service: electronic Medicare summary notice (e-MSN), so that the beneficiary can examine the MSN on his/her computer and print out copies. (The e-MSN is in addition to and does not replace the MSN mailed each month.)

VIII. DENIAL NOTICES.

See *Medicare/Denial Notices*.

IX. APPEALS.

The regular appeals process for appealing claims is explained in detail in *Appeals (Standard)/Medicare Appeal*. The expedited determination procedures relating to appeals of hospital discharges and termination of services by non-hospital provider are set forth in *Appeals (Expedited) discharge of hospital patient/Medicare;* and *Appeals (Expedited) non-hospital provider services termination/Medicare.*

X. MEDICARE PRIVATE CONTRACTS (OPTING OUT OF MEDICARE).

Physicians and certain other practitioners can opt out of Medicare, and ask their Medicare patients to sign private contracts if beneficiaries want to receive these services. The providers who enter into such contracts include doctors of medicine and osteopathy, podiatrists, dentists, optometrists, clinical social workers, clinical psychiatrists, physicians' assistants, nurse practitioners, clinical nurse practitioners, clinical nurse specialists, certified nurses, nurse anesthetists and certified nurse midwives. These private contracts are treated as outside the Medicare system. As such, a physician or practitioner may not receive from Medicare, or from an organization that receives Medicare reimbursement, any payment for any item or services furnished to a patient. In other words, Medicare will not pay nor reimburse, directly or indirectly, for health services under a private contract.

Private contracts are subject to requirements which are set forth in *Medicare/Private Contracts.*

XI. MEDICARE AS SECONDARY PAYER.

When another health plan covers benefits for a plan participant who is also a Medicare beneficiary entitled to such benefits under Medicare Part A and/or Part B, Medicare considers that such other plan is the primary payer for the benefits and that Medicare is only the secondary payer in such cases. Accordingly, should Medicare make payment for the benefits that should have been made by primary payer, Medicare may obtain recovery against the primary payer. Medicare is empowered to recover payments it incorrectly made if recovery is sought within three (3) years after the rendition of the services covered by the payment. Medicare may make conditional payments under the Medicare secondary payer provisions if a primary plan such as a group health plan, or a workmen's compensation plan, has not made or cannot reasonably be expected to promptly make payment; any such payment is conditional on reimbursement to Medicare by the primary plan. The United States government may bring an action against any and all entities responsible for payment under a primary plan. When such conditional payment is made, the government may receive double damages under such circumstances.

XII. COORDINATION OF COVERAGE -- MEDICARE AND EMPLOYER PLANS.

A. Employees 65 or Older.

Employer group health plans or Medicare group health plans of employers with twenty (20) or more employees, are required to offer to Medicare eligibles age 65 or over and working spouses who are age 65 or over, the same health insurance benefit under the same conditions offered to younger workers and spouses. In such situations the beneficiary's spouse has the option to accept or reject the employer's health plan. If an employee accepts the employer's health plan, it will be the first payer of employee health claims. Medicare will become the secondary payer. If the beneficiary rejects the employer health plan, Medicare will remain the primary health insurance payer. If an employee elects Medicare to be the primary payer, the employer cannot offer coverage that supplements Medicare.

B. Medicare Retired/Eligible Employees.

Many companies provide health insurance benefits to their Medicare-eligible retirees as part of the company retirement package. In order to avoid a duplication or overlapping between benefits of a company plan and Medicare, the plans often coordinate the two sets of benefits by provision in the company plan for carve-out coverage, wrap-around coverage, coordination of benefits coverage and exclusion coverage. The several types of coordination of Medicare coverage and employer plans coverage are set forth below:

Carve-out Coverage.

The plan deducts the amount that Medicare pays for services from a scheduled amount set forth in the plan representing a charge for the same services, and the plan pays the difference.

Wrap-Around Coverage.

This is somewhat like Medigap insurance and will typically cover Medicare cost-sharing requirements and supplemental benefits, such as prescription drugs, preventive care and dental care.

Coordination of Benefits Coverage.

The plan in most cases will pay the difference between the actual charge and the Medicare-allowed charge up to an amount scheduled in the plan. The effect of this coverage is that Medicare will pay for Medicare-covered service, and to the extent that Medicare does not cover such service, it will be subject to the plan's coinsurance requirements.

Exclusion Coverage.

Medicare payments are subtracted from the actual charge for services, and the plan will pay the balance subject to the beneficiary's responsibility for the plan's cost-sharing and deductible provisions.

XIII. PROGRAM FOR ALL-INCLUSIVE CARE OF THE ELDERLY (PACE).

This program began as a Medicare and Medicaid demonstration project initially tested at ten (10) sites. The Balanced Budget Act of 1997 (BBA) expanded PACE to become an option open to all states. PACE targets frail elderly persons living at home who are eligible for nursing home care. The program integrates health and long-term care services in an adult day care setting and uses a multidisciplinary case management team of providers, including physicians, nurses, social workers, nutritionists, occupational and speech therapists, and health and transportation personnel. PACE participants are required to attend an adult day care center regularly.

The BBA established PACE as a state option to furnish comprehensive health care to persons who are enrolled with an organization that has contracted to operate the PACE program, who are eligible for Medicaid, and who receive Medicaid solely through the PACE program. The salient characteristics of PACE offered as a state option are set forth below.

PACE providers may be public or private not-for-profit entities, except for those entities participating in the demonstration to test the operation of PACE by private, for-profit entities.

Persons eligible for PACE must be 55 years of age or older; require nursing facility level of care that would be covered under a state's Medicaid program; reside in the service area of the PACE program; and meet such other eligibility conditions as may be imposed under the PACE program agreement. Eligible individuals include both Medicare and Medicaid beneficiaries. Medicare participants not enrolled in the PACE program through Medicaid must pay premiums equal to Medicare capitation. PACE enrollees are reevaluated annually to determine if they continue to need nursing facility level of care.

Under a PACE agreement, a provider at a minimum must provide eligible persons all care and services covered under Medicare and Medicaid. The services must be provided without any limitation or condition as to amount, duration and scope and without application of deductibles, copayments, coinsurance or other cost sharing that would otherwise apply under Medicare or Medicaid. The services must be provided twenty-four (24) hours per day, every day of the year through a comprehensive multi-disciplinary health and social services delivery system which integrates acute and long-term services.

Primary medical care for a PACE enrollee must be furnished by a primary care physician who serves as a gatekeeper for access to treatment by specialists. CMS may grant waivers of this requirement. A primary care physician, registered nurse, medical director, program director, other health professionals and a governing body to guide the operation must be part of the multi-disciplinary team.

XIV. CONSOLIDATED OMNIBUS BUDGET RECONCILIATION ACT (COBRA) OF 1985.

This legislation requires that the employer continue to provide medical insurance to an employee for a specified time (e.g., eighteen (18) months if the employee's services were terminated) after the employee has left his/her employment. The COBRA coverage is for medical insurance that the employer then has in effect, and is at the employee's sole expense.

If a Medicare eligible has COBRA coverage when he/she first enrolls in Medicare, the coverage may end. The employer has the option of canceling the coverage if the first enrollment in Medicare is after the date the employee elected the COBRA coverage. Alternatively, after the employee attains age 65 or older, and he/she has COBRA coverage, the employer group plan may require the Medicare eligible to sign up for Part B.

XV. MEDICARE OUTPATIENT DRUG PROGRAM.

The Medicare Prescription Drug and Improvement Act of 2003 (MMA) enabled Medicare eligibles commencing January 1, 2006, to obtain prescription drug benefits (see *Medicare/Outpatient Prescription Drug Program – Medicare Part D*).

(continued on next page)

MEDICARE/DENIAL NOTICES

INTRODUCTION

Notices of denial of service are delivered by providers (hospitals, skilled nursing facilities, home health agencies and hospices) to beneficiaries as set forth below.

I.   HOSPITALS.

Hospitals (customarily through, their utilization review committee) issue notices of non-coverage of continued stay to beneficiaries when they believe that Medicare coverage of continued stay is not warranted.   Before making such determination, the utilization review committee (URC) will afford the beneficiary and attending physician an opportunity to present his/her claim.   If the URC decides that Medicare coverage should be denied, written notification will be given within two (2) days to the beneficiary and the attending physician.   The quality improvement organization (QIO) then automatically will review the URC claim denials, and if the QIO affirms the URC's determination, the patient may request a redetermination by the QIO, and should the QIO reaffirm its denial, the beneficiary may then pursue the regular appeal process.

A patient who has received a notice of non-coverage has the right to obtain and may request an expedited determination by the QIO (see *Appeal (Expedited), discharge of hospital patient/Medicare*).

II.   SKILLED NURSING FACILITIES.

The SNF provider may also make decisions about continuation of Medicare coverage of requested services.   Those decisions are made by the SNF through its URC.   The URC is made up of at least two (2) physicians and a registered nurse.   The nurse, as a matter of practice, will make the decision following a review by the URC.   Should the decision be to deny/reduce terminate services, the SNF must provide a patient a notice of non-coverage stating its decision that further care will not be covered by Medicare. The notice must explain that although the SNF believes that Medicare will not pay for the care, the patient may request a demand bill requiring that the care be provided and that the SNF submit bills to the fiscal intermediary; but the beneficiary must agree to pay if Medicare does not pay. If the fiscal intermediary determines that the claim is not covered by Medicare, the patient, if dissatisfied with such decision, may request reconsideration by the fiscal intermediary. If the intermediary reaffirms its decision, the patient may then pursue the regular appeals process. The beneficiary may not be billed by the SNF until the fiscal intermediary issues an initial determination regarding the claim.

Before any complete termination of services, the SNF must deliver to the beneficiary a written notice informing the beneficiary of its decision to completely terminate services. The beneficiary then has the right to request an expedited determination by the QIO (see *Appeal (Expedited), non-hospital provider's service termination/Medicare*)

III. HOME HEALTH AGENCIES.

Prior to a denial, reduction or a termination of services, the home health agency (HHA) must give the beneficiary an advance notice. This notice informs the patient of the HHA's opinion that Medicare will (or may) not cover certain services. The notice informs patients of their rights to cause the CMS to submit bills (no payment billing) to the fiscal intermediary to obtain an initial determination by the intermediary about Medicare coverage, and thereafter to a reconsideration by the intermediary, and then to pursue the regular appeal process. The beneficiary may require the HHA to submit bills to the fiscal intermediary covering such care; he/she must agree to pay if Medicare denies pay for the care. As opposed to the SNF context, beneficiaries can be required to pay for services pending review by the fiscal intermediary of the no payment billing.

IV. PHYSICIANS.

Physicians may require Medicare patients to sign a Medicare advance beneficiary notice as a condition to rendering services. It states the understanding of the patient that Medicare may not pay for the services, and constitutes a request by the patient, that the physician submit his/her claim to Medicare and that the patient agrees to pay the bill for services if Medicare determines not to cover and pay for the services. The patient may be required to pay the bill while Medicare is making its decision; the physician will reimburse the patient the amount of the payment made by the patient if Medicare does pay the physician. The patient has the right to pursue the regular appeals process should Medicare deny coverage.

(continued on next page)

MEDICARE/DURABLE MEDICAL EQUIPMENT (DME)

INTRODUCTION

Durable medical equipment (DME) is furnished to a beneficiary for use in the patient's home and is covered under Part B, whether furnished on a rental basis or purchased, as set forth below.

I.   DEFINITION OF DURABLE MEDICAL EQUIPMENT.

DME: (i) can withstand repeated use; (ii) is primarily and customarily used to serve a medical purpose; (iii) generally is not useful to a person in the absence of illness or injury; and (iv) is appropriate to use in the home.   An item is considered durable if it can withstand repeated use (i.e., the type of equipment that normally could be rented).   Medical supplies with expendable nature such as catheters and bandages are not considered to be durable equipment.   Other items, though they may be durable in nature, may fall into other Medicare coverage categories such as braces, prosthetic devices, or artificial arms, legs and eyes (see *section III.B*).

An item is considered medical equipment that is primarily and customarily used for medical purposes and is not generally useful in the absence of illness or injury (i.e., items such as hospital beds, wheelchairs, hemodialysis equipment, iron lung respirators, intermittent positive fresh breathing machines, medical regulators, oxygen tents, crutches, canes, trapeze bars, walkers, inhalators, nebulizers, commodes, suction machines, and traction equipment).   Seat-lift chairs are covered only for the seat-lift mechanism, not for the chair itself.   The following items are excluded from coverage as DME when furnished by a home health agency: (i) intraocular lenses and (ii) medical supplies (including canisters, catheter supplies, ostomy bags and supplies related to ostomy care).

II. REQUIREMENTS FOR COVERAGE.

Use in Patient's Home. An item of DME must be used in the patient's home in order to be covered for purposes of rental or purchase of DME. A patient's home may be the patient's own dwelling or apartment, a relative's home, a home for the aged or some other type of home. Neither a hospital nor a skilled nursing facility may be considered a patient's home.

Necessary and Reasonable. Coverage is subject to the requirement that the equipment be reasonable and necessary for the treatment of illness or injury or to improve the functioning of a body member.

Prescription. Medicare requires a physician's prescription for DME, prosthetics or products and other supplies.

Certificate of Medical Necessity (CMN). When DME items or services are billed to Medicare, the supplier must receive a signed certificate of medical necessity from the treating physician. The CMN can serve as the physician's order if the narrative description is sufficiently detailed.

III. REPAIRS, MAINTENANCE, REPLACEMENT AND DELIVERY.

Payment may be made by Medicare for repair, maintenance, and replacement of medically required DME that the beneficiary owns or is purchasing, including the equipment which has been in use before the user enrolled in Medicare Part B.

Repairs. Repairs to equipment that beneficiary is purchasing or already owns are covered when necessary to make the equipment serviceable. The expense of repairs may not exceed the estimated expense of purchasing or renting another item of equipment.

Maintenance. Medicare pays for maintenance and servicing of DME in the following categories: inexpensive or frequently purchased items, customized items, other prosthetic and orthotic devices, and capped rental items. Maintenance and service of items that require frequent, substantial servicing such as oxygen equipment are not reimbursed. Routine periodic servicing such as testing, cleaning, regulating and checking of the beneficiary's equipment is not covered.

Replacement. Replacement is covered in the case of loss, irreparable damage, or when required, should there be a change in the person's condition.

Delivery. Delivery and service charges are covered.

IV. SUPPLIES AND ACCESSORIES.

Reimbursement may be made for supplies – for example, oxygen – necessary for the effective use of DME. Such supplies include those drug and biologicals that must be put directly into the equipment in order for the achieved therapeutic benefit of the DME or to insure the proper functioning of the equipment.

V. OXYGEN SERVICES IN THE HOME.

Oxygen and oxygen equipment provided in the home are covered by Medicare. Initial claims for oxygen services must include a completed certificate of medical necessity to establish where the coverage criteria are met and to insure the oxygen services are provided consistent with a prescription order or other medical documentation.

VI. PURCHASE OPTION FOR CAPPED RENTAL ITEMS.

In the case of capped rental items (i.e., the rental may not exceed the monthly fee schedule amounts prescribed by Medicare), Medicare must offer a purchase option to a Medicare beneficiary to purchase these items. Beneficiaries have one month from the date the supplier makes the offer to accept the purchase option. For power-driven wheelchairs, the supplier must also make permissible a purchase option to beneficiaries at the time the equipment is initially furnished.

VII. PROSTHETIC DEVICES (OTHER THAN DENTAL).

A. Prosthetic Devices.

Prosthetic devices (other than dental) that replace all or part of an internal body organ, or replace all or part of the function of a permanently inoperative or malfunctioning internal body organ are covered by Medicare when furnished incident to a physician's services or on a physician's order. Examples of prosthetic devices are: artificial limbs, parenteral and enteral nutrition, cardiac pacemakers, prosthetic lenses, breast prostheses (including a surgical brassiere) for post-mastectomy patients, maxillo-facial devices and devices that replace all or part of the ear or nose. Chucks, diapers, rubber sheets, etc. are supplies that are not covered. Colostomy (and other ostomy) bags and other items supplied directly related to ostomy care are covered as prosthetic devices.

The term "internal body organ" includes the lens of an eye. Prostheses replacing the lens of an eye include post-surgical lenses customarily used during convalescence from eye surgery in which the lens of the eye was removed. In addition, permanent lenses also are covered when required by the individual lacking the organic lens of the eye because of surgical removal or congenital absence.

B.   Dentures.

Dentures are excluded from coverage. However, when a denture or a portion of the denture is an integral (built-in) part of a covered prosthesis (e.g., an obturator to fill an opening in the palate), it is covered as part of that prosthetic.

C.   Supplies, Repairs, Adjustments, and Replacement.

Supplies are covered that are necessary for the effective use of a prosthetic device (e.g., the batteries needed to operate an artificial larynx). Adjustment of prosthetic devices required by wear or by a change in the patient's condition is covered when ordered by a physician. Replacement of conventional eyeglasses or contact lenses furnished is not covered.

Necessary supplies, adjustments, repairs, and replacements are covered even when the device had been in use before the user enrolled in Part B of the program, so long as the device continues to be medically required.

(continued on next page)

MEDICARE/HOME HEALTH CARE

INTRODUCTION

Home care services permit a physically impaired older person to live at home independently, in a familiar environment, rather than in the institutional setting of a nursing home, or in a board-and-care facility. As a general rule, any person who is not acutely ill can be adequately cared for in the home provided his/her resources, governmental assistance and/or community-based services are available.

An organized home care program can be provided through a combination of informal caregivers, especially family members, as well as formal caregivers such as a geriatric case manager and providers from a home health agency. Under direction of a physician, the care can be oriented to a patient's needs. It may be similar to the level of skilled care provided in a skilled nursing facility (nursing nutritional services, physical, occupational and speech therapy), and more often than not it can be unskilled care in the nature of custodial or personal care.

Services may be provided by medical or other trained persons such as doctors, nurses, home health aides, therapists, geriatric care managers and social workers. Non-medical services may be provided by personal care aides, homemakers, family members, community volunteers and city or state agency personnel.

Family members and friends are the largest single source of support and care for older persons who continue to live at home, but are limited in one or more activities of daily living (ADL). ADLs consist of activities usually performed for oneself in the course of a normal day and are usually considered to be mobility (e.g., transfer from, or to a bed or chair), dressing, bathing, eating and toileting. Assistance to a person limited in his or her ADLs is customarily performed by a family member, home-health aide or attendant, or a nurse's aide in a nursing facility. The assistance is of a non-medical nature (physical) commonly characterized as personal care, or custodial. Assistance provided in a home setting goes beyond ADLs to non-medical activities commonly referred to as instrumental activities of daily living such as housekeeping (homemaker's chores) (e.g. cleaning, cooking, laundry and shopping). Medicare cannot be looked to, except to a limited extent if and when related to dependent services (described in *section I.B* below), for coverage of assistance with ADLs or instrumental ADLs. Medicare pays for acute care services but does not provide coverage for chronic care, personal (physical) care or custodial care. Medicare, as one of the hospice care benefits, will pay for respite care or temporary care by a surrogate caregiver to allow the primary caregiver some short-term relief from day-to-day responsibilities. Medicare will not pay for homebound meals (Meals on Wheels) or nutritional services at a senior center.

A wide array of resources provide assistance with information about or the actual delivery of home health care and related services, including hospital discharge planners, home health agencies, public health and welfare departments, area agencies on aging, non-profit voluntary agencies (e.g., United Way), adult day care centers, senior centers and churches and synagogues.

Home health agencies are the major source for obtaining home health care services. They provide nursing services, home health aide services, medical supplies and equipment, physical, occupational and speech therapy, nutritional counseling and social work services.

As indicated above, home care is a broadly based term whose meaning encompasses both (i) non-medically oriented services and (ii) the more restrictive, medically oriented term "home health care" which is restricted to skilled services (see *section I* below). The two terms should not be confused. As described below, Medicare basically covers only limited home health care and carefully defines home health care and the conditions for coverage.

The salient topics of home health care are described below.

I.   COVERAGE.

Medicare Part B covers the following home health care services (Medicare Part A post-institutional home health services are described in section III.)

A.   Part B Home Health Services.

These services are characterized by Medicare as qualifying skilled services and comprise (a) intermittent skilled nursing care (except private duty nursing, which Medicare will not cover), (b) physical and occupational therapy and (c) speech-language pathology. Occupational therapy is counted as a qualifying skilled service only if it is part of a care plan which also includes intermittent skilled nursing and occupational and physical therapy or speech-language pathology services.

B.   Dependent Services.

These services consist of the following:

Intermittent or part-time home health aide services (item 1 below);

Medical social services (item 2 below);

Durable medical equipment (item 3 below);

Medical supplies (other than drugs and biologicals) (item 4 below);

Intern and resident services (item 5 below); and

Medical nutrition therapy (item 6 below).

These supportive dependent services are incidental to the qualifying skilled services and are covered by Medicare only if one qualifying skilled service is required. The dependent services are described and defined as follows:

1.   **Home Health Aide Services**. This is one of the six dependent services.

1.1   *General*. A home health aide provides home health aide services and/or personal care services for a disabled person at home. A home health aide — sometimes incorrectly referred to as a home attendant or personal care aide — has more training than a home attendant or personal care aide and may perform more skilled tasks than a home attendant or personal care aide (e.g., giving an injection). A home health aide must successfully complete an approved training program and is required to receive at least twelve (12) hours of in-service training during each twelve- (12) month period.

1.2   *Conditions to obtaining Medicare home health aide services.*

The services of a home health aide must be obtained from a certified home health agency, not a non-Medicare-certified agency.

A person is not eligible to obtain these services through Medicare as a single, stand-alone service. Medicare eligibility is conditioned on the need for a skilled service which may be one of those performed by a home health aide.

> The services must be reasonable and necessary.
>
> The services must be ordered by a physician in a care plan.
>
> Written patient care instructions for the home health aide must be prepared by a registered nurse or other appropriate professional responsible for the supervision of the aide.
>
> Supervision of the aide is required periodically by a registered nurse.

1.3 *Part-time or Intermittent as a Coverage Limitation of Home Health Aide and Skilled Nursing Services.* The duration of the covered services of a home health aide and skilled nurse is limited to part-time or intermittent. The Balanced Budget Act of 1997 (Act) defines intermittent as an <u>eligibility factor.</u> However, for purposes of determining the extent of coverage of home health care — a coverage factor as contrasted with eligibility for such care — the Act does not define intermittent separately. Instead it refers to the statutory terms "part-time or intermittent nursing care" and "part-time or intermittent services of a home health aide." In this context as a coverage limitation, part-time or intermittent services are defined to mean skilled nursing and home aide services (combined) furnished any number of days per week so long as they are provided within the following time frames:

> less than eight (8) hours a day, and twenty-eight (28) or fewer hours a week;
>
> or
>
> on a case-by-case basis (subject to review as to the need for care), less than eight (8) hours a day and thirty-five (35) or fewer hours per week.

The Secretary of HHS is authorized under the Act to establish normative guidelines for the frequency and duration of these and other home health services.

Medicare frequently may limit the extent of the foregoing covered services due to the application of the reasonable and necessary standard, although use of home health aides may be available theoretically for extended periods. Medicare frequently will limit the visits of home health aides to three or four hours per day.

1.4 *Duties of Home Health Aide.* Services of the home health aide include, but are not limited to:

help that is supportive of skilled nursing or therapy;

hands-on personal care if it is prescribed by a physician and is incidental to regular home health aide services. The care is assistance in the activities of daily living such as bathing, dressing, eating, toileting, and transferring from bed to chair. Housekeeping tasks or homemaker services, such as cooking meals, dishwashing, doing laundry or shopping, generally are not covered by Medicare. However, under the Medicare hospice benefit, a home health aide may furnish homemaker services.

simple dressing changes that do not require the skills of a licensed nurse;

assistance with medications that are ordinarily self-administered and that do not require the skills of a licensed practical nurse to be provided safely and effectively;

assistance with activities that are directly supportive of skilled therapy services but do not require the skills of a therapist;

assistance in ambulation or exercise; and

routine care of prosthetic and/or orthotic devices.

1.5 *Supervision of Home Health Aide.* Several supervisory requirements apply to the duties of a home health aide.

If the patient is receiving skilled care as well as aide services, a registered nurse, or other appropriate professional, must make a supervisory visit to the patient's home at least once every two (2) weeks. This supervising visit must be made by a registered nurse, not by a licensed practical nurse (LPN).

If the patient is receiving home health aide services but not skilled care, the supervisory visit must occur at least once every sixty-two (62) days. If the aide is an employee of a home health agency or hospice, at least one of these visits must be made while the aide is providing care to the patient.

A registered nurse must assign the home health aide to a specified patient. This does not preclude the use of a substitute aide when illness or other unforeseen circumstances prevent the regularly scheduled aide to perform the regularly scheduled services.

2. **Medical Social Services.** This is one of the six (6) dependent services. Medical social services must be furnished by a qualified social worker or a qualified social worker assistant under the supervision of a social worker.

Medical social services are necessary to resolve social or emotional problems that are expected to be an impediment to the effective treatment of the beneficiary's medical condition or to his/her rate of recovery. Family counseling services by a physician are covered when the primary purpose is the treatment of the beneficiary's condition and not the treatment of a family member's condition. Family visits may be furnished only on a short-term basis to a beneficiary's family member or caregiver when it can be demonstrated that a brief intervention (i.e., two or three visits) by a medical social worker is necessary to remove an impediment which clearly and directly impedes a beneficiary's medical treatment. An example of such an impediment is the failure of a family member to provide necessary care or his/her engaging in an abusive, neglectful behavior.

Medical social services must be ordered by and under the direction of a physician, and included in the plan of care.

3. **Durable Medical Equipment.** This is one of the six (6) dependent services. Durable medical equipment must:

> be able to be used over again by other patients and primarily serve a medical purpose;

> be appropriate for use, and be used in the patient's home; and

be reasonable and necessary for the patient's illness or injury or to improve the functioning of his/her malformed body member.

The patient is required to pay twenty (20%) percent of the approved charges as a coinsurance payment. Examples of durable medical equipment include iron lungs, canes, oxygen tents, hospital beds, wheelchairs, walkers, and seat lift chairs. Under certain conditions, a beneficiary may elect to purchase an item of equipment rather than rent it.

4. **Medical Supplies.** This is one of the six (6) dependent services. Two types are covered by Medicare, the cost of which is included in the Medicare coverage of a home visit.

Routine. These supplies are customarily used during the course of most home care visits by home health agency staff and are not designated for a specific patient (for example, swabs, thermometers, and masks).

Non-routine. These supplies must be specifically ordered by a physician for use in treating a specific patient. Included in non-routine supplies are catheters, splints, syringes, and sterile dressings.

Drugs and biologicals are not considered medical supplies.

5. **Services of Interns and Residents.** This is one of the six dependent services. The services of interns and residents are covered by Medicare as part of home health care, if they are part of a physician's plan of care, ordered by the physician who is responsible for the plan, and obtained through a home health agency that is affiliated with or under the common control of an approved teaching hospital furnishing the medical services of interns and residents.

The need for such services must be reasonable and necessary for the diagnosis of or treatment for a beneficiary's illness or injury, or to improve the functioning of a malformed body member.

6. **Medical Nutrition Therapy.** This is one of the six dependent services. Medicare will cover medical nutrition therapy for beneficiaries with diabetes or renal disease. The covered services include nutritional diagnosis, therapy and counseling services for the purpose of disease management that are

furnished by a registered dietician or nutrition professional pursuant to a physician's referral.

II. ELIGIBILITY (QUALIFYING CRITERIA) FOR HOME HEALTH CARE SERVICES.

To qualify for home health care benefits, a Medicare beneficiary must meet the following home health requirements:

Be homebound (item 1 below);

Need one of the qualifying skilled services: (i) intermittent skilled nursing care (item 2.1 below), or (ii) physical therapy, speech-language pathology therapy and also occupational therapy if part of a plan includes at least one of the qualifying skilled services (item 3 below);

Obtain the services from a Medicare-certified home health agency (item 4 below); and

Obtain from his/her physician a plan of care prescribing the needed services (item 5 below).

The foregoing requirements are defined and described below:

1.   **Homebound.** The homebound beneficiary is an individual who is confined to home, not necessarily bedridden, and has a condition due to an illness or injury that restricts his/her ability to leave the home without the aid of another person or supportive device, such as crutches, a cane, a wheelchair, a walker, or specialized transportation. A person's "home" is any place in which a beneficiary resides that does not meet the definition of a hospital, skilled nursing facility or rehabilitation facility. Services can be provided in an outpatient setting if: (a) equipment is required that could not be made available in a beneficiary's home, or (b) services were furnished while the beneficiary is at a facility to receive services requiring equipment that cannot be made available at home; and the outpatient setting is in an approved hospital, skilled nursing facility, or rehabilitation facility. Such sources may include medical services provided at adult day care centers.

The medical services and treatment provided to the homebound individual must be in accordance with a physician's order and are performed under the supervision of a licensed health professional for the purpose of diagnosis or treatment of an illness or injury.

An absence of an individual from home will not disqualify an individual from being considered confined to home if the absence is of an infrequent or relatively short duration; for example, a trip to the barber or an occasional drive. Absences to attend a religious service are considered to be absences of infrequent or short duration.

2.   Intermittent Skilled Nursing Care

2.1   *Skilled Nursing Care Defined.* The Medicare decision as to whether skilled nursing services are covered depends upon whether they are reasonable and necessary. To be considered reasonable and necessary, the services must be consistent with the nature and severity of the beneficiary's illness or injury, his/her particular medical needs, and accepted standards of medical and nursing practice. The determination of whether skilled nursing care is reasonable and necessary must be based solely upon the beneficiary's unique condition and individual needs, without regard to whether the illness or injury is acute, chronic, terminal or expected to last a long time.

Skilled nursing care must be performed by a registered nurse or licensed practical (vocational) nurse, and meet the criteria for skilled nursing services. Examples of what constitutes skilled nursing care include: (i) observation and assessment of a patient's condition, (ii) management and evaluation of the patient's care plan, (iii) hands-on nursing services such as wound care, injections, tube feeding, kidney dialysis, colostomy care, changing specific dressings, (iv) patient education, and (v) the management and evaluation of the plan.

2.2   *Exclusion of Non-skilled Care.* If a service can be safely and effectively performed by the average non-medical person without direct supervision of a licensed nurse, then the service is a non-skilled nursing service. A non-skilled service does not become a skilled service because there is no competent person to perform such service.

Skilled nursing excludes any service that could be safely and effectively performed or self-administered by the average non-medical person without the direct intervention of a licensed nurse. It makes no difference if a patient's condition is acute, chronic or terminal.

2.3 *Skilled Nursing Visits*. When a nurse furnishes several services in the course of a single visit, this constitutes only one visit. The fact that the nurse also provides incidental unskilled services in addition to the skilled nursing care does not constitute that service as more than one visit.

In a situation in which a nurse and a home health aide are required to furnish a service, Medicare will pay for two visits so long as two individuals were needed to furnish a service (e.g., a bath, wound care, or a certain exercise). The clinical notes required of the home health agency should describe why it is necessary for two individuals to furnish the services.

The use of telehealth is not considered a home health visit for purposes of eligibility or payment. A beneficiary whose only skilled nursing service is provided via telecommunication by a home health agency is not eligible for home health services or payment; the beneficiary is not considered as having received a skilled nursing service.

2.4 *Intermittent Defined*. The need for skilled nursing care must be intermittent. The word "intermittent" as it relates to skilled nursing is used both as a condition of eligibility for home health services and as a coverage limitation as relates to the duration of coverage.

As an eligibility requirement (which is the subject of paragraph 3.1), the term "intermittent" determines health benefits of a patient because of his/her need for intermittent nursing care. In this context, intermittent is defined by the Balanced Budget Act of 1997 (Act) to mean nursing care that is needed for the following durations:

> fewer than seven (7) days each week; or

> less than eight (8) hours of each day for periods of twenty-one (21) days or less, with extensions in exceptional circumstances when the need for additional care is finite and predictable.

Note: As a coverage limitation, the word "intermittent" is part of the term "part-time or intermittent," and the term is separately and differently defined by the Act. The term describes the extent (i.e., duration) of coverage. (See *Intermittent care/Medicare*. See also *section I.B.1.3* above)

3. Physical Therapy, Speech-Language Pathology Services and Occupational Therapy

3.1 *Eligibility*. Skilled therapy services may be furnished to a Medicare beneficiary as a home health service. To qualify for at-home therapy services, the following requirements must be met:

> The services must be reasonable and necessary for the treatment of the patient's illness or injury or for the restoration or maintenance of function affected by the patient's illness or injury.

> The patient must be homebound.

> The therapy services must be obtained through a Medicare-certified home health agency.

> The services must be provided according to a physician's plan of care.

To be covered by Medicare, all skilled therapy services must relate directly and specifically to a treatment regimen, established by the physician after any needed consultation with the qualified therapist, that is designed to treat the beneficiary's illness or injury. Services related to activities for the general physical welfare of beneficiaries — for example, exercises to promote overall fitness — do not constitute physical therapy, occupational therapy, or speech-language pathology services for Medicare purposes. Occupational therapy services will qualify for Medicare coverage only if they are part of a plan that also includes intermittent skilled nursing care, physical therapy or speech-language pathology services. A patient who initially only needs occupational therapy will not qualify for home health service. However, if the patient's eligibility was already established by a prior need for skilled nursing care or speech or physical therapy, then the patient will qualify for a continued need of occupational therapy.

3.2 *Reasonable and Necessary Requirement for Therapy Services*. To be covered by Medicare, rehabilitation services must be reasonable and necessary. To be considered reasonable and necessary, the following four (4) conditions must be met:

> Each service must be considered under accepted standards of medical practice to be specific, safe, and effective treatment for the beneficiary's condition.

Each service must be sufficiently complex and sophisticated, or the condition of the beneficiary must be such, that the services required can safely and effectively be performed only by a qualified physical therapist or assistant, qualified speech-language pathologist, or qualified occupational therapist or assistant.

In the case of each service, there must be an expectation that the beneficiary's condition will improve materially in a reasonable and generally predictable period of time based on the physician's assessment, or the services must be necessary to establish a safe and maintenance program.

In the case of each service, its amount, frequency and duration must be reasonable.

4. **Certified Home Health Agency.** A certified home health agency (CHHA) is a public or private organization that specializes in providing skilled nursing services, therapeutic services (such as physical therapy) and home health aide services.

4.1 *Services.* Persons requiring home health care and seeking Medicare or coverage may acquire the following services from the CHHA: nursing services; home health aide services; medical supplies and equipment; physical, speech-language pathology and occupational therapy; nutritional counseling; social work services; and assessment. Skilled nursing services and home health aide services must be obtained from the CHHA.

4.2 *Assessment.*

(a) <u>Initial Assessment Visit</u>. A registered nurse provided by a CHHA must conduct an initial assessment visit to determine the immediate care and support needs of homebound patients as well as their eligibility for the Medicare home health benefit, including homebound status. The initial assessment visit must be held either within forty-eight (48) hours of referral or within forty-eight (48) hours of the patient's return home, or on the physician's start-up care date.

When rehabilitation therapy service (speech-language pathology, physical therapy or occupational therapy) is the only service ordered by the physician and if the need for that service establishes program eligibility, the initial assessment visit may be made by the appropriate skilled professional.

(b) Comprehensive Assessment. A patient-specific comprehensive assessment (identifying the patient's need for home care, and his/her medical nursing, rehabilitative, social and discharge planning needs) must be made and completed in a timely manner, no later than five (5) calendar days after the start of care. A registered nurse, except when a rehabilitative therapy service is the only health care needed, must complete the comprehensive assessment, and determine (in addition to a similar determination by the registered nurse or therapist at the time of the initial assessment) eligibility of the Medicare home health benefit, including homebound status.

When physical therapy, speech-language pathology or occupational therapy is the only service ordered by the physician, a physical therapist, speech-language pathologist or occupational therapist may complete the comprehensive assessment and determine eligibility for the Medicare home health benefit, including homebound status. An occupational therapist may complete the comprehensive assessment if the need for occupational therapy establishes program eligibility.

The comprehensive assessment must include a review of all medications that the patient is currently using in order to identify any potential adverse effects in drug reactions. The comprehensive assessment must be updated and revised, including the administration of the Outcome and Assessment Information Set Items (OASIS), as frequently as the patient's condition warrants, but not less frequently than every second calendar month, beginning with start of care date; within forty-eight (48) hours of the patient's return to the home after a hospital admission of twenty-four (24) hours or more, for any reason other than diagnostic test; or, at discharge. The OASIS data items are determined by the Secretary of HHS, and must be incorporated into the CHHA's assessment.

(c) Services Must be at Patient's Home. The CHHA must furnish at least one of the covered home health services (except durable medical equipment) through its agency employees in a place of residence used as the patient's home, but may furnish the second and additional services under management with another CHHA organization.

(d) Patient Rights. All CHHAs must give clients written notice of their rights either before the care relationship begins or during the initial evaluation visit before treatment. The following special requirements apply to clients who are beneficiaries under Medicare Part A and Part B; however, the requirements do not apply to a Part C managed care enrollee. If a CHHA expects Medicare to deny payment for home health services requested by a beneficiary and ordered by his/her physician, the beneficiary must be given a notice of non-coverage before home health care is initiated or continued, stating that in the CHHA's opinion Medicare will not cover the requested care, and therefore, payment will be required from him/her, and not from Medicare. The CHHA will state in this notice that it expects Medicare will stop paying for: any home health services for the patient; some of the patient's home health services; or all home health services for the patient. The expectation of Medicare denial may be for one or more reasons, including the facts that: (i) the requested services are not medically reasonable and necessary, and are custodial; (ii) the beneficiary is not homebound; or (iii) the beneficiary does not require part-time or intermittent services. Such notice must be issued by the CHHA and signed by the beneficiary each time. As soon as the CHHA makes the assessment that it believes that Medicare payment will not be made for the services ordered by the client's physician, the CHHA is required to submit a demand bill to the regional home health intermediary when requested by the patient.

(e) Rights of Incompetent Patients. The rights of patients who are adjudged incompetent can be exercised on their behalf by the court-appointed guardian or by family members. The rights include: respect for the patient's property; right to voice grievances about quality of care, and to have the grievance investigated by the CMS, without reprisals (if the state has a home health hotline for questions and complaints, the patient must be informed of its telephone number and hours of operation);

participation in treatment planning; and notification of any change in the plan of care.

(f) Other Requirements. A CHHA must inform the patient of the right to make a living will or other advance directive. If the patient has done so, or chooses to do so in response to the information, the existence and content of the advance directive must be made part of the patient's medical record. However, no health care provider can condition provision of its services on a person either signing or refraining from signing an advance directive.

Patient medical records must be kept confidential.

Patients must be advised in advance of the cost of care, the portion payable by Medicare and Medicaid; the individual's own payment responsibility, and any changes in charges or payment allocation.

CHHAs must abide by all relevant state and Federal laws and regulations.

CHHAs must disclose the names and addresses of everyone with an ownership or control interest, or who serves as an officer, director, agent or managing employee.

CHHAs must be organized and managed consistently with Federal requirements.

5.   **Plan of Care.** In order for any home health service to be covered under Medicare, the services must be furnished under a plan of care established and periodically reviewed by a physician. The physician must certify that the beneficiary satisfies the following criteria, namely that he/she is:

under a physician's care;

under a plan of care established and periodically reviewed by a physician; and

in need of qualifying skilled services, namely, skilled nursing care on an intermittent basis, physical therapy or speech-language pathology services, and in addition occupational therapy, provided the need for such services has been established because of a prior need for intermittent skilled nursing care, speech-language pathology or physical therapy.

The beneficiary must be under care of the physician who established the plan of care. This requirement does not preclude the patient's treatment by physicians other than the one who establishes the plan of care.

A therapist or other personnel of a home health agency may participate in developing a plan of care, but the physician is responsible for developing the plan.

The plan must be signed and dated by the physician. Verbal orders are permissible. However, they must be countersigned by the physician in a timely fashion and dated by the physician before the home health agency bills for the care.

The plan does not require a narrative description of the services ordered. It need only specify the medical treatment(s) to be furnished, a discipline which will furnish them, and the frequency with which they will be furnished.

Appropriate specificity of medical treatments would include such orders as "observe and evaluate surgical site" or "perform sterile dressing changes," and for home health aide services, "assist in personal care."

The number of visits ordered generally is required to be specified. However, a physician may limit the order to a specific range in the frequency of services "as ordered" or to a private registered nurse (PRN) when necessary.

Home health agencies do not have carte blanche on private registered nurse visits. The physician must impose a specific limit on the number of PRN visits; this can be accomplished by the physician describing and prescribing PRN visits only in specific instances as, for example, by describing the medical signs and symptoms of a PRN visit (e.g., a plugged urinary catheter).

The physician must review the plan of care at least once every sixty-two (62) days. Each review must contain the signature of the physician and the date of review.

The plan will be considered terminated when the beneficiary no longer requires for a sixty-two- (62) day period at least one of the qualifying skilled services such as skilled nursing, physical therapy, speech-language pathology, or occupational therapy.

III.   PAYMENTS BY MEDICARE.

Prior to the enactment of the Balanced Budget Act of 1997 (Act), Medicare prohibited payments for home health services to be made under Part B if the beneficiary was covered under Part A and Part B for the same services; in such event Part A was required to make the payment.

The Act significantly changed Part A payment for home health services rendered to Medicare beneficiaries enrolled under both Part A and Part B. Beginning in 1998, payments to eligible beneficiaries for post-institutional home health services (as defined below) were transferred gradually from Part A to Part B for services (referred to as "post-institutional home health services") after the first one-hundred (100) visits during a home health spell of illness that (i) required those services and (ii) followed the beneficiary's stay in a hospital (of at least three (3) days) or a skilled nursing facility. Hence, after such individual exhausts one-hundred (100) visits of Part A post-institutional home health services, Part B finances the balance of the home health spell of illness. To the extent that visits are not part of the first one-hundred (100) visits following a stay in the hospital (of at least three (3) days) or a skilled nursing facility, they are considered to be Part B home health services.

The transfer of payment of post-institutional home health services from Part A to Part B rendered to enrollees under both Part A and Part B was phased in over a period of six (6) years between 1998 and 2003. By a prescribed formula, a portion of visits was transferred each year. After January 1, 2003, Part A pays for post-institutional home health services for no more than one-hundred (100) visits during a home health spell of illness.

Post-institutional home health services are defined to be those that are furnished to a Medicare beneficiary within fourteen (14) days of being discharged from an inpatient hospital or rural primary hospital after a stay of at least three (3) days or from a skilled nursing facility.

A home health spell of illness is the period beginning when a patient first receives post-institutional home health services and ending when a beneficiary has not received inpatient care in a hospital or skilled nursing facility or received home health services for sixty (60) days.

Persons enrolled only in Part A will be covered for post-institutional home health care services under Part A without regard to post-institutional limitations. If a person is only enrolled in Part B and qualifies for Medicare home health care services, then all such services are covered under Part B.

IV. EXCLUSIONS.

Medicare will not cover non-medical care such as:

Personal (custodial) care, customarily rendered by a personal care aide. This is an unskilled service that assists elderly persons with activities of daily living such as bathing and eating. To a limited extent, these services may be covered by Medicare when performed by a home health aide, if prescribed by the patient's physician, and only if incidental to Medicare home health services.

Non-skilled services to assist with instrumental activities of daily living, such as preparing meals, shopping and light housework.

Community-based services such as meals to homebound individuals (Meals on Wheels) or congregate meals.

Management and coordination of services such as case management.

V. PRIOR HOSPITALIZATION.

There is no requirement of prior hospitalization, as a condition to a patient obtaining Part B home health services.

VI. NUMBER OF HOME HEALTH VISITS.

There is no limitation on the number of home health visits per year. However, the part-time or intermittent requirement and the reasonable and necessary requirement impose a practical limit on the number of visits.

(continued on next page)

MEDICARE/MENTAL HEALTH SERVICES

Mental disorders can be classified into three categories: psychosis, personality disorder, and neurosis. Mental illnesses are commonly characterized by depression, anxiety, mania or paranoid disorders.

Medicare will help to pay for mental health conditions as set forth below.

Medicare Part A will help to pay up to one-hundred ninety (190) days of inpatient psychiatric care in a participating psychiatric hospital. Psychiatric care provided at general hospitals is not subject to the one-hundred ninety- (190) day limit. Inpatient care in a participating psychiatric hospital is subject to the same terms and conditions, deductible and copayments as those for other Medicare inpatient hospital care.

Medicare Part B helps to pay for partial hospitalization for mental health services furnished by a hospital outpatient unit and by qualified community mental health centers. Partial hospitalization means an ambulatory program of active care that lasts less than twenty-four (24) hours a day.

In addition, Medicare Part B helps to pay for services received for non-hospital outpatient treatment of mental illness. This includes services from doctors, comprehensive outpatient rehabilitation facilities, physician assistants, psychologists and clinical social workers. Services for non-hospital treatment of mental illness and treatment for substance abuse and lab tests are subject to certain limits and conditions. What the outpatient will pay depends on whether he/she is being diagnosed or getting treatment:

(i)   For visits to a doctor or other health care professional to diagnose a condition, the outpatient pays twenty (20%) of the Medicare-approved amount;

(ii)   For outpatient treatment of the outpatient's condition (such as counseling or psychotherapy), he/she must pay forty (40%) of the approved amount (2012). This coinsurance amount will decrease until it reaches twenty (20%) in 2014.

403

The Part B deductible applies for both visits diagnose and treat the outpatient's condition. Partial hospitalization services for treatment of mental illness are not subject to this special payment rule.

(continued on next page)

MEDICARE/OUTPATIENT DEPARTMENT HOSPITAL SERVICES

INTRODUCTION

Medicare Part B helps pay for the salient outpatient department hospital services set forth below.

I.   COVERAGE.

Blood transfusions furnished to a person as an outpatient;

Drugs and biologicals that cannot be self-administered;

Laboratory tests billed by the hospital;

Mental health care if a physician certified that inpatient treatment would be required without it;

Medical supplies such as splints and casts;

Services in an emergency room or outpatient clinic, including same day surgery; and

X-rays and other radiology services billed by a hospital.

II.   COINSURANCE/COPAYMENT.

If an individual receives outpatient department (OPD) services at a hospital, other than for mental health, he/she is responsible for paying twenty (20%) percent of whatever the hospital charges not to exceed the standard Medicare hospital inpatient deductible – not merely the customary and lesser twenty (20%) percent of the Medicare-approved amount for Part B services rendered in other settings. According to CMS rules issued as a result of the Balanced Budget Act of 1997, this disparity in the amount of coinsurance for OPD services is scheduled to diminish gradually and become the same as the standard copayment. Under these rules, the copayment for hospital OPD services is subject to a cap equal to the hospital inpatient deductible ($1,156 in 2012).

If an individual receives outpatient mental health services, his/her coinsurance share is fifty (50%) percent of the Medicare-approved amount.

(continued on next page)

MEDICARE/OUTPATIENT PRESCRIPTION DRUG PROGRAM (MEDICARE PART D)

INTRODUCTION

Prescription drug coverage benefits are available to Medicare eligibles under a newly enacted Medicare Part D Program of Title XVIII of the Social Security Act. (Section 101 of the Medicare Prescription Drug and Improvement Act of 2003 ("Act")), also known as the Medicare Modernization Act (MMA).

The Centers for Medicare and Medicaid Services (CMS) has overall responsibility for implementing the Medicare Part D prescription drug benefits of the Act.

The salient topics of Medicare Part D program are discussed below.

I. GENERAL.

An individual is eligible for the Medicare prescription drug program if he or she is entitled to Medicare Part A and/or enrolled in Medicare Part B. Beneficiaries must take affirmative steps to enroll and get Part D coverage except that dual eligibles (see *section III.A.6* below) are entitled to automatic enrollment.

The Act provides for premium and cost-sharing subsidies of prescription drug coverage for certain individuals with low income and resources. The purpose of the subsidy program is to assist Medicare beneficiaries with limited financial means to pay for Medicare prescription drug coverage under Medicare Part D. Individuals with low incomes and limited resources may be eligible for a subsidy (referred to as extra help subsidy) to help pay for monthly premiums, coinsurances and the annual deductible under Medicare Part D.

Medicare beneficiaries are able to obtain prescription drug coverage either through (i) a stand-alone prescription drug plan (PDP), available to enrollees in original Medicare fee for services, or (ii) a comprehensive Medicare Advantage plan with prescription drug coverage (MA-PDP) available to Medicare eligibles who enroll in Medicare Advantage plans. The prescription drug coverage is operated through private insurance entities that contract with CMS.

Insurance companies are no longer able to sell existing Medigap policies that provide drug coverage to Medicare beneficiaries who are enrolled in or eligible for Medicare outpatient prescription drug coverage. They are, however, able to renew the Medigap drug policies issued prior to January 1, 2006 for beneficiaries who do not opt for the Medicare prescription drug plan (PDP); their Medigap policy will be modified to eliminate drug coverage, and premiums will be adjusted. Beneficiaries with the new Medicare drug coverage can purchase Medigap policies that do not cover drugs.

Medicare may not negotiate drug discounts. The MMA prohibits the government from negotiating discounts on drug purchases or otherwise interfering in drug pricing decisions.

Medicaid does not cover Part D drugs.

II.   PART D DRUGS.

A Part D drug is a drug that is approved by the U.S. Food and Drug Administration, for which a prescription is required, and for which Medicare requires payment. Biological products, including insulin and insulin supplies (syringes, needles, alcohol swabs and gauze), and smoking cessation drugs are also covered under Part D. The MMA excludes from coverage those categories of drugs for which Medicare payment is optional, such as drugs for weight gain, barbiturates, benzodiazepines and over-the-counter medications. MMA also excludes from Part D coverage those drugs for which payment could be made under Medicare Part A and Part B.

A plan's drug formulary must include at least one drug (but often two) in each approved category and class. Pharmacies will distribute or post notices that instruct enrollees to contact their Medicare PDP if they need a certain drug and the pharmacist informs them that the drug is not included in the plan's formulary.

All drug plan sponsors must establish an exceptions process whereby individuals enrolled in a drug plan can seek a non-formulary drug, or have a covered drug assigned to a lower tier to reduce their cost-sharing. CMS has developed appeals procedures which ensure that enrollees quickly receive decisions regarding medically necessary medications.

The plans may change their formularies any time upon giving a sixty- (60) day notice to the enrollee, his/her prescribing physician, pharmacist and CMS, of formulary changes. The notice must explain how an enrollee may request an exception.

III. ENROLLMENT.

A. Introduction.

Enrollment in Part D requires the beneficiary to take affirmative steps to enroll and get Part D coverage. The beneficiary must first choose a drug plan from the options available in his/her area. Then, the beneficiary must enroll through the plan that he/she chooses. If the beneficiary may be eligible for a low-income subsidy, he/she must file a second affirmation.

In order to be eligible to enroll in a PDP, the individual must reside in the plan's service area and cannot be enrolled in a MA plan (other than a medical savings account, or a private fee-for-service plan) that does not provide qualified prescription drug coverage.

PDP enrollees are locked in to their plan for the remainder of the calendar year, even though the plan in which they enroll may change the formulary or cost-sharing arrangements during the year. Enrollees in PDPs must wait until the next annual coordinated enrollment period to switch plans, with enrollment in the new plan becoming effective on January 1 of the following year.

B. Enrollment Periods.

There are three (3) coverage enrollment periods: (i) the initial enrollment period; (ii) the annual coordinated election period; and (iii) special enrollment period, as set forth below:

> *Initial Enrollment Period.* The initial enrollment period for individuals who are first eligible to enroll in Part D, corresponds to the initial enrollment period for Part B, i.e., the seven-month period running from three (3) months before the month when individual first becomes eligible and ending three (3) months after the first month of eligibility.

Annual Coordinated Enrollment Period. The annual coordinated enrollment period corresponds to the annual coordinated enrollment period for Part C and runs from October 15 through December 7.

Special Enrollment Period. Individuals may be eligible for a special enrollment period if:

> they did not enroll in Part D during their initial enrollment because they had other prescription drug coverage deemed to be "creditable coverage," and they lose the creditable coverage which is defined in section III. G below);

> they were given incorrect information concerning the status of their other prescription drug coverage as creditable coverage;

> they were given incorrect information about enrollment by a Federal employee;

> they have Medicare and full Medicaid coverage or a Medicare Savings Program (MSP);

> they move out of a plan's service area;

> their PDP's contract with Medicare is terminated;

> they enrolled in a MA-PDP during the first year of eligibility and want to return to traditional Medicare and a PDP; or

> they move into or out of a nursing home.

5-Star Special Enrollment Period. A Medicare eligible can switch to a 5-star Medicare PDP at any time during the year, but only if it is available in the individual's area. The Medicare-eligible person can use this special enrollment period to switch to a 5-star plan one time each year.

C.   Effective Date of Enrollment.

Part D coverage becomes effective:

> the same month that Part A and/or Part B coverage becomes effective for individuals who enroll before their month of entitlement to Part A or enrollment in Part B;

the first day of the next calendar month after enrollment for individuals who enroll after the first month of entitlement for Part A or enrollment in Part B;

the following January 1, for individuals who enroll during the annual coordinated enrollment period; and

at the time specified by CMS for individuals who enroll during a special enrollment period.

D. Involuntary Disenrollment.

An individual may be involuntarily disenrolled from a drug plan for one of several reasons. These include no longer living in the plan's service area, loss of eligibility for Part D, death of the individual, termination of the PDP, failure to pay premiums on a timely basis, and/or engaging in disruptive behavior that substantially impairs the ability of the plan to arrange for or provide services.

E. Ability to Change Plans Mid-Year.

Individuals may switch plans once during the annual coordinated enrollment period, which runs from October 15 to December 7. Enrollment becomes effective on January 1 of the next year.

Individuals enrolled in a Medicare Advantage plan with prescription drug coverage (MA-PDP) may change plans during the open enrollment period during the first three (3) months of each year (January 1 to March 31). An enrollee in a MA-PDP may use this period (January through March) to change to another MA-PDP or to disenroll from the MA-PDP and return to traditional/original Medicare and a PDP. Someone who enrolls in an MA plan that does not offer prescription drug coverage may not change to a MA-PDP or to an original Medicare and a PDP during this period. The beneficiary must wait to change plans until the next annual coordinated enrollment period.

Enrollees in original Medicare without drug coverage may enroll in a MA-PDP during the open enrollment period. Enrollees in original Medicare with a PDP may only enroll in an MA-PDP during the open enrollment period.

Individuals are eligible to change plans mid-year if they qualify for a special enrollment period described above.

Individuals who obtain Medicare due to a disability can join a plan during the three (3) months before to three (3) months after their 25th month of disability. They will have another chance to join three (3) months before the month they turn age 65 to three (3) months after the month they turn age 65.

F.   Enrollment Process for Individuals Who Are Full-Benefit Dual Eligible.

A full-benefit dual eligible individual means an individual who is determined eligible by the state for (i) medical assistance for full-benefits under Title XIX of the Social Security Act, under any eligibility category covered under a state plan; or (ii) medical assistance under the Act authorized for the medical need, or permitted by states that use more restrictive eligibility criteria than are used by the SSI program.

The MMA established an enrollment process involving automatic assignment into drug plans for individuals who are full-benefit dual eligibles, who are eligible for Medicare and Medicaid and who do not choose their own PDP or MA-PDP during their initial enrollment period. Full-benefit dual eligibles are automatically eligible for a continuous special enrollment period and therefore are not ever locked into a prescription drug plan. CMS must automatically enroll full-benefit dual eligible individuals who fail to enroll in Part D plan into a PDP offering basic prescription drug coverage in the area where the individuals reside that has a monthly beneficiary premium that does not exceed the low-income premium subsidy amount.

Nothing prevents a full-benefit dual eligible individual from: (i) affirmatively declining enrollment in Part D; or (ii) disenrolling from the Part D plan in which the individual is enrolled and electing to enroll in another Part D plan during the special enrollment period.

Enrollment of full-benefit dual eligible individuals is effective as follows: (i) the first day of the month the individual is eligible for Part D for individuals who are Medicaid eligible and subsequently become newly eligible for Part D; and (ii) for individuals who are eligible for Part D and subsequently become newly eligible for Medicaid after January 1, 2006. (Enrollment is effective as soon as practicable after being identified as a newly full-benefit dual eligible individual.)

G.   Failure to Enroll on a Timely Basis.

A beneficiary who does not enroll in a Part D plan within sixty-three (63) days of his/her initial enrollment period, and who does not have other creditable prescription drug coverage, must pay a late penalty if he/she subsequently enrolls in a Part D plan. Creditable coverage is other coverage, equivalent to Medicare basic drug benefit (e.g., VA coverage, Medigap coverage, and most employer (or union) sponsor retiree plans). Should a beneficiary's existing drug coverage end or change and thus cease to be creditable, he/she has up to sixty-three (63) days to enroll in a Medicare drug plan.

The penalty is assessed at one (1%) percent of the national average premium for each month of delayed enrollment, for the remainder of the time in which the beneficiary is enrolled in a Part D plan. Thus, a beneficiary who first becomes eligible for Part D at age 65, but who delays enrolling until age 70 may be assessed a sixty- (60%) percent penalty on his/her premium (5 years x 12 months x 1%). Since the penalty is based on a percentage of the average premium each year, the dollar value of the penalty changes as the national average premium changes.

IV.   STANDARD PART D DRUG COVERAGE.

All Medicare beneficiaries have access to the standard drug benefit. The drug plans – PDP (stand-alone prescription drug plan) or MA-PDP (Medicare Advantage plan) – are allowed to provide limitations and restrictions on available drugs and other specifications, but the benefit offered must be at least equal to the standard benefit. For the standard benefit in 2012, the individual will pay:

> A monthly premium (which varies depending on the plan chosen). (See *Medicare, section V.C.2.*)
>
> A yearly deductible of $320 (2012);
>
> Twenty-five (25%) percent of the yearly drug costs of $2,610 (2012), representing the costs between $320 and $2,930 (initial coverage limit) which amounts to $652.50). The plan pays the other seventy-five (75%) (plan cost-share) which represents $1,957.5 (2012);
>
> One-hundred (100%) percent of the next additional out-of-pocket expenses of $3,725.50 (2012) in drug costs (sometimes referred to as the doughnut hole or coverage gap). The beneficiary must pay the plan's premiums while in the coverage

gap. The most the Part D eligible must pay out-of-pocket is $3,725.50 (2012);

After having spent $4,700 (2012) out of pocket (out-of-pocket threshold) – the total of the annual deductible ($320), the 25% copay of costs between the deductible and the initial coverage limit ($652.50), and the additional out-of-pocket expenses ($3,727.50) – the Part D beneficiary will have catastrophic coverage. The individual during this entire period of coverage will only have to pay $2.60 copayment for a generic or preferred brand Part D drug and $6.50 for other drugs or five-(5%) percent coinsurance, whichever is greater. The plan pays for the rest.

The deductible, initial coverage limit and annual out-of-pocket threshold increase (i.e., indexed for inflation) each year.

Rephrased for ready understanding, the foregoing payments of $4,700 by the beneficiary in 2012 are set forth in the table below:

Annual Deductible	$320.00
25% copay of costs between the $320 deductible and the initial coverage limit of $2,930	$652.50
Subtotal (annual deductible + copay)	$972.50
Additional out-of-pocket expenses (doughnut hole)	$3727.50
Out-of-pocket threshold	$4,700.00

V. ALTERNATIVE PRESCRIPTION DRUG COVERAGE PLAN.

Part D drug plans are not required to offer the standard benefit plan, but can offer alternative prescription drug coverage. Alternative coverage must be "actuarially equivalent" to the standard benefit. In an actuarially equivalent plan, the cost sharing varies through the use of such mechanisms as tiered copayments. However, a plan that offers an alternative benefit package cannot impose a higher annual deductible ($320 in 2012) or require a higher out-of-pocket threshold ($4,700 in 2012) than required by the standard benefit. Plans can offer enhanced alternative coverage that may include changes to the deductible and the initial coverage limit, though the deductible cannot be higher than $320 (2012).

Enhanced alternative coverage under Part D might include coverage of some drugs that are excluded under Part D, or that are in the coverage gap (doughnut hole). A PDP that wants to offer a drug plan with enhanced alternative coverage in a service area must also offer a PDP with a basic benefit prescription package in that area.

Note: In addition to the above drug coverage plan, Part D eligibles are offered a wide variety of drug plans which must abide by the requirements of the foregoing plans but may have variations such as gap coverage insurance, no deductibles, higher or lower premiums and/or copayments.

Note: The cheapest plan is not necessarily the best. Among things to consider are whether a plan carries a deductible, what it charges for copayments on individual drugs, whether it covers drugs in the doughnut hole, the amount of the premiums, and whether there are restrictions on some drugs.

VI. SUBSIDY PROGRAM.

The MMA provides for premium and cost-sharing payments (deductibles and copayments) subsidies of prescription drug coverage for certain individuals with low-income and resources (*see section VII* below). The purpose of the subsidy program is to assist Medicare beneficiaries with limited financial means, to pay for Medicare prescription drug coverage under Medicare Part D.

Resources include savings and stocks, but not an individual's home or car. If an individual qualifies, he/she will receive help paying for the Medicare drug plan's monthly premium, yearly deductible, and prescription copayments.

If an individual lives in Alaska or Hawaii, or pays more than half of the living expenses of dependent family members, income limits are higher. Puerto Rico, the Virgin Islands, Guam, the Northern Mariana Islands, and American Samoa have their own rules for providing extra help to their residents.

VII. SUBSIDIES FOR LOW-INCOME INDIVIDUALS.

A. Low-Income Beneficiaries.

A low-income beneficiary is a subsidy-eligible individual and according to income or status is (i) a full-subsidy-eligible individual (full-benefit dual eligible), (ii) an individual treated (deemed) as a full-subsidy dual eligible, or (iii) a partial-subsidy individual. These individuals are discussed below:

1.   **Subsidy-eligible individual**

A subsidy-eligible individual is eligible for Part D and (i) is enrolled in or seeking to enroll in a Part D plan, (ii) has an income below one-hundred fifty (150%) percent of the Federal poverty level, and (iii) has resources at or below the thresholds set forth below.

There are two groups of subsidy eligible low-income individuals. The first group is composed of persons who either:

> are enrolled in a prescription drug plan;
>
> have incomes below one-hundred thirty-five (135%) percent of the Federal poverty level; and
>
> have resources in 2012 below $8,440 for an individual (including $1,500 burial exclusion) and $13,410 (including $3,000 burial exclusion) for a couple (increased in future years by the percentage increase in the consumer price index (CPI); or
>
> are full-benefit dual eligibles without regard to income resources and without regard as to whether they meet other eligibility standards.

The second group of subsidy-eligible individuals is persons meeting the same requirements as above, except that the income level is above one-hundred thirty-five (135%) percent but below one-hundred fifty (150%) percent of the Federal poverty level, and an alternative resources standard is used. The alternative resource standard in 2012 is $13,070 for an individual (including burial exclusion) and $26,120 for a couple (including burial exclusion), increased in future years by the percentage increase in the CPI.

2.   **Full-subsidy eligible individuals**

A full-subsidy eligible individual has full Medicaid status (full-benefit dual eligible) and has (i) income below one-hundred thirty-five (135%) percent of the Federal poverty level and (ii) resources of not more than $8,440 (single person, 2012) or less than $13,410 (married couple), including $1,500 per person for burial expenses.

3. Individuals deemed as full-subsidy eligible

Individuals who are treated or deemed as full-subsidy eligibles are: i) recipients of Supplemental Security Income without Medicaid; ii) individuals with incomes below one-hundred thirty-five (135%) percent of individuals with incomes below one-hundred thirty-five (135%) percent of the Federal poverty level and countable resources of not more than $8,440 for an individual, and $13,410 for a couple, including $1,500 per person for burial expenses; and/or iii) individuals enrolled in one of the following Medicare Savings Programs (also called buy-in programs): Qualified Medicare Beneficiary (QMB); Specified Low-income Medicare Beneficiary (SLMB); or Qualifying Individual (QI) under a state's plan.

4. Partial-subsidy eligible individuals (non-deemed)

Partial-subsidy eligible individuals have income above one-hundred thirty-five (135%) percent of the Federal poverty Level, but income less than one-hundred fifty (150%) percent of the Federal poverty level and have resources that in 2012 do not exceed $13,070 if single, or $26,120 if married, including $1,500 for burial expenses.

B. Part D Drug Subsidies.

Subsidies for Part D drugs are provided to full-subsidy individuals (full-benefit dual eligibles), individuals deemed to be full-subsidy eligibles, and partial subsidy individuals as follows:

1. Full-subsidy eligible individuals.

The cost-sharing benefit for these eligible Medicaid recipients includes the following:

> No premiums;
>
> No deductible;
>
> No doughnut hole (i.e., continuation of coverage through the doughnut hole);
>
> Copayments:
> - Full benefit dual eligibles with incomes up to one-hundred (100%) percent of the Federal poverty level with copays of no more than $1.10 (2012) for generic or preferred brands or $3.30 for non-preferred brands up to the out-of-pocket threshold of $4,700 (2012).

- All other full subsidy individuals_will copay no more than $2.60 (2012) for generic or preferred brand or $6.50 (2012) for non-preferred brand name drugs, up to the out-of-pocket threshold of $4,700 (2012).

2.   **Deemed full-subsidy eligible individuals**

The cost-sharing benefit of these individuals includes the following:

No premiums;

No deductible;

No doughnut hole;

Copayment of $2.60 (2012) for generic or preferred brand drugs and $6.50 (2012) for non-preferred brand drugs, up to the out-of-pocket threshold of $4,700 (2012).

3.   **Partial-subsidy eligible individuals**

The cost-sharing benefit of the following individuals is set forth below:

(a)   Medicare beneficiaries, who are not eligible for Medicaid, with resources in 2012 less than $13,070 (for a single person) or less than $26,120 (for a married couple) and income below one-hundred thirty-five (135%) percent of the Federal poverty level. The cost-sharing benefit of these individuals include the following:

No premiums;

No deductible;

No doughnut hole;

Copayments (2012) of $2.60 for each generic drug and $6.50 for each brand name drug, after the out-of-pocket limit is reached ($4,700).

(b)   Medicare beneficiaries with resources in 2012 below $13,070 (for a single individual) or $26,120 (for a married couple), and income between one-hundred thirty-five (135%) percent and one-hundred fifty (150%) percent of the Federal poverty level. The cost-sharing benefit of these individuals includes the following:

A sliding scale monthly premium namely:

A premium subsidy equal to seventy-five (75%) percent of the premium subsidy for individuals with income greater than one-hundred thirty-five (135%) percent but at or below one-hundred forty (140%) percent of the Federal poverty level.

A premium subsidy equal to fifty (50%) percent of the premium subsidy standard for individuals with income greater than one-hundred forty (140%) percent but at or below one-hundred forty-five (145%) percent of the Federal poverty level.

A premium subsidy equal to twenty-five (25%) percent of the premium subsidy for individuals with income greater than one-hundred forty-five (145%) percent but below one-hundred fifty (150%) of the Federal poverty level applicable to family size.

No doughnut hole;

A $65 (2012) deductible;

Coinsurance of fifteen (15%) percent after the deductible, up to the out-of-pocket threshold of $4,700 (2012); and

Copayments (2012) of $2.60 for each generic or preferred brand drug or $6.50 for each non-preferred brand name drug, after the out-of-pocket limit of $4,700 (2012) is reached.

Note: There is no cost sharing for subsidy-eligible individuals residing in a medical facility which is defined as a nursing home, psychiatric center, residential treatment center, developmental center, intermediate care facility. Other group residences such as assisted living programs, group homes and adult homes are subject to copayments.

VIII. EMPLOYER-SPONSORED DRUG BENEFIT PROGRAMS FOR RETIREES.

Plans have been made available to employer-sponsors to prompt them through special subsidy payments to continue to provide retirees drug benefits. The special subsidy payment amount for a coverage year for a qualifying covered retiree enrolled with the sponsor of a qualified retiree prescription drug plan equals twenty-eight (28%) percent of the retiree's gross covered retiree plan-related prescription drug costs for a year greater than a "cost threshold" ($250), but not greater than the cost limit ($5,000) for plans that end in 2006. Such amounts are adjusted annually by the percentage increase in Medicare per capita prescription drug costs.

Some employer-sponsored health plans help retirees pay medical expenses which are not covered by Medicare. Those expenses could include copayments and deductibles, the catastrophic costs of severe illness and the cost of preventive care and prescription drugs, beyond what Medicare might pay. In an adverse turn for retirees, the Equal Employment Opportunity Commission has voted to allow employers to reduce or eliminate such health benefits for retirees when they become eligible for Medicare at age 65. The Commission approved a rule saying that such cuts do not violate the civil rights law banning age discrimination. The rule creates an explicit exemption to the Age Discrimination in Employment Act of 1967; in practice, it allows employers to reduce health benefits for retirees when they become eligible for Medicare at the age of 65. However, for the moment, due to the pressures exerted by AARP, which represents millions of Americans age 50 and older, the Commission is holding back in enforcing its ruling. It is important to note that a Federal Appeals Court ruled in 2000 that such age-based distinctions were unlawful.

IX. MEDIGAP INSURANCE POLICIES – PROHIBITED USE.

Starting in January 1, 2006, insurance companies may not sell existing Medigap policies that provide drug coverage to Medicare beneficiaries who are enrolled in or eligible for the new Medicare out-patient prescription drug coverage. They are, however, able to renew the Medigap drug policies issued prior to January 1, 2006 for beneficiaries who do not opt for the new Medicare outpatient prescription drug coverage. For Medicare beneficiaries with Medigap drug policies who enroll in a new Medicare outpatient prescription drug plan, their Medigap policy will be modified to eliminate drug coverage, and premiums will be adjusted. Beneficiaries with the new Medicare drug coverage can purchase Medigap policies that do not cover drugs.

X.   MEDICARE CANNOT NEGOTIATE DRUG DISCOUNTS.

The MMA prohibits the government from negotiating discounts on drugs purchases or otherwise interfering in drug pricing decisions.

(continued on next page)

MEDICARE/OUTPATIENT SKILLED THERAPY

INTRODUCTION

Generally Medicare will pay for outpatient physical and occupational therapy, including speech-language pathology services, received as part of a patient's treatment in a doctor's office or as an outpatient of a participating hospital, skilled nursing facility, or through a home health agency, approved clinic, rehabilitative agency or public health agency, if the services are furnished under a plan established by a physician or therapist and the following conditions set forth in sections I – IV below are satisfied; and payment for the services is made as specified in sections V and VI below. A more definitive description of the foregoing is set forth below.

I. HOMEBOUND NOT A REQUIREMENT.

Skilled therapy services may be furnished to a Medicare beneficiary, whether or not homebound, on an outpatient basis by a participating hospital, skilled nursing facility, clinic, rehabilitation center, comprehensive outpatient rehabilitation facility, public health agency, or also, if the beneficiary is not homebound, by a home health agency. The provided services are covered as one of the "medical and other health services" under Medicare Part B.

Instead of obtaining skilled therapy services from a participating Medicare facility, patients can receive services directly from private practicing, Medicare-approved therapists performing such services in their office or in the patient's home, if such treatment is prescribed by a doctor.

II. REASONABLE AND NECESSARY REQUIREMENT.

The therapy services, to be covered by Medicare, must be reasonable and necessary. To be considered such, the services must be a specific, safe and effective treatment for the beneficiary's condition. The required services must be sufficiently complex or the condition of the beneficiary such that the services can be performed only by a qualified therapist. There also must be an expectation that the beneficiary's condition will improve materially in a reasonably predictable period of time or that such services are necessary to establish a safe maintenance program. The services must relate directly and specifically to a treatment regimen established by a physician, after any needed consultation with the qualified therapist, and designed to treat the beneficiary's illness or injury. The therapy services cannot merely relate to activities for the general physical welfare of the beneficiary.

III.   PHYSICIAN'S CARE PLAN AND CERTIFICATION.

In addition to being reasonable and necessary, outpatient therapy services must meet the following conditions:

The outpatient must be under the care of a physician.

Services must be furnished and related directly to and specifically under a written plan of care established by a physician or the therapist who will provide the therapy services. The plan must be established before the treatment is begun and reviewed by the attending physician in consultation with the therapist at least every thirty (30) days.

The physician must certify at intervals of at least every thirty (30) days that a continuing need exists for such services and should estimate how long the services will be needed.

Recertification should be obtained at the time the plan of treatment is reviewed.

IV.   APPLICABLE STANDARDS .

Medicare will not make payment for outpatient occupational therapy services or outpatient physical therapy, furnished as an incident to a physician's professional services, that do not meet the standards applicable to a therapist furnishing such services in a clinic, rehabilitation agency or public health agency.

V.   AMOUNT OF PAYMENT BY PATIENT.

The provider of therapy services, other than a hospital outpatient department, may charge the patient any part of the Medicare Part B annual deductible not met, and the twenty- (20%) percent copayment of the Medicare-approved charge. However, if an individual receives outpatient services at a hospital outpatient department, as opposed to the other settings, his/her copayment is twenty (20%) percent of the hospital bill – a much higher amount than the standard copayment of twenty (20%) percent. However, this disparity gradually will diminish so that the copayment in time will equal the standard copayment.

VI. FINANCIAL LIMITATIONS (CAP).

Until December 31, 2001, payments by Medicare to beneficiaries for outpatient physical therapy services, which include speech-language pathology, were not subject to any charge limit. Beginning in 2002, an annual limit of $1,500 was applied to all outpatient physical therapy services, including speech language pathology, except services in a hospital outpatient department (which has no cap). A separate $1,500 limitation applied to occupational therapy. Thereafter these limitations were suspended for the period between December 8, 2003 and December 31, 2005; the suspension ended on December 31, 2005. Financial limitations on outpatient therapy services resumed on those services effective January 1, 2006. The annual limit on the allowed amount for outpatient physical therapy and speech pathology combined is $1,870 (2012); the limit for occupational therapy is $1,870 (2012). The limits apply to outpatient Part B therapy services in all settings except outpatient hospital services and hospital emergency rooms.

VII. TYPES OF THERAPISTS.

The types of therapists are set forth below:

Physical Therapist. A physical therapist has a bachelor's degree and also some postgraduate training. Physical therapy is frequently needed by a patient who has lost some use of his or her limbs or muscles because of an illness or accident.

After reviewing the physician's medical diagnosis and treatment plan, a physical therapist may visit the patient at home, as required under a plan of care. The therapist generally prepares a treatment schedule

and visits the patient on a routine basis until determining, after consultation with the physician, that therapy is no longer necessary or advisable.

Speech-language Pathologist. A speech-language pathologist has a graduate degree and is certified by the American Speech Language Hearing Association. A speech-language pathologist can assess the patient's problem, design a treatment program, and provide therapy to help the patient regain or maintain speech or language skills.

Occupational Therapist. An occupational therapist has either a bachelor's or master's degree with special training in occupational therapy. Such a therapist may be needed by a patient who has suffered an illness or injury which has affected daily activities, movement or perceptual abilities. The occupational therapist evaluates the patient's ability to dress, wash, walk or perform other routine functions and, when necessary, provides devices which add to the patient's comfort. Examples include using larger buttons on clothes to facilitate dressing; adding a board to the arm of a wheelchair to help support a patient's paralyzed arm; and providing a leg or ankle splint to aid in walking.

(continued on next page)

MEDICARE/PREVENTIVE DISEASE

INTRODUCTION

Medicare Part B covers the preventative disease management services set forth below.

I. ANNUAL PROSTATE CANCER SCREENING TESTS.

Annual prostate cancer screening tests for men age 50 or over, including digital rectal exam and prostate-specific antigen (PSA) blood tests. Neither the Part B $140 (2012) annual deductible nor the twenty- (20%) percent coinsurance apply to the PSA test, but they do apply to the digital rectal exam.

II. SCREENING PAP SMEARS, SCREENING PELVIC EXAM.

Screening pap smears for early detection of cervical cancer is covered every three (3) years. The coverage is authorized on a yearly basis for women at high risk if developing cervical or vaginal cancer and for women of child bearing age who have had a negative test in the three (3) preceding years. The Part B annual deductible is waived for screening pap smears and pelvic exams, but the twenty- (20%) percent coinsurance must be paid by the beneficiary.

III. SCREENING MAMMOGRAPHY.

Screening mammography, which is defined as a radiologic procedure provided to a woman for the early detection of breast cancer, including a physician's interpretation of the results of the procedure. For women age 40 and over, screening under normal circumstances is covered every twelve (12) months. For women age 30-39, Medicare will help pay for one baseline mammogram. The Part B annual deductible is waived, but not the twenty- (20%) percent coinsurance amount.

IV. CARDIOVASCULAR SCREENING BLOOD TESTS.

Cardiovascular screening blood tests to patients at risk every two (2) years, services for which beneficiaries would not have to meet a deductible or co-pay. At-risk individuals eligible for screening include those with hypertension, dyslipidemia, obesity or a family history of diabetes. This benefit provides blood tests for the early detection of cardiovascular disease or elevated risk of cardiovascular disease by testing total cholesterol levels, high-density lipoprotein, and triglycerides levels. There is no coinsurance on Part B deductible for lab tests. For all other tests, the beneficiary must pay twenty (20%) percent of the Medicare-approved amounts, after the Part B deductible.

V.   DIABETES SCREENINGS.

Diabetes screenings for certain beneficiaries who are considered at high risk for developing the disease. The screenings include a fasting plasma glucose test. Patients who meet the at-risk criteria can be screened up to twice each year, and are not required to meet a deductible or co-pay for the tests. There is no coinsurance or Part B deductible for diabetes screening tests. For all other tests and services, the beneficiary must pay twenty (20%) percent of the Medicare-approved amount after the yearly Part B deductible.

VI.   COLORECTAL CANCER SCREENING TESTS.

Fecal-occult blood tests (FOBT) annually; flexible sigmoidoscopies (FSO) every four (4) years, and colonoscopy (CO) once every two (2) years (if at high risk) for beneficiaries age 50 and older to screen for colorectal cancer. No Part B deductible, or coinsurance for FOBT. For FSO and CO, the beneficiary must pay twenty (20%) percent of the Medicare-approved amount, and, in the case of FSO only, and not CO, the yearly Part B deductible. If the test is done in a hospital outpatient department, the beneficiary must pay twenty-five (25%) percent of the Medicare-approved amount after (where applicable) the yearly Part B deductible.

VII. GLAUCOMA SCREENING.

Glaucoma screening is covered once in every twelve (12) months for people who are at high risk for glaucoma, including people with diabetes, a family history of glaucoma, or African Americans age fifty (50) or older. The beneficiary must pay twenty (20%) percent of the Medicare-approved amount after the yearly Part B deductible.

VIII. ULTRASOUND SCREENING FOR ABDOMINAL AORTA ANEURISM.

Screening of abdominal aortic aneurisms for Medicare beneficiaries as of January 1, 2007: (i) who receive a referral for an ultrasound screening as a result of an initial preventive physical examination, (ii) who have not been previously furnished such an ultrasound screening, and (iii) who either have a family history of abdominal aortic aneurisms or manifest risk factors included in a beneficiary category recommended for screening by the United States Preventive Services Task Force regarding abdominal aortic aneurisms. There is no required Part B deductible.

IX.   PREVENTIVE PHYSICALS.

Beneficiaries are eligible, within twelve (12) months of first becoming eligible for Medicare, for a "Welcome to Medicare Physical," consisting of a comprehensive exam (not including lab tests). This initial one-time preventive physical also includes education, counseling, and referrals to other preventive services.

A Medicare beneficiary who had had Medicare Part B for longer than twelve (12) months can get a yearly Wellness Visit to develop or update a personalized prevention plan based on his/her current health and risk factors. The first year wellness exam cannot take place within twelve (12) months of the Welcome to Medicare physical exam. The beneficiary need not pay anything for this exam if the doctor accepts assignment. The exam is covered once every twelve (12) months.

NOTE:

(i) Many vascular specialists say two diagnostic tests – carotid ultrasound and the ankle-brachial test – can provide a clear window into artery disease that can lead to strokes, heart attacks and related lethal events. Despite being two decades old, the carotid ultrasound and ankle-brachial tests often are overlooked. Many general practitioners haven't embraced the tests, in large part because Medicare and insurers do not pay for them as screening tools. However, if a doctor writes a referral for one based on the patient's risk-factor profile, the cost of the screening, if done at a hospital vascular laboratory, usually may be reimbursed.

(ii) The Centers for Medicare and Medicaid Services (CMS) has expanded Medicare coverage of positron emission tomography (PET scan) when used to confirm Alzheimer's disease diagnosis, to include some Medicare beneficiaries with suspected Alzheimer's disease and to include other beneficiaries at risk for Alzheimer's disease who are enrolled in a large and easily accessible clinical trial. Medicare beneficiaries who meet specific criteria may participate in the clinical trial and receive a PET scan.

X.   OBESITY SCREENING AND COUNSELING.

If a beneficiary has a body mass index of thirty (30) or more, Medicare covers intensive counseling to him/her lose weight. This counseling may be covered if obtained in a primary care setting, where it can be coordinated with his/her comprehensive prevention plan.

XI.   DEPRESSION SCREENING.

Medicare covers one depression screening per year for all beneficiaries. The screening must be done in a primary care setting that can provide follow-up treatment and referrals. The outpatient beneficiary pays nothing if the doctor or other health care professional accepts assignment.

XII.   ALCOHOL MISUSE COUNSELING.

Medicare covers one alcohol misuse screening per year for adult beneficiaries (including pregnant women) who misuse alcohol but aren't alcohol dependent and are competent and alert during counseling. Beneficiaries who screen positive can get up to four (4) brief face-to-face counseling sessions per year. A qualified primary care doctor or other primary care provider must provide the counseling in a primary care setting. The patient pays nothing if the doctor or other health care provider accepts assignment.

(continued on next page)

MEDICARE/PRIVATE CONTRACTS

INTRODUCTION

Physicians and certain other practitioners can opt out of Medicare and ask their Medicare patients to sign private contracts if beneficiaries want to receive these services. The providers who enter into such contracts include doctors of medicine and osteopathy, podiatrists, dentists, optometrists, clinical social workers, clinical psychiatrists, physicians' assistants, nurse practitioners, clinical nurse practitioners, clinical nurse specialists, certified nurses, nurse anesthetists and certified nurse midwives. These private contracts are treated as outside the Medicare system. As such, a physician or practitioner may not receive from Medicare, or from an organization that receives Medicare reimbursement, any payment for any item or services furnished to a patient. In other words, Medicare will not pay nor reimburse, directly or indirectly, for health services under a private contract. Private contracts are subject to the requirements that are set forth below.

I.   BENEFICIARY PROTECTIONS.

A private contract:

     (i)   must be written and signed by the beneficiary before any item or service is provided pursuant to the contract

     (ii)   may not be entered into at a time when a beneficiary is facing an emergency or urgent health care situation

     (iii)   must fully indicate that a beneficiary, by signing the contract: (i) agrees not to submit a claim for services even if they were otherwise covered under Medicare; (ii) agrees to be responsible whether through insurance or otherwise for payment of such items of services and understands that no Medicare reimbursement will be provided; and (iii) acknowledges that: no Medicare limiting charges apply (i.e., no limit to balance billing). (Medigap plans do not, and other supplemental insurance plans may not elect not to, make payment for items of services rendered. The Medicare beneficiary has the right to have such items or services provided by other physicians or practitioners to whom Medicare payment will be made.); and

(iv) must indicate whether the physician or practitioner is excluded from Medicare participation.

II. NO LIMITING CHARGES.

Medicare limiting charges (charge limits) do not apply to private contracts. In other words, there are no balance billing restrictions.

III. PHYSICIAN'S OR PRACTITIONER'S REQUIRED AFFIDAVIT.

At the time services are provided under a private contract, the physician or practitioner must have a signed affidavit in effect. It must state that the physician or practitioner will not submit any Medicare claim for any item or service provided to any Medicare beneficiary, and will not receive any reimbursement for any such item of service, for a two- (2) year period beginning on the date the affidavit is signed. A copy of the affidavit must be filed with the Secretary of HHS within ten (10) days after the first private contract to which the affidavit applies is entered into.

Should a physician or practitioner signing the affidavit knowingly and willfully submit a Medicare claim, or receive Medicare reimbursement, for an item or service during such two- (2) year period, the ability to provide services under the private contract will cease for the remainder of the period. Further, the physician or practitioner may not receive any Medicare payments during such period.

(continued on next page)

MEDICARE/PROSPECTIVE PAYMENT SYSTEM

INTRODUCTION

Medicare requires that a predetermined prospective payment system (PPS) as opposed to a retrospective cost-based system of payment, be used to determine Medicare reimbursement for the following covered services: inpatient hospital, skilled nursing, hospital outpatient department and home health services. Outpatient rehabilitation services are excluded as covered services under the outpatient PPS. The prospective payment for outpatient rehabilitation services and for services at a comprehensive outpatient rehabilitation facility (CORF) is the Medicare physician fee schedule.

I. INPATIENT HOSPITAL SERVICES.

Medicare pays for most inpatient hospital care under a prospective payment system. Under it, hospitals, excluding certain specialty hospitals such as cancer hospitals), are paid a predetermined rate for each hospital discharge regardless of costs incurred for inpatient services furnished to Medicare beneficiaries. The predetermined rates are based on payment categories called "diagnosis-related groups" (DRGs). Hence, upon an individual being admitted to a hospital, he/she is assigned a DRG. Medicare will pay the hospital a flat fee as a prospective payment, based upon the diagnosis of the patient, instead of paying retrospectively on a day to day individualized basis.

Medicare pays for the inpatient services on the basis of a rate per discharge that varies by the DRG to which a beneficiary's stay is assigned. The formula used to calculate payment for a specific case takes an individual hospital's payment rate per case and multiplies it by the weight of the DRG to which the case is assigned.

Each DRG weight represents the average resources required to care for cases in that particular DRG relative to the average resources used to treat cases in all DRGs.

When a beneficiary has a medically necessary stay that is much longer and more expensive for the hospital than an average case covered by the appropriate DRG, the hospital must receive additional Medicare coverage, called outlier payments.

II. SKILLED NURSING FACILITY SERVICES.

Historically, Medicare reimbursed most SNF care on a retrospective costs basis. Thus, after services were delivered, SNFs were paid for reasonable costs that they incurred for the care provided. These costs were divided into three major categories – routine services (e.g., nursing, room and board); ancillary services (e.g., therapy and laboratory services); and capital-related costs (e.g., lease payments, taxes). With the advent of the Balanced Budget Act of 1997, Medicare payments to SNFs over three (3) years were gradually shifted from cost-based reimbursement to prospective payment.

Under the prospective payment system, SNFs are paid through prospective Federal per diem payment rates applicable to all SNF services. These rates cover all the costs of furnishing covered skilled nursing services – that is, routine service costs (including Part A skilled nursing care benefits as well as services for which payment may be made under Part B), ancillary and capital-related costs. The prospective payments methodology does not cover the services of health care professionals such as physicians, nurse practitioners, physician assistants and psychologists.

The Federal per diem rate incorporates adjustments to account for the relative resource utilization of different patient types. This classification system, known as Resource Utilization Groups, Version III, is based on a beneficiary's assessment, using the minimum data set to assign beneficiaries to one of forty-four (44) groups. The Federal rates are further adjusted by a hospital wage index to account for geographic variations in wages and by use of a SNF market basket.

III. HOSPITAL OUTPATIENT DEPARTMENT SERVICES.

A system of prospective payment governs hospital outpatient department (OPD) services such as hospital outpatient surgery, radiology and other diagnostic services covered by Medicare upon admission to a hospital. This system does not apply to physical and occupational therapy and speech-language pathology or to ambulance services which are paid under a Medicare physician fee schedule. To implement this system, the Secretary of HHS is required to: establish a classified system for the covered OPD services, relative payment rates for these services and an annual conversion factor to determine OPD fee schedule amounts and to compute for each covered service an amount equal to the product of the conversion factor determined by CMS for the year, and the relative payment rate for the service.

CMS has classified all covered OPD services into groups called Ambulatory payment classifications (APC). Each APC consists of clinically similar services requiring comparable resources. A payment rate is established for each APC.

IV. OUTPATIENT REHABILITATION SERVICES.

Since 1999, the Medicare physician fee schedule (MPFS) has been the method of prospective payment for outpatient physical therapy (which includes outpatient speech-language pathology) and occupational therapy services furnished by:

> Hospitals to outpatients and inpatients whose stay is not covered by Medicare Part A;

> SNFs to residents whose stay is not covered by Part A to non-residents who receive outpatient rehabilitation services from the SNF;

> Home health agencies to individuals who are not homebound or otherwise are not receiving services under a home health plan of treatment; and

> Rehabilitation agencies (e.g., outpatient physical therapy providers and CORFs).

Therapy services are billed to the appropriate fiscal intermediary; assignment is mandatory.

The MPFS does not apply to outpatient rehabilitation services furnished by critical access hospitals which are paid on a reasonable cost basis.

V HOME HEALTH SERVICES.

Medicare historically reimbursed home health agencies (HHA) on a retrospective cost basis under Part A and Part B. After delivery of the services, the agencies were paid for the reasonable costs incurred for the care they provided, subject to certain limits. The Balanced Budget Act of 1997 required the Secretary of HHS (now CMS) to establish a prospective payment system (PPS) for home health services provided by HHAs. In establishing the home health PPS, the Secretary was required to consider an appropriate number of units of service and the characteristics of services provided within each unit.

Under the PPS rules adopted by CMS, Medicare is required to pay HHAs for all home health services (including medical supplies) except osteoporosis drugs which continue to be paid on a reasonable cost basis. Durable medical equipment (DME) continues to be paid under the DME fee schedule in an amount that is additional to the PPS payment rate for home health services.

Medicare's unit of payment to HHAs under the PPS is a sixty- (60) day episode. The payment is referred to an unadjusted national prospective sixty- (60) day episode payment. This is a predetermined rate that is subject to certain adjustments and additions such as schedule changes, geographic differences in wage levels, and annual updating of episode payment rates.

Home health resource groups (HHRG) are the basis of payment of each episode. The appropriate HHRG is determined after the results of a comprehensive assessment of a beneficiary, based on the outcome and assessment information set, are input into a computer software package. If the number of therapy services delivered during an episode does not meet a threshold of ten (10) therapy visits, the HHRG will be adjusted downward.

So that HHAs can maintain their cash flow, payments are split in two in each sixty- (60) day episode, one billed at the beginning of an episode and the other as a residual payment at the end of an episode. For the initial episode, the initial payment by Medicare is sixty (60%) percent of the anticipated payment, and the final residual payment is forty (40%) percent. For subsequent episodes, the payments are split equally in half.

A HHA may request CMS to make the initial payment based on the verbal orders of the beneficiary's physician provided that they are recorded in the plan of care and included a description of the patient's condition and the services to be provided by the HHA. The plan of care must be reviewed by the physician at least every sixty (60) days, or more frequently when a beneficiary has elected to transfer from one HHA to another or when there is a significant change of conditions or upon discharge.

---

*Medicare Advantage Plans/Medicare

A Medicare Advantage Plan (like an HMO or PPO) is another Medicare health plan choice you may have as part of Medicare. Medicare Advantage Plans, sometimes called "Part C" or "MA Plans," are offered by private companies approved by Medicare.

If you join a Medicare Advantage Plan, the plan will provide all of your Part A (Hospital Insurance) and Part B (Medical Insurance) coverage. In all types of Medicare Advantage Plans, you're always covered for emergency and urgent care. Medicare Advantage Plans must cover all of the services that Original Medicare covers except hospice care. Original Medicare covers hospice care even if you're in a Medical Advantage Plan. Medicare Advantage Plans aren't supplemental coverage.

Medicare Advantage Plans may offer extra coverage, such as vision, hearing, dental, and/or health and wellness programs. Most include Medicare prescription drug coverage (Part D). In addition to your Part B premium, you usually pay one monthly premium for the services included.

Medicare pays a fixed amount for your care every month to the companies offering Medicare Advantage Plans. These companies must follow rules set by Medicare. However, each Medicare Advantage Plan can charge different out-of-pocket costs and have different rules for how you get services (like whether you need a referral to see a specialist or if you have to go to only doctors, facilities, or suppliers that belong to the plan for non-emergency or non-urgent care). These rules can change each year.

There are different types of Medicare Advantage Plans:

> *Health Maintenance Organization (HMO) Plans.*
>
> *Preferred Provider Organization (PPO) Plans.*
>
> *Private Fee-for-Service (PFFS) Plans.*
>
> *Special Needs Plans (SNP).*

<u>*There are other less common types of Medicare Advantage Plans that may be available:*</u>

> ***HMO Point-of-Service (HMOPOS) Plans*** *– An HMO plan that may allow you to get some services out-of-network for a higher cost.*

Medical Savings Account (MSA) Plans – *A plan that combines a high deductible health plan with a bank account. Medicare deposits money into the account (usually less than the deductible). You can use the money to pay for your health care services during the year.*

As with Original Medicare, you still have Medicare rights and protections, including the right to appeal.

You can join a Medicare Advantage Plan even if you have a pre-existing condition, except for End-Stage Renal Disease.

You can only join or leave a plan at certain times during the year.

If you go to a doctor, facility, or supplier that doesn't belong to the plan, your services may not be covered, or your costs could be higher, depending on the type of Medicare Advantage Plan. In most cases, this applies to Medicare Advantage HMOs and PPOs.

If the plan decides to stop participating in Medicare, you will have to join another Medicare health plan or return to Original Medicare.

You usually get prescription drug coverage (Part D) through the plan. In some types of plans that don't offer drug coverage, you can join a Medicare Prescription Drug Plan. If you're in a Medicare Advantage Plan that includes prescription drug coverage and you join a Medicare Prescription Drug Plan, you will be disenrolled from your Medicare Advantage Plan and returned to Original Medicare. You can't have prescription drug coverage through both a Medicare Advantage Plan and a Medicare Prescription Drug Plan.

You can generally join a Medicare Advantage Plan if you meet these conditions:

You have Part A and Part B.

You live in the service area of the plan.

You don't have End-Stage Renal Disease (ESRD) (permanent kidney failure requiring dialysis or a kidney transplant) except as previously explained.

(continued on next page)

MEDICARE ADVANTAGE (MA) PROGRAM

INTRODUCTION

In the early 1980s Congress enacted the Tax Equity and Fiscal Responsibility Act of 1982 (TEFRA). TEFRA authorized Medicare to offer the voluntary option to Medicare beneficiaries to receive Medicare benefits (Parts A and B) through private health maintenance organizations (HMOs), as an alternative to, rather than from, Medicare (traditional or original Medicare). The TEFRA program is described in section I below. (See also *Health Maintenance Organization (HMO)*)

The Balanced Budget Act of 1997 (BBA) established a new Part C of the Medicare program, known as the Medicare+Choice (M+C) program (see section II).

In 2003, Congress enacted the Medicare Prescription Drug Improvement and Modernization Act (MMA) replacing the Medicare+Choice program with the Medicare Advantage (MA) Program (see section III).

The following MA subjects mentioned in this overview are discussed in detail in the next eleven (11) successive Overviews:

> Common Features of MA Plan;
> Coordinated Care Plans – Common Features;
> Eligibility and Enrollment, Medicare Advantage Plans
> HMO plans with and without point-of-service option;
> Preferred Provider Organization Plan;
> Provider-sponsored Organization Plan;
> Religious Fraternal Benefit Plan;
> Regional Preferred Provider Organization Plan;
> Medical Savings Account Plans;
> Private Fee-for-Services Plans; and
> Outpatient Prescription Drug Plans

I. TEFRA HMO PROGRAM – REPLACED BY M+C PROGRAM (MEDICARE PART C).

Three (3) types of HMOs were created by TEFRA: (i) a private entity commonly known as a risk HMO, sometimes as a TEFRA risk contract, that entered into a risk contract with Medicare to provide Medicare benefits to Medicare beneficiaries; (ii) an entity, commonly known as a cost-basis HMO or which cost-reimbursement HMO, sometimes as a TEFRA cost-basis contract, that had a cost contract with Medicare to furnish Medicare benefits to Medicare beneficiaries; and (iii) a health care prepayment plan, a form of Medicare managed care that consisted of cost contracts for only Medicare Part B service to Medicare beneficiaries. These contracts with Medicare are described below (see *sections A, B, and C*):

A. Risk HMO Plans.

The word "risk" in the term risk HMO referred to the contractual arrangement a health plan had with Health Care Finance Administration (HCFA, now known as the Centers for Medicare and Medicaid Services, CMS). Medicare risk HMOs agreed to accept a set amount from HCFA to care for a Medicare beneficiary. The classic risk HMO was responsible for delivering broad care, at least the services Medicare covers, and it accepted the risk that if costs for a particular beneficiary be higher than the set amount, it bore the loss.

These risk HMOs provided Medicare Part A and B benefits, other than hospice, to Medicare enrollees who were entitled to both programs. Thus, inpatient hospital care and some skilled nursing facility care were available to Medicare enrollees. The same coverage time limits that applied to the traditional fee-for-service Medicare plan applied to Medicare HMO coverage.

Medicare HMO enrollees were locked into risk HMOs, except for emergency and urgent care. To receive care, to see specialists, or to be admitted to a hospital, the enrollee was required to get prior approval from his/her primary care doctor, sometimes called the gatekeeper. Enrollees were limited to doctors associated with the HMO. All services, except emergency and urgent care, received by the risk enrollee which were outside the HMO medical network were required to be paid for by the enrollee and were not paid for or reimbursed by Medicare. Commencing in 1996, these HMOs were authorized to provide an out-of-network option known as point of service (POS) under which beneficiaries were not locked into network providers but could use a non-network provider.

Medicare paid risk HMOs a fixed capitated amount (capitation) for each Medicare beneficiary enrolled in the HMO to cover Part A and Part B benefits customarily provided by Medicare.

Although a risk HMO was permitted to charge for deductibles and copayments, customarily it waived both. In lieu of such charges, the HMO could, but usually did not, charge the enrollee a premium or membership fee. Risk HMO plans usually offered supplemental benefits not covered by Medicare for little or no additional cost. In large part, these benefits took the place of those provided by a Medigap policy. Benefits could include preventive care, prescription drugs, dental care, hearing aids and eyeglasses. In contrast with traditional Medicare, enrollees in Medicare HMO plans avoided the need to complete claims forms, and deductibles and coinsurance payments were usually not required of beneficiaries.

B. Cost-Basis HMO Plans.

If, among other reasons, an otherwise eligible HMO did not have the capacity to bear the risk of potential losses under a risk-sharing contract, the Secretary of Health and Human Services was authorized to enter into a cost-basis contract pursuant to which the organization would be reimbursed on the basis of its reasonable costs.

As with risk HMO enrollees, enrollees of most cost-basis HMOs were entitled to all Part A and Part B services except hospice care. Unlike risk HMO enrollees, cost-basis enrollees were not locked in and could seek services either through the HMO or other sources. If outside providers were used, then the out-of-pocket costs of the enrollee were higher.

Medicare paid cost-basis HMOs the reasonable costs that they might incur in providing Medicare beneficiaries services customarily covered under Parts A and B, less the estimated charges of beneficiary cost sharing.

Enrollees in cost-basis HMOs paid a considerably higher premium than did risk enrollees. Unless the plan provided otherwise, cost-basis HMO enrollees were required to pay for supplemental services obtained from the HMO above those covered by Medicare. However, a plan was not allowed to charge a Medicare beneficiary more than a maximum amount set by Medicare.

C. Health Care Prepayment Plan.

A private health care prepayment plan was a form of Medicare managed care that consisted of cost contracts for Medicare Part B services only. The contracting private health plan was paid by Medicare for all reasonable costs for Part B services that were provided under the plan.

The foregoing TEFRA plans were impacted, and additional private managed care plans were authorized, by the Medicare+Choice program under the Balanced Budget Act of 1997 (BBA). The Medicare+Choice program is briefly described in section II below.

II. MEDICARE+CHOICE (M+C) PROGRAM (MEDICARE PART C).

A. BBA Established the M+C Program.

The Balanced Budget Act of 1997 (BBA) established a new Part C of the Medicare program, known as the Medicare+Choice (M+C) program.

While, with the advent of BBA, no new TEFRA risk HMO contracts could be made, existing contracts could continue through 1998, and effective January 1, 1999, they could contract with HCFA (now known as CMS) only as Medicare+Choice plans. Cost-basis HMO contracts could not be extended or renewed beyond December 31, 2002 (later extended by subsequent legislations), unless two (2) other Medicare+Choice plans entered the cost-basis contracts' service area. Health care prepayment HMO plans were extinguished effective August 5, 1997.

The primary goal of the M+C program was to provide Medicare beneficiaries with a wider range of private health plan choices through which to obtain their Medicare Part B benefits. The BBA authorized Medicare to contract with private organizations offering a variety of private health plan options for beneficiaries, including certain traditional managed care plans (such as HMOs that had been offered under TEFRA, mentioned above).

All Medicare eligibles entitled to Medicare Part A and enrolled under Medicare Part B, except for individuals with end-stage renal disease, could elect to receive the basic Part A/B Medicare benefits either through the traditional (original) Medicare program, or the M+C plans.

All Medicare eligibles were given the continuing opportunity to switch among Medicare+Choice plans described below, or to original Medicare during the annual election period.

B. Types of M+C Plans.

BBA created three general categories of M+C plans:

Coordinated Care Plans. These consist of the following:

Health maintenance organizations (HMOs) with or without point of service options;

Provider-sponsored organizations (PSOs);

Preferred provider organizations (PPOs);

Religious fraternal benefit plans (RFBs).

Medical Savings Accounts (MSAs).

Private Fee-for-Service (PFFS).

C. Capitation.

Historically, contributions to Medicare HMOs by Medicare under risk contracts were calculated by using the average adjusted per capita cost payment formula (AAPCC) of providing health care to Medicare beneficiaries. AAPCC is an estimate of the average per capita amount spent by Medicare for each beneficiary in receipt of care under a traditional/original Medicare plan.

The BBA, in replacement of AAPCC, established a new administered pricing system of reimbursement to M+C organizations:

> Under the BBA, M+C capitation payments were made to all plans and were determined in the same manner. The HHS was required to make payments a month in advance to each M+C organization for each M+C beneficiary in the plan's payment area, in an amount equal to one-twelfth (1/12) of the annual M+C capitation rate.
>
> The actual rate was a new 50/50 blended capitation under an adjusted community rate (ACR) process, and represented a blend of the local historical per capita cost in each county and the national average per capita costs, adjusted for local differences in the price of care. All plans, except MSAs, were required to reflect and be based upon the ACR. In the event the ACR was lower than the annual capitation payment, then the plan was required to offer additional benefits at no additional charge or return the excess to Medicare. The blended rate was phased in over six (6) years.
>
> Capitation payments were adjusted for age, gender, Medicare eligibility and the institutional status of the individual beneficiary.
>
> In the instance of MSAs, if the premium under the MSA plans was less than one-half of the Medicare+Choice capitation rate, HHS was required to deposit an amount equal to the difference into the individual's MSA.

All plans, except PFFS and MSAs, were required to accept the Medicare+Choice capitation as payment in full for the Medicare basic (Part A/B) benefit package.

With the advent of subsequent legislation (see section III.D below), the foregoing pricing system to calculate the capitation payment to Medicare+Choice plans was replaced by a bidding methodology.

III. MEDICARE ADVANTAGE PROGRAM.

See *Medicare Advantage plan (MAP)/Common Features*

On December 8, 2003, Congress enacted the Medicare Prescription Drug, Improvement and Modernization Act of 2003 (MMA) (i) replacing the M+C program (albeit retaining most of the key features of the M+C program), with the Medicare Advantage program, and its array of private managed care plans and establishing Medicare Part D (prescription drug coverage).

The highlights of the Medicare Advantage (MA) program are set forth below (A – F).

A. Prescription Drug Coverage (Medicare Part D).

MMA allows (and in some cases requires) most MA plans to offer Part D prescription drug coverage. (See *Medicare Advantage/Outpatient Prescription Drugs.*)

B. Additional Coordinated Care Plans.

Under the MMA, beneficiaries have expanded M+C managed care plans with two (2) additional choices of coordinated care plan options: Regional Preferred Provider Organization (PPO) plans and Specialized MA Plans for Special Needs Individuals (SNPs):

Regional Plans

MMA expanded the single type of Medicare + Choice PPO into two types under the Medicare Advantage program of the MMA, by including regional and local coordinated PPOs.

In the enactment of the MMA, MA regional plans represent an effort to increase beneficiaries' choice of plans across all regions of the country, including rural areas. Prior to MMA, each local PPO Medicare plan selected the area (on a county-to-county basis) in which it offered service. Most MA plans were offered only in urban areas. (Local PPOs are popular health plan options in the under-65 market, because they offer the advantage of cost savings from care coordination combined with the ability to see any provider.)

To foster the formation of regional PPO plans, a moratorium was imposed in the first two (2) years of the formation of regional plans, on the formation or expansion of new local plans that operated as PPOs. However, until December 31, 2007, local PPO plans in the current demonstration areas were authorized.

The regional plans are subject to different payment and other rules than MA local PPO plans, but are structured as PPOs. While local PPO plans may choose the counties in which they wish to operate as MA plans, Regional plans must cover an entire region; regions are designated by CMS.

Specialized Plans for Specialized Needs Beneficiaries (SNPs)

The SNPs may limit their enrollment to special needs beneficiaries, or they may serve a disproportionate percentage of special needs beneficiaries, thus ensuring that the health care needs of these special populations are met as effectively as possible. SNPs may be of any type of coordinated care plan, including local and regional.

C. Types of Medicare Advantage Plans.

There are three (3) basic types of MA plans open to all MA-eligible Medicare beneficiaries if offered in the service area in which they reside: coordinated care plans (CCPs), Medical Savings Account (MSA) plans, and private fee-for-service (PFFS) plans. These plans as prescribed by MMA are set forth below:

> **Coordinated Care Plans**. These include the following six (6) plans:
>
>> *Health Maintenance Organizations (HMOs)*. Point of service (POS) is an option in some coordinated care plans that allows enrollees to obtain non-network services, with the plan providing some limited level of reimbursement for such services.
>>
>> *Local Preferred Provider Organizations*
>>
>> *Regional Preferred Provider Organizations*

Provider-sponsored Organizations

Religious Fraternal Benefits Plans

Specialized MA Plans for individuals with special needs (SNP) – An SNP includes any type of coordinated care plan that meets CMS' SNP requirements and either exclusively enrolls special needs individuals, or enrolls a greater proportion of special needs individuals that occur nationally in the Medicare population as defined by CMS; and

Medical Savings Account (MSA) Plans (network or non-network). Under the MMA, MA organizations are authorized to offer MSA plans as a permanent option with no enrollment cap. Under the MMA, MSA plans are local plans.

Private Fee-for-Service (PFFS) Plans.

D. Bidding Methodology.

The MMA mandated a new plan payment system which incorporates principles of competition by moving from an administered pricing system to a bidding methodology. Payments for local and regional MA plans will be based on competitive bids rather than administered pricing. The MA organizations submit an annual aggregate bid amount for each MA plan. An aggregate plan bid is based upon the MA organization's determination of expected costs in the plan's service area for the national average beneficiary for providing (i) non-drug benefits (that is, original Medicare Part A and Part B benefits), (ii) Part D basic prescription drugs, and (iii) supplemental benefits if any (including reductions in cost sharing). CMS will negotiate bid amounts with the plans.

CMS payment to an MA organization for an MA plan's coverage of Original Medicare benefits depends on the relationship of the plan's basic Part A and Part B (A/B) bid to the plan benchmark. For a plan with a basic A/B bid below its benchmark, CMS will pay the MA organization the basic A/B bid amount, adjusted by the individual enrollee's risk factor, plus the rebate amount. (The rebate is seventy-five (75%) percent of the difference between the plan bid and benchmark, and is used to provide mandatory supplemental benefits or reductions in Part B or Part D premiums. The government retains the other twenty-five (25%) percent.) For a plan with a bid equal to or above its benchmark, Medicare will pay the MA organization the plan benchmark, adjusted by the individual enrollee's risk factor. In addition, CMS will pay the bid amount, if any, for Part D basic coverage.

E. Comparison – Medicare Advantage/Original Medicare.

Compared to the original Medicare program, an enrollee under a Medicare Advantage plan will:

Be part of the Medicare program and entitled to receive Medicare Part A and Part B coverage;

Receive prescription drug coverage (Part D) under the MA plan. If the plan offers prescription drug coverage, the enrollee must obtain that coverage from the Medicare Advantage Plan;

Fill the gaps in 0riginal Medicare coverage, generally covered by a Medigap policy (Medicare Supplemental Insurance), without the necessity of buying such policy;

Be required to pay the Part B premium, in addition to the plan's premium for Part A and Part B benefits, prescription drug coverage (if offered), and other benefits that may be offered; and

Receive more benefits or lower cost-sharing than in the original Medicare program.

MEDICARE ADVANTAGE PLANS (MAP)/ELIGIBILITY AND ENROLLMENT

I.   ELIGIBLE PERSONS.

Beneficiaries entitled to Medicare Part A and Part B are eligible to elect a Medicare Advantage plan, except those with ESRD. (However, an individual who develops ESRD if enrolled in a Medicare Advantage plan is entitled to continue such enrollment.)

Certain limitations exist in enrolling in a Medical Savings Account (MSA) plan, one of the MA plans.

> Certain low-income Medicare beneficiaries are not eligible to participate in an MSA plan; namely, qualified Medicare beneficiaries, qualified disabled working individuals, specified low-income Medicare beneficiaries, or individuals otherwise entitled to Medicaid cost-sharing assistance under the Medicaid program.
>
> In addition, certain other classes of Medicare beneficiaries are not eligible to choose an MSA plan:
>
> –   Beneficiaries who have coverage benefits under high-deductible policies, including an employer's group plan that provides this coverage.
>
> –   Beneficiaries who are retired Federal government employees and part of the Federal Employee Health Benefits Program.
>
> –   Individuals who are retired Department of Defense or Department of Veterans Affairs employees.

A beneficiary's choice of Medicare Advantage plan coverage is deemed to continue until: (a) the beneficiary changes his/her election; (b) the Medicare Advantage plan is discontinued; or (c) the Medicare Advantage plan no longer serves the geographic area where the beneficiary resides.

II.   ENROLLMENT PERIODS (ELECTION OF PLANS).

The periods during which elections may be made by individuals are set forth below:

Initial Enrollment (Initial Coverage Election) Period.

Upon attaining eligibility for Medicare, individuals have a choice between original fee-for-service Medicare (Medicare FFS) or any Medicare Advantage plans available in their area. Any individual failing to make an election during the initial election year will be deemed to have chosen the Original Medicare FFS option. An election becomes effective on the date a beneficiary becomes entitled to benefits under Part A and enrolls in Part B.

The initial election period of seven (7) months begins one month before the month that the beneficiary is first entitled to both Parts A and B and ends on the last day of the individual's Part B initial enrollment period. As instructively rephrased in the CMS handbook *Medicare and You 2012: When you first become eligible for Medicare, you can join a Medicare Advantage plan during the 7-month period that begins 3 months before the month you turn 65, includes the month you turn 65, and ends 3 months after the month you turn 65.*

Open Enrollment Period.

Between October 15 and December 7 of each year (open enrollment period), an individual can join, switch, or drop a Medicare Advantage plan. Coverage will begin on January 1.

The election made during an open enrollment period will become effective on the first day of the first month after enrollment. More specifically, an individual can:

(i)   can change original Medicare to a Medicare Advantage plan;

(ii)   change from a Medicare Advantage plan to original Medicare; and

(iii)   switch Medicare Advantage plan for another.

A Medicare Advantage organization must accept eligible beneficiaries who elect that organization's plan during an open enrollment period without restrictions, waiting period, or pre-existing medical exclusion.

A beneficiary can elect an MSA plan only during the initial enrollment period or the annual coordinated election period.

Annual Coordinated Election Period.

If an individual does not enroll for Part A and/or Part B when first eligible, he/she may enroll, subject to a late enrollment penalty, during the annual coordinated election period. This period runs from October 15 to December 7 each year. Enrollment becomes effective on the following January 1.

During the annual coordinated election period, all Medicare beneficiaries are free to elect among all available options, including Original Medicare, MA plans, MA-prescription drug plans (MA-PDP), or prescription drug plans (PDPs). They may choose to enroll in an MA plan, change a default MA plan, or return to Original Medicare.

Special Enrollment Periods (SEP).

An individual may disenroll from a Medicare Advantage plan, other than during the annual coordinated election period, and may make a new choice of plans, in certain events: (i) the individual's plan has been terminated (see below), (ii) the individual has moved ((i.e., changed place of residence) (see below), (iii) the organization has breached its contract or made material misrepresentations, or (iv) other special circumstances (e.g., for cause).

In cases of termination or discontinuance of an organization, the SEP begins when the organization is required to give notice to beneficiaries and ends three months after the notification.

For a beneficiary who has moved, the SEP runs for three (3) months starting with the month prior to the permanent move and ending the month after the move. The beneficiary may choose an effective date of up to three (3) months after the month when the Medicare Advantage plan receives the beneficiary's completed enrollment form, but the effective date may not be prior to the date the beneficiary moved or the date the Medicare Advantage organization received the completed enrollment form.

In the case of breach of contract or material misrepresentations by the organization, the SEP begins once CMS agrees that a violation occurred. The length of the SEP depends on whether the beneficiary immediately elects a new Medicare Advantage plan on disenrollment from the original, or whether the beneficiary first elects Original Medicare before choosing a new Medicare Advantage plan.

5-Star Special Enrollment Period

Medicare and You 2012 instructively explains this new enrollment period as follows; *Medicare uses information from member satisfaction surveys, plans, and health care providers to give overall performance star ratings to plans. A plan can get a rating between one and five stars. A 5-star rating is considered excellent. These ratings help you compare plans based on quality and performance. Starting December 8, 2011, you can switch to a 5-star Medicare Advantage plan at any time during the year. The overall plan star ratings are available at* www.medicare.gov/find-a-plan. *You can only join a 5-star Medicare Advantage plan if one is available in your area. You can only use this special enrollment period to switch to a 5-star plan one time each year. You can't use this period to join a Medicare cost plan.*

Special Enrollment Periods for Employees.

There is a special enrollment period (SEP) available for individuals who elect their Medicare Advantage plans through their employers. The SEP may be used during the open enrollment period if the employer group health plan is not open for enrollment at the same time as the Medicare Advantage open enrollment. The SEP may also be used when the employer group health plan would permit a beneficiary to change elections based upon personal or life changes. The special enrollment period is only available to Medicare beneficiaries who are members of an employer group health plan that has an arrangement with a Medicare Advantage organization which offers a Medicare Advantage plan to the members of the employer group health plan.

Special Rules for Enrolling in an MSA.

A beneficiary (as stated above) can elect to enroll in an MSA plan only during: (i) an initial enrollment period upon attaining Medicare eligibility; or (ii) the annual coordinated election period. New enrollees may revoke their election if they do so before December 15 of the year they make an election.

Change of Election.

An enrollee of a Medicare Advantage plan may leave the plan and switch to Original Medicare between January 1 and February 14. Coverage will begin the first day of the following month.

As instructively stated the CMS handbook *Medicare and You 2012: Between January 1-February 14, if you're in a Medicare Advantage plan, you can leave your plan and switch to Original Medicare. If you switch to Original Medicare during this period, you will have until February 14 to also join a Medicare prescription drug plan to add drug coverage. Your coverage will begin the first day of the month after the plan gets your enrollment form.*

During January 1 to February 14, an enrollee of a MA plan cannot switch Original Medicare for a MA plan, or join, switch, or drop a Medical Savings Account.

(continued on next page)

MEDICARE ADVANTAGE PLANS (MAP)/COMMON FEATURES

INTRODUCTION

The common features (with related definitions) of Medicare Advantage (MA) plans, except where noted, are set forth below.

(See also *Medicare Advantage (MA)/Coordinated Care Plans – Common Features; Medicare Advantage (MA)/Medicare Savings Account (MSA) Plans; Medicare Advantage (MA)/Private Fee-for-Service (PFFS) Plans*)

I. DEFINITIONS.

MA Regional Plan. A coordinated care plan structured as a preferred provider organization (PPO) that serves one or more entire region. An MA regional plan must have a network of contracting providers that have agreed to a specific reimbursement for the plan's covered services and must pay for all covered services whether the benefits are provided within the network of providers. MA Regional plans may be joint enterprises where each health plan in the joint enterprise holds a state license in the state in which it does business and meets all applicable Medicare requirements.

MA Local Plan. A MA local plan is a MA plan that is not a MA regional plan.

MA Local Area. A payment area consisting of a county or equivalent area specified by CMS.

Specialized MA Plans for Special Needs Beneficiaries (SNPs). SNPs are coordinated care plans that exclusively or disproportionately (as defined below) serve special needs individuals and provide Part D benefits to all enrollees. CMS has designated these plans as meeting the requirements of a SNP, as determined on a case-by-case basis. The establishment of SNPs allows MA plans to exclusively enroll special needs individuals (as defined below). The SNPs have targeted clinical programs for these individuals.

CMS has defined a disproportionate percentage SNP as one that enrolls a greater proportion of the target group of special needs individuals than occur nationally in the Medicare population based on data acceptable to CMS.

A special needs individual means an MA-eligible individual who is institutionalized, is entitled to medical assistance under a state plan, or has a severe or disabling chronic condition and would benefit from enrollment in a specialized MA plan. For the purposes of a special needs individual, institutionalized means continuously residing or being expected to continuously reside for ninety (90) days or longer in a long-term care facility that is a skilled nursing facility (SNF), nursing facility (NF), SNF/NF, an intermediate care facility for the mentally retarded, or an inpatient psychiatric facility. CMS may also consider as institutionalized those individuals living in the community but requiring a level of care equivalent to that of those individuals living in these long-term facilities.

Annual Aggregate Bidding (see also *section V* below). Payments by Medicare to MA organizations will be based on competitive bids rather than (as provided in BBA) administered pricing. MA organizations will submit an annual aggregate bid amount for each MA plan. An aggregate plan bid is based upon its determination of expected costs in the plan's service area for the national average beneficiary for providing (i) non-drug benefits, that is, original Medicare (Part A and Part B) benefits, (ii) Part D basic prescription drugs, and (iii) supplemental benefits if any. To determine the amount of payment to a plan by Medicare, CMS will compare the non-drug portion of the aggregate bid to the local or regional plan benchmark (an amount which is an average of county rates, if the plan is in a plan's service area). For a plan with a bid below the benchmark, CMS will pay the MA organization the total plan bid (for Parts A, B, and D benefits plus any supplemental bid amount), risk adjusted for the plan risk profile, plus the rebate amount (an amount equal to seventy-five (75%) percent of the difference between the plan bid and benchmark); the remaining twenty-five (25%) percent is retained by the government. For a plan with a bid equal to or above its benchmark, CMS will pay the MA organization the plan benchmark, risk adjusted. Hence, Medicare payments to a local or regional plan will depend on the benchmark determined by competitive bidding. The benchmark is the most that Medicare will pay for Medicare Part A and Part B services.

Prescription Drug Plans. A prescription drug plan (PDP), authorized by Medicare Part D, is prescription drug coverage that is offered under an approved contract or policy, by a prescription drug sponsor that has a contract with CMS. A prescription drug sponsor is a private, non-governmental entity that is certified as meeting the requirements that apply to prescription drug plans, including fallback entities. They may offer multiple plans throughout the country or in a region, but they must maintain an individual bid for each plan. An MA prescription drug plan (MA – PDP) is an MA plan that provides qualified prescription drug coverage under Part D. An organization offering a coordinated care MA plan must have a PDP plan in each of the service areas in which it operates.

Medicare+Choice (M+C). This term does not apply after 2005.

Mandatory Supplemental Benefits. These are health care services not covered by Medicare that an MA enrollee must purchase as part of an MA plan. Supplemental benefits may include reductions in cost sharing for benefits under the original Medicare fee-for-service program, and are paid for in the form of premiums and cost sharing, or by an application of the beneficiary rebate rule (see section I, *Annual aggregate bidding*; and section VI.E *Savings rebate*), or both.

Optional Supplemental Benefits. These are the health services not covered by Medicare that are purchased at the option of the MA enrollee and paid for in full, directly by the enrollee, in the form of premiums or cost sharing. These services may be grouped or offered individually. The phrase "supplemental benefits" refers to both mandatory and optional supplemental benefits; the terms "mandatory supplemental" and "optional supplemental" are used when referring specifically to one of the types of supplemental benefits.

Basic Benefits. Basic benefits means all Medicare-covered Part A and B benefits, except hospice services. The term "additional benefits" has been eliminated from the definition of "basic benefits."

Benefits. Benefits means health care services that are intended to maintain or improve the health status of enrollees, for which the MA organization incurs a cost or liability under an MA plan (not solely an administrative processing cost). Benefits are submitted and approved through the annual bidding process.

Coinsurance. Coinsurance is a fixed percentage of the total amount paid for a health care service that can be charged to an MA enrollee on a per-service basis.

Copayment. Copayment is a fixed amount that can be charged to an MA plan enrollee on a per-service basis.

Cost sharing. Cost sharing includes deductibles, coinsurance, and copayments.

Continuation Area. A continuation area is an additional area (outside the service area) within which the MA organization offering a local plan furnishes or arranges to furnish services to its continuation-of-enrollment enrollees. MA plan continuation areas are available to MA local plans only. An MA organization may offer a continuation-of-enrollment option to MA local plan enrollees when they no longer reside in the service area of a plan and permanently move into the geographic area designated by the MA organization as a continuation area.

Service Area. "Service area" was revised to incorporate the concept of the new MA regional plan's service area that consists of an entire region.

II.   ELIGIBILITY.

Any beneficiaries entitled to Medicare Part A and Part B are eligible to choose a Medicare Advantage plan, except those with ESRD. (An individual who develops ESRD if enrolled in a Medicare Advantage plan is entitled to continue such enrollment.)

III.   ELECTION OF PLANS (ENROLLMENT).

A.   General.

Beneficiaries may make their choice to join a MA plan or terminate their choice by filing an appropriate form with a Medicare Advantage organization.

A beneficiary's choice of Medicare Advantage plan coverage is deemed to continue until: (a) the beneficiary changes his/her election; (b) the Medicare Advantage plan is discontinued; or (c) the Medicare Advantage plan no longer serves the geographic area where the beneficiary resides.

An individual who is a Qualified Medicare Beneficiary, a Qualified Disabled and Working Individual, a Specified Low-income Medicare Beneficiary, or otherwise eligible for Medicare and entitled to Medicare cost-sharing under state Medicaid programs, is not eligible to enroll in an MSA plan.

B.   Election Periods.

The periods during which elections may be made by individuals are set forth below:

Initial Enrollment (Initial Coverage Election) Period. Upon attaining eligibility for Medicare, individuals have a choice between traditional/original fee-for-service Medicare (Medicare FFS) or any Medicare Advantage plans available in their area. Any individual failing to make an election will be deemed to have chosen the Medicare FFS option. An election becomes effective on the date a beneficiary becomes entitled to benefits under Part A and enrolls in Part B.

An individual who enrolls in a Medicare Advantage plan upon first becoming eligible at age 65 may at any time during the first twelve (12) months of coverage (commencing on the effective date of enrollment) disenroll from the Medicare Advantage plan and enroll in the original Medicare program.

The initial election period begins three (3) months before the month that the beneficiary is first entitled to both Parts A and B. It ends the last day of the month preceding the individual's entitlement.

Open Enrollment Period.   In addition to initial enrollment, beneficiaries are able to enroll in a Medicare Advantage plan (other than an MSA), on an annual basis. In other words, they are able to switch between Original

Medicare and Medicare Advantage once every year. The open enrollment period is the first three (3) months of each year.

An election made during an open enrollment period will become effective on the first day of the first month after the election is made.

A Medicare Advantage organization must accept eligible beneficiaries who elect that organization's plan during an open enrollment period without restrictions, waiting period, or pre-existing medical exclusion.

A beneficiary can elect an MSA plan only during the initial enrollment period or the annual coordinated election period.

Annual Coordinated Election Period. Selection of a Medicare plane may be made each November. The month of November is considered the annual, coordinated election period. Enrollment is effective the following January.

During the annual coordinated election period, all Medicare beneficiaries are free to elect among all available options, including original Medicare, MA plans, MA-prescription drug plans (MA-PDP), or prescription drug plans (PDPs). They may choose to enroll in a MA plan, change a default MA plan, or return to original Medicare, and an above-stated enrollment is effective the following January.

Special Enrollment Periods (SEP). An individual may disenroll from a Medicare Advantage plan, other than during the annual coordinated election period, and may make a new choice of plans, in certain events: (i) the individual's plan has been terminated; (ii) the individual has moved ((i.e., changed place of residence); (iii) the organization has breached its contract or made material misrepresentations; or (iv) other special circumstances (e.g., for cause). The time frames for commencement of the SEP upon the occurrence of such events are set forth below.

In cases of termination of an organization, the SEP begins when the organization is required to give notice to beneficiaries and ends three (3) months after the notification.

For a beneficiary who has moved, the SEP runs for three (3) months starting with the month prior to the permanent move and ending the month after the move. The beneficiary may choose an effective date of up to three months after the month when the Medicare Advantage plan receives the beneficiary's completed enrollment form, but the effective date may not be prior the date the beneficiary moved or the date the Medicare Advantage organization received the completed enrollment form.

In the case of breach of contract or material misrepresentations by the organization, the SEP begins once CMS agrees that a violation occurred. The length of the SEP depends on whether the beneficiary immediately elects a new Medicare Advantage plan on disenrollment from the original, or whether the beneficiary first elects original Medicare before choosing a new Medicare Advantage plan.

Special Enrollment Period for Employees. There is a special enrollment period available for individuals who elect their Medicare Advantage plans through their employers. This special period may be used during the open enrollment period if the employer group health plan is not open for enrollment at the same time as the Medicare Advantage open enrollment; and may also be used when the employer group health plan would permit a beneficiary to change elections based upon personal or life changes. The SEP is only available to Medicare beneficiaries who are members of an employer group health plan that has an arrangement with a Medicare Advantage organization which offers a Medicare Advantage plan to the members of the employer group health plan. Beneficiaries will still have the opportunity to participate in the annual elections. The election period starts November 15 and ends December 31.

Special Rules for Enrolling in an MSA. A beneficiary can elect to enroll in an MSA plan only during: (i) an initial enrollment period upon attaining Medicare eligibility; or (ii) the annual coordinated election period. New enrollees may revoke their election if they do so before December 15 of the year they make an election.

Change of Election. A beneficiary may only change an election made during open enrollment periods, from one MA plan to another MA plan if it is the same type of MA plan in which the beneficiary is already enrolled. For example: a beneficiary in an MA plan that does not provide drug coverage may change only to another similar MA plan, or to original Medicare, but may not enroll in a plan that provides Part D coverage. Similarly, a beneficiary enrolled in an MA plan that includes Part D coverage may enroll only in another MA plan with Part D coverage, or change to Original Medicare coverage with an election of a Part D plan.

Disenrollment by the MA Organization. CMS has changed the grace period after which a plan may disenroll a Medicare beneficiary for failure to pay plan premiums from ninety (90) days to no sooner than one month from the date the premium was due. Because it is a minimum grace period, MA organizations have the option of offering a more generous grace period.

In addition to providing the grace period, an MA organization also must provide proper notice to individuals before it takes any disenrollment action, and it must demonstrate that it has made reasonable efforts to collect unpaid premium amounts.

Disenrollment for Disruptive Behavior. Disruptive behavior is a ground for disenrollment. An MA plan enrollee is disruptive "if his behavior substantially impairs the plan's ability to arrange for or provide services to the individual or plan members."

CMS requires that MA organizations provide such individuals reasonable accommodation. A beneficiary cannot be considered disruptive if such behavior is related to the use of medical services or compliance (or non-compliance) with medical advice or treatment. Additionally, the MA organization must make a serious effort to resolve the problem, and must inform the individual of the right to use the organization's grievance procedures. CMS staff with the appropriate medical expertise will be involved in the case-by-case review of the MA organization's request for disenrollment.

The MA organization may request approval to decline future enrollment by the individual if it submits sufficient documentation and information and makes a serious effort to resolve the problems that the behavior presents. However, CMS rejected the proposed provision for expedited disenrollment in cases where the behavior poses an immediate threat of health and safety to others.

IV. PART D (OUTPATIENT PRESCRIPTION DRUGS) COVERAGE.

(See also *Medicare Advantage (MA) Outpatient Prescription Drugs.*)

Access by a Medicare Advantage plan enrollee to prescription drug coverage differs, depending on the MA plan chosen, as follows:

Coordinated Care Plans. In order to offer an MA coordinated care plan in an area, the MA organization offering the coordinated care plan must offer Part D prescription drug coverage in that plan or in another MA plan in the same area.

MSA Plans. MA organizations offering MSA plans are not permitted to offer prescription drug coverage, other than that required under Medicare Parts A and B. If a beneficiary enrolls in an MSA plan that does not offer Part D coverage; he/she may also enroll in a prescription drug plan (PDP).

PFFS Plans. MA organizations offering private fee-for-service plans can choose to offer Part D coverage. If a beneficiary enrolls in a PFFS plan, he/she may also enroll in a PDP.

V.   BIDDING PROCESS.

Submission of Bids.   MMA replaced the adjusted community rate proposal system (in effect under BBA's Medicare Part C) with a competitive bid submission process, in place of administered pricing.   No later than the first Monday in June, MA organizations must submit annual aggregate bids (aggregate bids) for each MA plan that they intend to offer in the following year (other than PFFS plans and MSA plans, which have separate requirements. In the case of PFFS plans and MSA plans, CMS will not review, negotiate, or approve amounts of bids.

Plan bids must meet specific bid requirements and provide specific information.

Aggregate Bid Defined. The aggregate plan bid is based upon the plan's determination of expected costs in the plan's service area for the national average beneficiary for providing: (1) the unadjusted non-drug bid to provide original Medicare benefits (Parts A/B); (2) the amount to provide basic prescription drug coverage; and/or (3) the amount to provide supplemental coverage, if any.

MMA Standards of Review. MMA established three (3) standards for the review of bids by CMS: First, a bid must be supported by the actuarial basis. Second, the bid amount must reasonably and equitably reflect a plan's revenue requirements for providing the benefit package. Third, the actuarial value of plan cost sharing applicable on average to plan enrollees cannot exceed the actuarial value of cost sharing applicable on average under original Medicare FFS.

VI.   PAYMENTS TO THE PLAN (CAPITATION).

A. Payments - Relationship of Bid to Benchmark.

MA plans. MA plans (except MSA plans) will be paid based on the relationship of the plan's risk-adjusted (as defined in section D below) basic Part

A/B benefit (i.e., the non-drug portion of the bid) to a monthly benchmark (as defined in section B below), calculated by CMS, representing one-twelfth (1/12) of the annual capitation rate (ACR) (as defined in section C below).

If a plan's risk-adjusted basic Part A/B bid is less than the risk-adjusted benchmark, CMS will pay the MA organizations the total plan bid. It is the amount bid (for Parts A, B and D benefits), plus (i) any supplemental bid amount, (ii) adjustment for the plan risk profile, and (iii) the rebate amounts (which amount is equal to seventy-five (75%) percent of the difference between the plan bid and the benchmark – the remaining twenty-five (25%) percent is retained by the government.

If the plan's risk-adjusted basic bid is equal to zero percentage above the benchmark, CMS will pay the MA organization the benchmark risk adjustment. The benchmark is the most that Medicare will pay for Medicare Part A and Part B services.

CMS will deposit into an individual's Medical savings account (MSA), for the calendar year commencing with the month in which the MSA coverage begins, a lump sum equal to the annual difference between the MSA premium and the capitation rate for the area.

B. Definition of Benchmark.

Local Area Plans. The MA area-specific non-drug monthly benchmark amount (used for local area plans) is equal to the monthly MA capitation rate for the local area. For a service area that is in more than one MA local area, the benchmark amount is calculated as a weighted average of the local MA monthly capitation rates (see section C below), using as weights the projected enrollment in each county used to calculate the bid.

Regional Area Plans. The MA region-specific non-drug monthly benchmark amount is the sum of a (i) statutory component and (ii) a plan-bid component for the year; the terms are described below.

The statutory component is the product of (x) the statutory region-specific non-drug amount for the region and the year, and (y) the statutory national market share percentage. The statutory region-specific non-drug amount, the first part of the statutory component, is an amount equal to the sum (for each local MA area within the region) of the product of the MA area-specific non-drug monthly benchmark amount for the area and the year, and the number of MA-eligible individuals residing in the local area, divided by the total number of MA-eligible individuals residing in the region. The statutory national market share percentage, the second part of the statutory component, is equal to the proportion of MA-eligible individuals nationally who were not enrolled in an MA plan during the most recent month during the previous year for which data are available.

The plan-bid component is the product of (x) the weighted average of MA plan bids for the region and the year and (y) the non-statutory market share percentage. The weighted average of plan bids for an MA region is calculated as the sum for MA regional plans of region and year of: (i) the unadjusted MA statutory non-drug monthly bid for the plan, and (ii) the plan's share of MA enrollment in the region.

MSA Plans. CMS will make monthly payments to MA organizations for MSA enrollees based upon (x) the area-specific non-drug benchmark amount (which is basically the amount submitted to the CMS by the MSA plan) less (y) one-twelfth (1/12) the annual lump sum amount, if any, deposited by CMS to the enrollee's Medicare savings account, adjusted for the enrollee's risk.

C. Definition of Capitation.

The CMS announces each year the annual capitation rate which, subject to certain statutorily prescribed factors, is an amount primarily based upon one-hundred (100%) percent of original Medicare annual costs for covered service (Parts A/B) for persons not enrolled in an MA plan. The monthly capitation rate is an amount equal to one-twelfth (1/12) of the annual capitation rate.

D. Risk Adjustment.

CMS will make a risk adjustment to the capitation rate for age, gender, disability status, and institutional status.

E. Savings Rebate.

If a plan's risk-adjusted basic Part A/B bid is less than the risk-adjusted benchmark, the plan is paid the benchmark and has savings equal to one-hundred (100%) percent of the difference between the bid and the benchmark. In such cases, the beneficiary is entitled to a rebate of seventy-five (75%) percent of the savings and CMS will retain the other twenty-five (25%) percent. If a plan's risk-adjusted basic Part A/B bid is equal to or greater than the risk-adjusted benchmark, the plan has no savings, and no beneficiary rebate is required. Rebate dollars cannot be used to fund supplemental benefits.

F. Payment Areas.

Under the M+C program, a payment area was defined as a county or equivalent area defined by the Secretary of Health and Human Services (with the exception of ESRD enrollees, for whom the payment area was a state). MMA establishes two (2) general types of payment areas: (i) for MA local plans, the payment area is an MA local area (defined as a county or equivalent specified by CMS); and (y) for MA regional plans, the payment area is an MA region.

VII. PREMIUMS.

MMA does not require a fixed premium amount. Premiums are determined by a bidding process and will vary from plan to plan. Premiums are determined by comparing the unadjusted statutory non-drug bid amount (the basic A/B bid) to the unadjusted benchmark amount. For an MA plan with a basic A/B bid that is less than the appropriate unadjusted non-drug benchmark amount, the basic beneficiary premium is *zero*. For an MA plan with a basic A/B bid that is equal to or greater than the unadjusted non-drug benchmark amount, the basic beneficiary premium (which the plan must charge) is the amount by which the bid amount exceeds the benchmark amount. All approved premiums must be charged; plans are not allowed to waive basic beneficiary premiums.

Monthly Supplemental Premiums. A monthly supplemental premium is the portion of the plan attributable to mandatory and/or supplemental health care benefits (less any applicable rebate).

Single Premiums. MA enrollees must be charged consolidated monthly premiums. An MA enrollee will pay a single premium consisting of the sum of all premiums a particular plan charges its enrollees, which will be one or more of the following: (i) the monthly basic beneficiary premium; (ii) the monthly supplemental premium; and (iii) the MA monthly prescription drug premium.

Premiums Charged. Enrollees in most coordinated care plans are not required to pay any premiums to the plan for Medicare basic benefits (i.e., Part A/B benefits).

PFFS plans and MSA plans may charge enrollees unlimited premiums for Medicare basic benefits.

Enrollees of all plans are required to pay the Medicare monthly Part B premium, which is deducted from their Social Security checks.

VIII.   BENEFITS.

A. Basic Benefits.

These are all services covered under Medicare Parts A/B benefits except hospice services, (if an enrollee is entitled to benefits under both Parts A and B; and Part B benefits only if enrollee is entitled to benefits only under Part B). A Medicare Advantage (MA) organization offering an MA plan must, at a minimum, provide enrollees with coverage of basic benefits. MA plans have an annual cap on how much an enrollee must pay for Part A and Part B during the year. The annual out-of-pocket amount cannot differ among plans. MA plans cannot charge enrollees more than Original Medicare for certain services like chemotherapy, dialysis, and skilled nursing care.

In the case of MSA plans, until the enrollee meets his deductible, he/she is generally responsible for payment for all covered services. Once the enrollee meets his/her MSA deductible, the MA organization offering the plan is responsible for payment of one-hundred (100%) percent of basic benefits.

Amongst the basic benefits covered under Part A of Medicare is post-institutional home health services. These services consist of the following: Homebound beneficiaries in need of skilled nursing care, or physical, speech, or occupational therapy are entitled to services of a home health agency according to a physician's treatment plan, after minimum three- (3) day hospitalization, or stay in SNF. Coverage is limited to one-hundred (100) visits in a spell of illness.

The MMA has extended this benefit in the case of MA-covered plans to provide that MA organizations may elect to furnish, as part of their Medicare covered benefits, coverage of post-hospital SNF care (as described above). Notwithstanding the absence of the prior qualifying hospital stay that would otherwise be required for coverage of such care, the CMS has issued a ruling to this effect: that if a MA organization so elects, an individual, who would be eligible for a skilled nursing facility (SNF) upon discharge from a hospital stay, would have the right to receive home SNF benefits in the absence of a hospital stay.

B. Additional Benefits.

These benefits have been removed by MMA from the definition of basic benefits. An MA plan no longer offers additional benefits.

C. Mandatory Supplemental Benefits.

These supplemental benefits are health care services not covered by Medicare that an MA enrollee must purchase as part of an MA plan. The benefits may include reductions in cost sharing for benefits under the original fee-for-service program and are paid for in the form of premiums and cost sharing, or by application of the beneficiary rebate rule or both. Subject to approval by CMS, an MA organization may require enrollees of an MA plan (other than an MSA plan) to accept or pay for services in addition to Medicare-covered basic services. If the MA organization imposes mandatory supplemental benefits, it must impose them on all beneficiaries enrolled in that plan. CMS approves mandatory supplemental benefits only if the benefits are designed in accordance with CMS written instructions.

D. Optional Supplemental Benefits.

Optional supplemental benefits are health services not covered by Medicare, are purchased at the option of an MA enrollee, and are paid for in full directly by the Medicare enrollee in a form of premiums and cost sharing. These services may be grouped or offered individually. MA regional plans are permitted to have only a single deductible related to combined Parts A and B services, to the extent that they apply a deductible.

IX. ACCESS TO SERVICES.

An organization offering an MA plan is authorized to select the providers from whom benefits are provided only if:

the organization makes available benefits under the plan with promptness and continuity; and, when medically necessary, available twenty-four (24) hours a day, seven (7) days a week.

coverage is provided for ambulance services, emergency and urgently needed services without regard to prior authorization or the emergency care provider's relationship with the organization.

X.   EMERGENCY SERVICES BASED ON A PRUDENT LAY-PERSON TEST.

Each MA plan must provide for emergency and urgently needed services for its enrollees regardless of whether the services are obtained within or outside the MA organization, and without prior authorization. The term emergency services means, with respect to an individual enrolled with a MA organization, those inpatient and outpatient services which are furnished by a qualified provider and needed to evaluate and stabilize an emergency medical condition. The term emergency medical condition means a medical condition manifesting itself by acute symptoms of sufficient severity, including severe pain, such that a prudent layperson who possesses an average knowledge of health and medicine could reasonably expect the absence of immediate medical attention to result in: (i) placing the health of the individual in serious jeopardy; (ii) serious impairment of bodily functions; and/or (iii) serious dysfunctions of bodily organ parts.

For emergency services obtained outside the plan's network, the organization may not charge an enrollee more than $50 of what it would charge the enrollee if he/she obtained the service through the MA plan, whichever is less.

XI.   ASSUMPTION OF FULL FINANCIAL RISK.

An MA organization -- other than PFFSs which assume no financial risk and PSOs which assume substantial financial risk -- must assume full financial risk on a prospective basis for the provision of health services, other than hospice services. The organization, however, may obtain insurance or make other arrangements for costs that exceed an amount that may be set by CMS from time to time.

XII.   LICENSED UNDER STATE LAW.

An MA organization, except a PSO, must be organized under state law as a risk-bearing entity eligible to offer health insurance or health benefits coverage in each state in which it offers a MA plan.

XIII.   ENROLLEE-PROVIDER COMMUNICATIONS.

An MA organization must not prohibit or otherwise restrict a health care professional from advising patients about health status, medical care or treatment options, regardless of whether benefits for such care or treatment are provided under the contract, if the professional is acting within the lawful scope of practice.

Health care professionals include physicians and other professionals such as podiatrists, optometrists, chiropractors, physiologists, dentists, physician assistants, physical or occupational therapists and therapy assistants, speech-language pathologists, audiologists, registered or licensed practical nurses, licensed certified social workers, registered respiratory therapists and certified respiratory therapy technicians.

XIV.   PHYSICIAN INCENTIVE PLANS.

An MA organization may not operate with any physician incentive plan unless the following requirements are met: No specific payment may be made to a physician or physician group as an inducement to reduce or limit medically necessary services. If the plan places a physician or physician group at substantial financial risk (as determined by the CMS) for services not provided by the physician or physician group, the organization must provide protection for the physician or group that is adequate and appropriate and that takes into account: (i) the number of physicians placed at such substantial financial risk in the group or under the plan; and (ii) the number of individuals enrolled with the organization who receive services from the physician or group.

Physician incentive plan means any compensation arrangement between the MA organization and a physician or physician group that may directly or indirectly have the effect of reducing or limiting services provided with respect to individuals enrolled with the organization.

XV.   MEDICARE AS SECONDARY PAYER.

When another health plan covered benefits for a plan participant who is also a Medicare beneficiary entitled to such benefits under Medicare Part A and/or Part B, Medicare considers that such other plan is the primary payer for the benefits and that Medicare is only the secondary payer in such cases. Accordingly, should Medicare make payment for the benefits that should have been made by the primary payer, Medicare can obtain recovery against the primary payer. The MA organization similarly may seek payments from primary payers.

Medicare may recover payments it incorrectly makes if recovery is sought within three (3) years after the rendition of the services covered by the payment.

XVI.   CONTINUITY OF CARE.

All MA organizations must ensure continuity of care through arrangements that include:

> policies that specify methods for coordination of plan services;

> offering to provide each enrollee with an ongoing source of primary care and providing a primary care source to each enrollee that accepts the offer;

> programs for coordination of plan services with community and social services generally available; and

> procedures to ensure the organization makes a "best effort" attempt to conduct an initial assessment of each enrollee's health care needs, including following up on unsuccessful attempts to contact an enrollee within ninety (90) days of the effective date of enrollment.

XVII.   QUALITY IMPROVEMENT PROGRAM.

Each MA organization (other than MA private fee-for-services plans and MSA plans) that offers one or more MA plans must have for each of those plans an ongoing quality improvement program administered by an independent review entity (IRE), referred to as a quality improvement organization (QIO). As part of the quality improvement program, a plan must develop criteria for a chronic care improvement program.

All MA coordinated plans (except for regional PPO plans), including local PPO plans that are offered by organizations that are licensed or organized under a state law as an HMO, as part of their quality improvement program, must comply with certain requirements specified by CMS (including processing requests for initial or continued authorization of services and the following of written policies and procedures that reflect current standard methods of medical practice). Local PPO-type plans that are offered by an organization that is licensed or organized under a state law as an HMO must follow the same quality improvement requirements as other MA coordinated care plans.

MA regional and local plans that are offered by an organization. that is not licensed to organize under a state law as an HMO, must follow certain requirements specified by CMS (including the measuring of performance under the plans using standard procedures required by CMS and reporting performance to CMS).

All MA plans must follow certain requirements specified by CMS (including the maintenance of a health information system that collects, analyzes and integrates the data necessary to implement its quality improvement program). There must be in effect a process for performance evaluation at least annually of the impact and effectiveness of the plans and quality improvement program.

There is no requirement in the case of any of the MA plans that a plan must contract with a QIO or other external review and improvement organizations to review appeals for patient claims; however, the QIO will still be involved in all appeals relating to hospital and nursing home discharges.

XVIII. GRIEVANCES.

See *Grievance procedures/Medicare Advantage Organization.*

XIX.   APPEALS.

See *Medicare Advantage/Notice of Non-Coverage of Hospital Care); Appeal (Standard)/Medicare Advantage; Appeals (Fast-track) termination of non-hospital services/Medicare Advantage Organization (MA);* and *Appeals (Expedited) discharge of hospital patient/Medicare Advantage Organization).*

XX.   OUTPATIENT DRUGS.

See *Medicare Advantage/Outpatient Prescription Drugs.*

MEDICARE ADVANTAGE (MA)/COORDINATED CARE PLANS – COMMON FEATURES

INTRODUCTION

The Medicare Prescription Drug Improvement and Modernization Act of 2001 (MMA), which replaced the Balanced Budget Act of 1997 (BBA), provides (as did the BBA) to every individual entitled to Medicare Part A and enrolled under Part B (except individuals with end-staff renal disease) Medicare benefits through several alternative Medicare Advantage plans, in lieu of traditional fee-for-service Medicare.

The various MA plans are classified into three (3) general types – coordinated care plans (CCP), Medical savings account plans (MSA), and private fee-for-service plans (PFFS). The features set forth below apply only to coordinated care plans.

I. DEFINITION OF MA COORDINATED CARE PLAN.

An MA coordinated care plan is a care plan offered by an MA organization that includes a network of providers that are under contract to or have an arrangement with organization to deliver at least the benefit package authorized by CMS. The network of providers must be approved by CMS to ensure that all applicable requirements are met, including access and availability standards, service area requirements, and quality standards. CMS has promulgated the following rules to access standards.

Provider Network. The organization must maintain a network of appropriate providers.

PCP Panel. A panel of primary care physicians (PCPs) must be established by the organization from which the enrollee may select a PCP. If an enrollee desires to change his/her PCP, the enrollee can request the plan for the names of the other plan doctors in the plan area. There is no requirement that a treatment plan be updated by a PCP; any health professional or team of health professionals may develop the treatment plan. If a specialist develops a treatment plan, he/she should be the one to update it.

Serious Medical Conditions. The organization must ensure it has in effect CMS approval procedures which (i) identify individuals with complex or serous medical conditions; (ii) assess and monitor those conditions; and (iii) establish a treatment plan which includes an adequate number of direct access visits to specialists.

Specialty Care. The organization must provide or arrange for necessary specialty care, and in particular for women enrollees the option of direct access to a women's health specialist within the network for routine and prevention health care services. The CMS regulations does not prohibit the organization from limiting the number of direct visits to the specialist, as long as the number is adequate and consistent with the treatment plan.

Hours of Operation. Plan services must be made available by the organization twenty-four (24) hours a day, seven (7) days a week, when medically necessary.

Initial Assessment. The organization must make a best effort attempt to conduct an initial assessment of each enrollee's health needs.

II. PREMIUMS.

Enrollees in most coordinated care plans are not required to pay the plan any premiums for Medicare basic benefits (Part A/B).

III. CHARGE LIMITS (BALANCE BILLING).

When a provider does not have a contract with the plan. A physician or other provider who does not have a contract establishing payment amounts for services furnished to an enrollee of one of the CCP organizations is required to accept a payment in full for covered services amounts that physicians or other providers could collect if the individual were not enrolled in such organization (i.e., the amount that original Medicare fee-for-services would have paid to an enrollee if enrolled in original Medicare).

When a provider does have a contract with the plan. A physician or other provider of services who has a contract with the plan establishing payment amounts for services furnished to an enrollee of a CCP organization is required to accept as payment in full for covered services the amount set forth in the plan's fee schedule.

IV. FLEXIBILITY OF CHOICE BY A MEDICARE ELIGIBLE AMONG COORDINATED CARE PLANS.

A Medicare eligible may choose from among a variety of CCPs. They include, but are not limited to, HMO organizations (with or without point-of-service options), plans offered by local preferred provider organization (PPO) plans, provider-sponsored organizations (PSOs), regional PPOs, religious fraternal benefits (RFB) plans, and specialized MA plans for special needs beneficiaries (SNPs).

V. STATE LICENSURE AND OTHER STATE REQUIREMENTS.

Except in the case of a PSO (granted a waiver of state licensing requirements), all organizations offering the CCP must meet state licensure requirements. Thus, the CCP must be offered by an entity that is (i) appropriately licensed as a risk-bearing entity by the state, and (ii) eligible to offer health insurance or health benefits coverage, in each state in which it offers an MA plan. The coverage which the entity provides may be on an indemnity basis, as in the case of a PPO, or a pre-capitated basis, as in the case of an HMO. The entity does not need to be licensed specifically as an HMO, PSO, or PPO to offer a CCP.

(continued on next page)

MEDICARE ADVANTAGE (MA)/HMO PLANS

INTRODUCTION

A Medicare Advantage HMO is one of the several coordinated care plans.

The special features of Medicare Advantage HMO plans are set forth below. (See also *Medicare Advantage (MA)/Coordinated Care Plans – Common Features.*)

I. DEFINITION OF HMO.

The HMO is a managed care arrangement between: (i) individual participants and the HMO, which provides to the participants through a network of doctors and other health providers an array of Medicare-covered medical services (physician services, and a range of laboratory, x-ray and ancillary services); and (ii) the HMO and Medicare which pays the HMO a fixed predetermined, periodic fee, known as a capitation fee.

II. LOCK-IN FEATURE.

The plan participants are locked-in to and may only use a network provider (except emergency or urgent care), unless the HMO has opted for a point of service option for its enrollees. Services received by a participant, other than through the HMO network, will not be paid for by the HMO; the participant is personally liable for these out-of-network services.

III. PRIMARY CARE PHYSICIAN – SPECIALIST.

An enrollee generally will be asked to choose a primary care doctor (commonly referred to as gatekeeper). Should the enrollee seek a specialist, he/she needs a referral from the primary care doctor, except that generally a woman does not need a reference for a yearly screening mammogram, or two in-network pap tests and pelvic exams (at least every other year), provided the specialist is in the network.

IV.   PRESCRIPTION DRUGS.

An enrollee who wants prescription drug coverage must get it from the HMO plan.

(continued on next page)

MEDICARE ADVANTAGE (MA)/HMO POINT OF SERVICE OPTION

INTRODUCTION

There has been an increasing use by HMOs of a program known as a point of service (POS) option, under which the enrollee is not locked into network providers, but may use non-network providers, at rates of coinsurance, copayment and deductibles set by the HMO.

The salient elements of the POS option are set forth below.

I. OPTION AVAILABLE UNDER A MEDICARE ADVANTAGE COORDINATED CARE PLAN OR NETWORK MSA PLANS.

A Medicare Advantage HMO may offer an option to a Medicare eligible through a coordinated care plan (CCP) or network Medical Saving Account (MSA) plan, to obtain outside the plan specified health care items and services from providers that do not have a contract with the MA organization. The plan with the POS option feature is required to provide, at a minimum, all Medicare-covered services available to beneficiaries under original Medicare fee-for-service coverage available through Medicare Parts A and B. Should a participant choose care outside of the plan's network, he/she is subject to paying coinsurance, copayment and deductibles, which are usually higher than in a typical CCP.

II. MANDATORY, SUPPLEMENTAL OR OPTIONAL SUPPLEMENTAL BENEFIT.

A coordinated care plan may offer a POS option as a mandatory supplemental benefit, or an optional supplemental benefit. A network MSA plan (one of the coordinated care plans) may offer the POS option but only as a supplemental benefit.

III.   CAP ON ENROLLEE'S LIABILITY.

There must be a plan cap placed by the plan on an enrollee's total annual financial liability under a POS benefit.   The enrollee must be clearly informed about all of the estimated potential costs when enrolling in the plan.

IV.   DIRECT ACCESS.

A Medicare beneficiary may not use a POS option to seek direct access to a specialist within the plan network.   The beneficiary must comply with the rules of the plan typically requiring prior authorization (pre-certification) by a primary care physician, or other network health professionals.

(continued on next page)

MEDICARE ADVANTAGE (MA)/PREFERRED PROVIDER ORGANIZATION (PPO) PLANS

INTRODUCTION

The Medicare Advantage PPO plan is one of the several coordinated care plans. Special features of PPO plans are set forth below. (See also *Medicare Advantage Plans (MAP)/Common Features; Medicare Advantage (MA)/Coordinated Care Plans--Common Features*)

I. DEFINITION OF PPO.

A PPO plan is an arrangement between an employer or insurance company and network of health care providers whereby the providers, called preferred providers, have agreed to a contractually specified reimbursement for covered services with the organization offering the plan. As part of the arrangement, the insurance company or employer negotiates discounted fees with the PPO so that the insured enrollees receive lower than the customary fee-for-services basis. A form of managed care, the PPO plan is a variant of the classic HMO; however, PPO enrollees may visit any doctor in the network without a referral, and choose doctors outside of the provider network, usually for higher fees and/or deductibles.

II. LICENSURE BY STATE AS A RISK-BEARING ENTITY.

In order for a PPO to offer a MA plan as a separate entity all unto itself, it is required to be licensed by the state as a risk-bearing entity. However, if a PPO is not so licensed, it may enter into partnership or contract with a state-licensed indemnity carrier, or state-licensed HMO and "rent" out its PPO network of health care products to that licensee. In such a case, the PPO may operate in conjunction with the licensed carrier or HMO under a PPO plan, and CMS will defer to the applicable licensing state, as to the issue of whether the PPO may accept partial capitation from the licensed carrier or HMO.

III. LIMIT OF ENROLLEE'S LIABILITY.

An enrollee's financial liability to providers under a PPO plan is limited in the same manner that liability is limited under an HMO plan or any other type of CCP. That is, the sum of the premium for basic benefits and the actuarial value of all out-of-pocket expenses for such benefits (including the actuarial value of cost-sharing for non-participating providers of the PPO) cannot exceed the actuarial value of deductibles and coinsurance for original Medicare fee-for-services.

Commencing January 1, 2006, the single type of PPO in the definition of CCP was expanded into two by including local and regional coordinated care plans. The regional plans are subject to several rules different from those of local plans but are structured as PPOs.

IV. PRESCRIPTION DRUGS.

An enrollee who wants prescription drug coverage must get it from the PPO plan.

(continued on next page)

MEDICARE ADVANTAGE (MA)/PROVIDER-SPONSORED ORGANIZATION (PSO) PLANS

INTRODUCTION

The Medicare Advantage PSO plan is one of the several coordinated care plans. (See also *Medicare Advantage (MA)/Coordinated Care Plans – Common Features.*) Special features of the PSO plans are discussed below.

I. OVERVIEW.

A variety of health care providers, such as physicians and hospitals, may integrate themselves into a provider-service network organization, and through that organization create and administer a managed care plan that provides a wide spectrum of medical services to patients. Unlike other coordinated care plans, a PSO directly enrolls individuals, and no insurance carrier participates in the arrangement.

II. DEFINITION.

A PSO is a public or private entity:

> that is established or organized under state law and operated by a health care provider or by a group of affiliated health care providers;

> that provides a substantial proportion of the required services under a contract directly through the provider or group of providers; and

> where the providers share substantial financial risk with respect to the provision of health services and have at least a majority stake in the entity.

III. MINIMUM NUMBER OF ENROLLEES.

In order to qualify as a provider for a risk-basis contract, a PSO must have at least 1,500 enrollees in urban areas, or in rural areas 500 enrollees.

IV. RISK-BEARING ENTITY.

Generally, a PSO must be organized under state law as a risk-bearing entity eligible to offer health insurance or health benefits in each state in which it offers a Medicare+Choice plan.

V. SERVICES TO ENROLLEES.

The plan is required to provide enrollees through its physicians, and other providers' services not less than those items and services available under Medicare Part A and Part B, other than hospice care.

In order for enrollees to receive coverage for services rendered by a provider outside the PSO, a referral from the enrollee's primary care physician typically is required.

VI. PAYMENT LIMITATIONS (CHARGE LIMITS).

Physicians under contract with the plan may not charge above the plan's fee-payment schedule. Physicians not under contract with the plan may not charge for basic benefits more than the total amount payable under original Medicare.

VII. PREMIUMS.

A PSO plan may not impose any additional premiums (above those established by the Secretary of HHS) for Medicare basic benefits (i.e., Part A and Part B) and must accept the Medicare capitation payment as payment in full for these benefits. Premiums for basic benefits charged in lieu of cost sharing may not exceed the actuarial value of cost-sharing in original Medicare.

VIII. PRESCRIPTION DRUGS.

An enrollee who wants prescription drug coverage must get it from the PSO plan.

IX.   PRIMARY DOCTORS – SPECIALISTS.

Enrollees who are not limited to service of primary doctors or specialists in the network may choose a doctor (including a specialist) outside of the network, but often for larger fees and/or deductibles.

(continued on next page)

MEDICARE ADVANTAGE (MA)/RELIGIOUS FRATERNAL BENEFITS (RFP) PLANS

INTRODUCTION

The Medicare Advantage religious benefits plan (RFP) is one of the several coordinated care plans. (See also *Medicare Advantage (MA)/Coordinated Care Plans -- Common Features.*) The special features of the RFB plans are set forth below.

I.   **DEFINITION.**

A RFB plan is one that:

is offered by a religious fraternal benefit society, only to the members of the church, convention, or affiliated group.

permits all members to enroll without regard to health status-related factors.

must be offered by a religious fraternal benefit society that:

is described under §501(c)(8) of the Internal Revenue Code and is exempt from taxation under §501(a) of that enactment;

is affiliated with, carries out the tenets of, and shares a religious bond with, a church or convention or association of churches or an affiliated group of churches;

offers, in addition to the MA religious fraternal benefits society plan, at least the same level of health coverage to individuals not entitled to Medicare benefits, who are members of such church, convention or group; and, does not impose any limitation on membership in the society based on any health status-related factors.

may be any type of MA plan, including PFFS plan or MSA.

II.   STATE LICENSE.

As with other types of coordinated care plans, an entity offering an RFB plan must be organized and licensed under the state law as a risk-bearing entity eligible to offer health insurance or health benefits coverage in each state in which it offers an MA plan. The RFB must meet all other of the state's licensing requirements.

III.   NETWORK OF HEALTH PROFESSIONALS IS REQUIRED.

An organization offering an RFB plan must do more than merely pay health care claims on behalf of its beneficiaries. The plan must meet the definition of a coordinated care plan. As such, the organization must have a network of health professionals and meet the applicable access, availability, service area and quality assurance requirements of a coordinated care plan.

IV.   ENROLLEES MAY BE LIMITED TO MEMBERS OF THE CHURCH.

RFP plans have a major distinguishing factor from other types of coordinated care plans. The plans are allowed to limit enrollment to members of the church. A religious fraternal benefit society offering an MA plan may restrict the enrollment of individuals in the plan to individuals who are members of the church, convention, or group with which the society is affiliated.

V.   PRESCRIPTION DRUGS.

An enrollee who wants prescription drug coverage must get it from the RFP plan.

VI.   PRIMARY DOCTORS – SPECIALISTS.

Enrollees who are not limited to service of primary doctors or specialists in the network may choose a doctor (including a specialist) outside of the network, but often for larger fees and/or deductibles.

MEDICARE ADVANTAGE (MA)/SPECIAL NEEDS BENEFICIARIES (SNP) PLANS

INTRODUCTION

The Medicare Advantage SNP is one of the several coordinated care plans. (See also *Medicare Advantage Plans (MAP)/Common Features;* and *Medicare Advantage (MA)/Coordinated Care Plans – Common Features*). The special features of SNP plans are set forth below.

I.   DEFINED TERMINOLOGY.

Commencing January 1, 2006, MMA has authorized SNPs as coordinated care plans that exclusively or disproportionately (as defined below) serve special needs individuals (as defined below) and provide Part D benefits to all enrollees. CMS has designated these plans as meeting the requirements of a SNP, as determined on a case-by-case basis. The establishment of SNPs allows MAPs that have targeted clinical programs for special needs individuals to exclusively enroll them.

CMS has defined a disproportionate percentage SNP as one that enrolls a greater proportion of the target group of special needs individuals than occur nationally in the Medicare population based on data acceptable to CMS.

A "special needs individual" means an MA-eligible individual who is "institutionalized," is entitled to medical assistance under a state plan, under Title XIX of the Social Security Act, or has a severe or disabling chronic condition and would benefit from enrollment in a specialized MA plan.

For the purposes of a special needs individual, "institutionalized" means continuously residing or being expected to continuously reside for ninety (90) days or longer in a long-term care facility that is a skilled nursing facility (SNF), nursing facility (NF), SNF/NF, an intermediate care facility for the mentally retarded, or an inpatient psychiatric facility. CMS may also consider as institutionalized those individuals living in the community but requiring a level of care equivalent to that of those individuals living in those long-term care facilities.

II. ELIGIBILITY.

To be eligible to elect a special needs MA plan (SNP), the beneficiary must:

> meet the definition of a special needs individual,
>
> meet the eligibility requirements for that specific SNP, and
>
> be eligible to elect an MA plan.

CMS may exclude beneficiaries with ESRD from eligibility. It also has the authority to designate certain MA plans as SNPs if they disproportionately serve special needs beneficiaries. Furthermore, the SNPs may restrict eligibility solely to those individuals who are in one or more classes of special needs individuals.

MMA provides for continued eligibility for a beneficiary enrolled in a SNP who no longer meets the eligibility criteria, but who can reasonably be expected to meet the criteria of the plan within a six- (6) month period. In such a case, the enrollee is deemed to continue to be eligible for the MA plan for a period of not less than thirty (30) days but not to exceed six (6) months. The MA organization may choose any length of time from thirty (30) days to six (6) months for deemed continued eligibility as long as it applies this period consistently among all members in its plan and fully informs its members of the time period.

Beneficiaries already enrolled in an MA plan that CMS later designates as an SNP may not be involuntarily disenrolled because they do not meet the definition of special needs individuals. They may continue to be enrolled in the plan or choose to elect another MA plan during the appropriate election periods provided to all MA eligible beneficiaries.

"Grandfathered" SNP beneficiaries are distinguished from beneficiaries who join a new SNP and then lose their special needs status on other than a temporary basis. Those special needs beneficiaries would be involuntarily disenrolled after losing their special needs status (and after any period of deemed continued eligibility, if appropriate, as explained above) and receiving proper notice.

III.   PAYMENTS TO SNPS.

SNPs are paid the same as other MA plans, based on the plan's enrollment. There are no special payment features specific to special needs plans. However, a risk adjustment payment methodology is being phased in for all MA plans. Under risk adjustment, payments are more accurate because they reflect the health status of an organization's enrollees. Therefore, to the extent that a SNP enrolls less healthy beneficiaries, it will receive higher payments to account for higher risk health status.

IV.   PRESCRIPTION DRUGS.

SNPs must provide prescription drug Part D coverage. An enrollee who wants prescription drug coverage must get it from the PPO plan.

V.   PRIMARY DOCTORS – SPECIALISTS.

Enrollees who are not limited to service of primary doctors or specialists in the network, may choose a doctor (including a specialist) outside of the network, but often for larger fees and/or deductibles.

(continued on next page)

MEDICARE ADVANTAGE (MA)/REGIONAL PREFERRED PROVIDER ORGANIZATION (PPO) PLANS

INTRODUCTION

The Medicare Prescription Drug Improvement and Modernization Act of 2003 (MMA) has expanded the single type of PPO in the definition "coordinated care plans" into two under the Medicare Advantage (MA) program, by including regional PPOs and local PPOs as defined below. (See also *Medicare Advantage (MA)/Coordinated Care Plans – Common Features;* and *Medicare Advantage Plans (MAP)/Common Features*)

I.   DEFINITIONS.

Regional Plan. An MA regional plan is a coordinated care plan, structured as a PPO, that: i) services one or more entire regions mean; (ii) that has a network of providers that have agreed to contractually specified reimbursement for covered benefits with the organization offering the plan; (iii) that provides for reimbursement for all covered benefits regardless of whether such benefits are provided within such network of providers; and (iv) that has a service area that spans one or more entire MA regions.

Regional PPOs can only be offered in an MA region, which is defined as an area within the fifty (50) states and the District of Columbia. Congress did not include Puerto Rico or the other U.S. territories in the areas in which organizations could offer regional PPOs.

An employer or union group health plan that is an "800-series" plan is open only to group enrollment and cannot be a regional PPO plan, with one exception. If the MA organization offering a regional PPO plan that is open to individual enrollment also offers an 800-series employer group health plan (EGHP) in the identical service area, this EGHP plan can be considered a regional PPO plan.

Local Plan. An MA local plan is an MA plan that is not an MA regional plan. Under current law, MA local plans are county or equivalent areas as specified by the Secretary of HHS.

II. STRUCTURED AS A PPO BUT SUBJECT TO SEVERAL SPECIAL RULES.

Regional plans are subject to several rules different than MA local plans as described below, but are structured as PPOs. While local PPO plans may choose the counties in which they wish to operate as Medicare Advantage plans, regional plans must cover an entire region.

III. MORATORIUM ON FORMATION AND EXPANSION OF LOCAL PPOS.

In the first two (2) years of formation of regional plans, there is a moratorium imposed on the formation or expansion of local plans that operate as PPOs. Starting in 2006, only local PPO plans in the current demonstration areas are authorized. Accordingly, an MA organization cannot offer a new PPO plan in a service area if the MA organization did not offer a PPO plan in that service area in 2005. The MA organization must have actually enrolled beneficiaries into the plan prior to January 1, 2006. The CMS will determine the boundaries for the regions in which regional plans will operate.

IV. SPECIAL RULES.

The following special rules apply to regional PPOs.

Single Deductible Out-of-Pocket Limit. MA regional plans have a single deductible for both Part A and Part B benefits. The single deductible may be applied differentially for in-network services and waived for preventive or other items and services.

Catastrophic Limits. MA regional plans are required to have a catastrophic limit on beneficiary out-of-pocket expenditures for in-network benefits under the original Medicare program. Similarly, MA regional plans must provide a total catastrophic limit on beneficiary out-of-pocket expenditures for in and out-of-network benefits under the original Medicare program. The total out-of-pocket catastrophic limit may be higher than the in-network catastrophic limit, but may not increase the limit applicable to in-network services. MA plans must track the deductible and catastrophic limits based on incurred, rather than paid, out-of-pocket beneficiary costs, and notify beneficiaries and providers when the limit has been reached.

State Licenses. CMS may temporarily waive state license requirements in order to facilitate the offering of MA plans in regions encompassing multiple states. However, MA plans will need to be licensed by at least one state in the region and are required to have submitted applications in all of the other states. The licensure waiver is temporary, and in most cases, CMS expects the waiver to be for less than a year.

(continued on next page)

MEDICARE ADVANTAGE (MA)/MEDICAL SAVINGS ACCOUNT (MSA) PLANS

INTRODUCTION

A private MSA, established by an employer, enables employees to obtain and pay for high-deductible catastrophic health insurance policies. The private MSA, still in effect, has stimulated development of Federal demonstration projects. (See also *Medicare Savings Account (MSA)*)

The Balanced Budget Act of 1997 created one of the Federal demonstration projects called Medicare Advantage Savings Account plan. Enrollment was available to a maximum cap of 390,000 Medicare beneficiaries. Under MMA, MA organizations are now authorized to offer Medicare Advantage MSA plans as a permanent option; the enrollment cap was eliminated. The salient special features of the Medicare Advantage MSA plans are set forth below. (See also *Medicare Advantage Plans (MAP)/Common Features.*)

I.   ELIGIBILITY.

Individuals (subject to the limitations mentioned below) who are entitled to Medicare Part A and enrolled under Part B, may elect to participate in an MSA plan. To be eligible for an MSA, an individual must reside in the U.S. for at least one-hundred eighty-three (183) days during the year, and must not have end-stage renal disease (permanent kidney failure), nor currently be receiving hospice care.

Certain low-income Medicare beneficiaries are not eligible; namely, Qualified Medicare Beneficiaries, Qualified Disabled Working Individuals, Specified Low-income Medicare Beneficiaries, or individuals otherwise entitled to Medicare cost-sharing assistance under the Medicaid program.

In addition, certain classes of Medicare beneficiaries (though they have Medicare Part A and Medicare Part B) are not eligible to choose an MSA plan:

>Beneficiaries who have coverage benefits that cover the high deductible of policies, including an employers' group plan that provides this coverage.

>Beneficiaries who are retired Federal government employees and part of the Federal Employee Health Benefits Program.

>Individuals who are retired Department of Defense or Department of Veterans Affairs employees.

II.   ENROLLMENT.

Eligible individuals may select an MSA plan at either of the following times: (i) at the time they become entitled to benefits under Part A and enroll in Part B (the selection will be effective at such time), and (ii) during the coordinated enrollment period October 15 – December 7 (the selection will be effective on January 1st of the following year). The first time an eligible individual enrolls, he/she has until December 15th of the same year to change his/her mind and choose another Medicare health plan. Otherwise, the enrolled individual must stay with the MSA plan for one (1) full year.

III.   MEDICAL SAVINGS ACCOUNT + HIGH-DEDUCTIBLE HEALTH POLICY (HDHP).

The MSA plan is basically divided into two main operational parts: a Medical Savings Account, and a high-deductible health policy (HDHP). Under the plan, Medicare contributes the following payments: (i) a lump-sum contribution (annual deposit) to the MSA (an account described in section IX below), which the account holder may use only for payment of qualified medical expenses, plus (ii) a monthly payment by Medicare to the insurance company of the company's premium, for the HDHP that the account holder has chosen. The money expended by the Medicare program for the annual deposit, plus the HDHP's monthly premiums, equals the same capitation amount that the Medicare would have spent if the account holder joined another MA health plan option.

IV.   ANNUAL DEDUCTIBLE.

The MSA pays for at least the items and services covered under Medicare Parts A and B, and such additional health services as the CMS may approve, but only after the enrollee meets the amount of the annual deductible of a required HDHP by first using the annual deposit or his/her own money.

For the year 2008, the annual deductible was limited to be not more than $10,500, nor less than $2,000. For subsequent contract years, the deductible may not exceed the maximum amount for the previous contract year, increased by the National Per Capita Medicare+Choice growth percentage as defined in Section 1853(C)(6) of the Social Security Act.

The MSA plan counts towards meeting the annual deductible all amounts that would have qualified for payment under Parts A and B by the enrollee as deductibles, or copayments (but not supplemental benefits), as if the enrollee had elected to receive benefits through those parts.

V.   TAX EXEMPT TRUST OR CUSTODIAL ACCOUNT.

The MSA is a tax-exempt trust or a custodial account created for the purpose of paying qualified medical expenses solely of the account holder. The account holder pays for the medical expenses, using the annual deposit in the MSA and his/her own money until the annual deductible is reached. After that, the HDHP will pay some or all of the enrollee's qualified medical expenses.

Qualified medical expenses are expenses defined as such under the Federal tax rules relating to itemized Federal tax deductions for medical care (see section VII below). The expenses cover a broader range than covered by Medicare (e.g., prescription drugs).

The trustees or custodians of an MSA may be a bank, insurance company or other financial institution satisfactory to the Secretary of HHS. They will provide a form of check or debit card to the account holder so that he/she can access the account; and they will report any deposits and withdrawals on the account to the IRS at the end of the year.

VI.   CHOICE OF HEALTH PROFESSIONALS – NETWORK OR NON-NETWORK MSA.

An enrollee's choice of health professionals depends on whether an MSA plan is a provider network plan or a non-network plan described as follows:

> Non-network MSA Plan This is a plan where the account holder has the free choice of doctors and other health professionals to whom payment is made for qualified medical services that they render.

Network MSA Plan This is a managed plan under which enrollees must receive services through a defined provider network consisting of providers with which the MA organization contracts to furnish health care services to Medicare enrollees under the MSA plan.

VII. QUALIFIED MEDICAL EXPENSES–ACCOUNT HOLDERS ONLY.

The MSA may only pay for qualified medical expenses of the account holder -- not those of a spouse or dependents. Expenses may not include any insurance premiums, other than those for: long-term care insurance, continuation insurance (so-called COBRA coverage) and coverage while an individual is receiving unemployment insurance. Qualified medical expenses cover a range of services not covered by Medicare -- e.g. prescription drugs, dental claims (including false teeth) and vision care (including eye glasses).

To the extent payments are made by the MSA for non-qualified medical expenses, these payments are included in the taxable income of enrollee.

VIII. PROHIBITION AGAINST COMMINGLING OF MSA FUNDS.

MSA assets may not be invested in life insurance contracts, nor commingled with other payments, except a common trust fund or common investment fund.

IX. CONTRIBUTIONS TO THE MSA -- BY MEDICARE ONLY.

The only contribution that may be made to an MSA is a specified contribution by the Secretary of HHS to the MSA.

The contribution begins, and is made in a lump sum, the month and year that an individual's election of the MSA plan is effective. The amount of the contribution for that month and all successive months in the year will be deposited in a single lump sum (annual deposit) during the first month. If an MSA is terminated before the end of the year, the proportionate share of the lump sum deposited by the Secretary of HHS must be refunded to Medicare.

If the amount of the required Medicare contribution to the plan (i.e., the capitation) is greater than the cost of the high-deductible health policy (HDHP), the difference must be deposited by Medicare in the MSA.

X. PROHIBITED SALES OF MEDIGAP AND OTHER POLICIES.

Insurers are prohibited from selling to an MSA plan enrollee a Medigap policy that duplicates benefits to which the beneficiary is eligible under Medicare.

Insurers are also prohibited from selling policies (other than those specified below) to persons covered under an MSA plan that would provide coverage for expenses that are otherwise required to be counted toward meeting the annual deductible amount of the HDHP. Thus, the account holder may not carry health insurance that covers the policy's deductible. This prohibition does not extend to HDHPs that provide coverage for any of the following: accidents; disability; dental care; vision care; long-term care; liabilities incurred under workers' compensation laws, tort liabilities, or liabilities relating to ownership or use of property; specified diseases or illnesses; and, a fixed amount per day of hospitalization.

XI. PREMIUMS.

Unlike all MA plans (other than PFFS plans), MSA plans are without limit on premiums that maybe charged enrollees for Medicare basic benefits (Parts A and B). The plan is required to accept the Medicare capitation (i.e. the amount of required Medicare contribution) to the plan as payment in full for such basic benefits.

If the premium under the MSA plan is less than one-half of the required amount of Medicare contribution to the plan, the Secretary of HHS must deposit an amount equal to the difference in the account holder's MSA.

XII. CHARGE LIMITS.

When a provider does not have a contract with the plan. A physician or other provider who does not have a contract establishing payment amounts for services furnished to an enrollee of an MSA organization is required to accept as payment in full for covered services amounts that physicians or other providers could collect if the individual were not enrolled in such organization (i.e., the amount that original Medicare fee-for-services would have paid to an enrollee if enrolled in original Medicare).

When a provider does have a contract with the plan. A physician or other provider of services who has a contract with the plan establishing payment amounts for services furnished to an enrollee of an MSA organization is required to accept as payment in full for covered services the amount set forth in the plan's fee schedule.

XIII. TAX TREATMENT OF MSA.

A.   Tax Treatment during Life of Account Holder.

The following are not included in taxable income of the account holder:

> Contributions by the HHS to the MSA are not included in taxable income.

> Transfers of one Medicare MSA from one trustee to another trustee are not included in taxable income. When multiple Medicare MSAs may have been created by an account holder, he/she must designate only one as the MSA.

> Distributions from an MSA used to pay qualified medical expenses of the account holder are not included in taxable income and cannot be taken into account as itemized tax deductions for medical expenses.

> Income earned on assets in the MSA is not included in taxable income.

The following are included in the taxable income of the account holder:

> Payments for medical expenses of the account holder's spouse or dependents, or any person other than the account holder are included in taxable income of the account holder; they are not qualified medical expenses.

> Distributions made for other than qualified medical expenses are included in income. To the extent that they exceed a prescribed limit, such excess distributions are subject to a statutory penalty; the limit can be different each year. (For example, for the year 2006, the limit is equal to the account balance of the MSA on December 31st of the prior year, less sixty (60%) percent of the annual deductible of the high-deductible health policy (HDHP)).

B.   **Tax Treatment upon Death of the Account Holder.**

The tax treatment of the MSA depends on which of three (3) alternatives applies:

Surviving spouse is designated beneficiary. The surviving spouse may continue the MSA, as if the spouse were the account holder. No new contributions may be made to the MSA. Earnings on the account balance are not included in taxable income.

Distribution of qualified medical expenses to the surviving spouse or spouse's dependents is not included in income.

Distributions other than for qualified medical expenses are included in income. They are subject to a penalty tax, unless the distributions are made after the surviving spouse attains age 65, dies or becomes incapacitated.

A beneficiary other than surviving spouse is designated. The MSA ceases to be treated as an MSA. The value of the MSA is included in the gross taxable income of the beneficiary for the taxable year in which the death occurs.

No beneficiary is designated. The MSA ceases to be treated as an MSA. The value of the MSA on the account holder's death is included in the gross income of the account holder's final income tax return.

(continued on next page)

MEDICARE ADVANTAGE (MA)/PRIVATE FEE-FOR-SERVICE (PFFS) PLANS

INTRODUCTION

There are several types of Medicare Advantage plans, which are alternatives to the original Medicare fee-for-service plan. The MA Private Fee-for-Service (PFFS) plan is one of the alternative plans.

Salient special PFFS features are set forth below (see also *Medicare Advantage Plans (MAP)/Common Features*).

I. DEFINITION.

A PPFS plan:

> reimburses hospitals, physicians and other providers at a rate determined by the plan on a fee-for-service basis without placing the providers at financial risk;
>
> does not vary its rates for such providers based on utilization of the PFFS plan by the providers;
>
> does not restrict the selection of providers by enrollees to only those who provide the services and agree to accept the terms and conditions of payment established by the plan;
>
> provides access to any Medicare-approved doctor or hospital that accepts the plan's payment; the plan rather than the Medicare program determines how much it will pay and what the beneficiary pays for the services he/she is rendered;
>
> may provide supplemental benefits (i.e., benefits in addition to items and services available under Parts A and B) and coverage

of additional services that the plan finds to be medically necessary; and,

unlike all other plans, except MSAs, may provide for payment by enrollees of an extra premium for Medicare basic benefits in addition to the regular Medicare premiums. Beneficiaries are liable for the full amount of any premium that the plan may charge.

II. PREMIUM.

Unlike all MA plans (other than MSA), PFFS plans do not limit the premiums that may be charged enrollees for Medicare basic benefits (Parts A and B). The plan is required to accept the Medicare capitation (i.e., the amount of required Medicare contribution) to the plan as payment in full for such basic benefits.

III. CHARGE LIMITS.

A. When a Provider Does Not Have a Contract with the Plan.

A physician or other provider who does not have a contract establishing payment amounts for services furnished to an enrollee of PFFS organizations is required to accept as payment in full for covered services amounts that physicians or other providers could collect if the individual were not enrolled in such organization (i.e., the amount that the original Medicare fee-for-services plan would have paid to an enrollee if enrolled in original Medicare).

B. When a Provider Has a Contract with the Plan.

A physician or other provider of services that has a contract, or is deemed to have a contract, with a PFFS plan must accept as payment in full for services that are furnished to enrollees an amount not to exceed (including deductibles, coinsurance, copayments or balance billing) one-hundred fifteen (115%) percent of the payment fee schedule rate as determined by the plan.

A health provider is treated ("deemed") as having a contract with the plan (i) if the provider furnishes services that are covered by the plan and (ii) if before furnishing the services the provider has been informed of the individual's enrollment under the plan and has also been informed of the terms and conditions for those services under the plan or is given the opportunity to obtain information on those terms and conditions.

IV.   SERVICES TO ENROLLEES.

The plan is required to provide its enrollees through its physicians and other providers of services not less than all those items and services, other than hospice care, available under Medicare Part A and Part B.

V.   ACCESS TO SERVICES – PRIMARY CARE DOCTOR -- SPECIALIST

The organization offering a PFFS plan must demonstrate to the CMS that it has a sufficient number and range of health care professionals and providers willing to provide services under the terms of the plan.

The plan must permit enrollees to obtain services from any entity authorized by Medicare to provide for Part A/B services, and agree to provide services under the terms of the plan.

An enrollee is not required to choose a primary care doctor or obtain a reference to see a specialist.

VI.   QUALITY ASSURANCE.

The plan is not required to meet prescribed quality assurance requirements.

VII.   EXPLANATION OF BENEFITS.

The plan must offer enrollees of the plan an appropriate explanation of benefits that includes a clear statement of the amount of an enrollee's liability, including balance billing, for services rendered.

VIII.   NOTICE TO ENROLLEES BY HOSPITALS.

The organization must require hospitals to provide notice to enrollees prior to receipt of inpatient hospital services, or other services, when the amount of balance billing could be substantial. The notice must include a good faith estimate of the likely amount of such balance billing.

IX.   PRESCRIPTION DRUGS.

A PFFS may choose to offer Part D prescription drugs, or not.

MEDICARE ADVANTAGE (MA)/OUTPATIENT PRESCRIPTION DRUGS*

INTRODUCTION

Section 101 of the Medicare Modernization Act (MMA), which was enacted into law December 8, 2003, established a new Medicare Part D program for voluntary outpatient prescription drug coverage (Part D drugs) under Medicare Advantage plan benefits described below.

Salient aspects of the Medicare Part D program are set forth below.

I.   ADMINISTRATION.

The Centers for Medicare and Medicaid Services (CMS) has overall responsibility for implementing the Medicare Part D prescription drug benefits and its published final rules.

II.   PART D DRUGS DEFINED.

A Part D drug is a drug that is approved by the Food and Drug Administration, for which a prescription is required, and for which payment is required under Medicaid. Biological products, including insulin and insulin supplies (syringes, needles, alcohol swabs and gauge) and smoking cessation drugs are also covered under Part D. MMA excludes from coverage those categories of drugs for which Medicaid payment is optional, such as drugs for weight gain, barbiturates, benzodiazepines and over-the-counter medications. MMA also excludes from Part D coverage those drugs for which payment could be made under Medicare Part A or Part B.

---

* This Overview is repetitive of matter contained in the Overview *Medicare/Outpatient Prescription Drug Program (Part D)*. The author believes that direct access to the subject will be convenient to the reader.

III.   PART D DRUG BENEFITS.

MMA established a standard drug benefit that MA plans may offer (see A below), or alternative prescription drug coverage (see B below) to Part D eligibles (individuals who are entitled to benefits under Part A or who are enrolled in Part B).

A.   Standard Drug Benefit.

The MMA established a standard drug benefit that Part D plans may offer, consisting of the following features:

i)   A yearly deductible of $320 (2012);

ii)   Twenty-five (25%) percent of the yearly drug costs of $2,610 (2012), representing the costs between $320 and up to $2,930 (initial coverage limit) which amounts to $662.50). The plan pays the other seventy-five (75%) percent (plan cost share) which represents $1,957.5 (2012);

iii)   One-hundred (100%) percent of the next additional out-of-pocket expenses of $3,725.50 (2012) in drug costs (sometimes referred to as the "doughnut hole" or coverage gap). The beneficiary must pay the plan's premiums while in the coverage gap.

iv)   After having spent $4,700 (2012) out of pocket (out-of-pocket threshold) – the total of the items i) ($320), ii) ($652.50) and iii) ($3,727.50) – the Part D-eligible individual will have catastrophic coverage. This means the individual during this entire period of coverage will only have to pay $2.60 (2012) copayment for a generic or preferred brand Part D drug and $6.50 (2012) for other drugs or five (5%) percent coinsurance, whichever is greater. The plan pays for the rest.

The deductible, initial coverage limit and annual out-of-pocket threshold amount are indexed for inflation each year.

Rephrased for ready understanding the foregoing payments of $4,700 by the beneficiary in 2012 are set forth in the table below:

- Annual Deductible	$320.00
- 25% co-pay of costs between the $320 deductible and the initial coverage limit of $2,930	$652.50
Subtotal (annual deductible + co-pay)	$972.50
- Additional out-of pocket-expenses (doughnut hole)	$3,727.50
Out-of-pocket threshold	$4,700.00

B.   Alternative Prescription Drug Coverage.

Part D drug plans are not required to offer the standard benefit, but can offer alternative prescription drug coverage. Alternative coverage must be actuarially equivalent to the standard benefit. In other words, the value of the benefit package must be equal to or greater than the value of the standard benefit package. In an actuarially equivalent plan, the cost sharing varies through the use of such mechanisms as tiered copayments. However, a plan that offers an alternative benefit package cannot impose a higher annual deductible ($320 in 2012) or require a higher out-of-pocket threshold ($4,700 in 2012) than required by the standard benefit. Plans can offer enhanced alternative coverage that may include changes to the deductible and the initial coverage limit, though the deductible cannot be higher than the $310. Enhanced alternative coverage under Part D might include coverage of some drugs that are excluded under Part D, or that are in the coverage gap (doughnut hole). A prescription drug plan (PDP) that wants to offer a drug plan with enhanced alternative coverage in a service area must also offer a PDP with the basic benefit prescription package in that area.

IV.   FORMULARY.

The MMA requires that a plan's drug formulary must include at least one (but often two) drugs in each approved category and class. CMS has developed appeals procedures which ensure that enrollees quickly receive decisions regarding medically necessary medications. Pharmacies will distribute or post notices that instruct enrollees to contact their Medicare prescription drug plan if they need a certain drug and the pharmacist informs them that the drug is not included in the plan's formulary. The plans may change their formularies any time upon giving a sixty- (60) day notice to the enrollee, his/her proscribing physician, pharmacist and

CMS, of formulary changes. The notice must explain how an enrollee may request an exception. If an enrollee requests an exception, the plan must make its decision as expeditiously as the enrollee's health condition requires after it receives the request, but no later than twenty-four (24) hours for an expedited coverage determination or seventy-two (72) hours for a standard coverage determination.

V. MEDIGAP INSURANCE POLICIES – PROHIBITED USE.

Insurance companies are no longer able to sell existing Medigap policies that provide drug coverage to Medicare beneficiaries who are enrolled in or eligible for the new Medicare outpatient prescription drug coverage. They are, however, able to renew the Medigap drug policies issued prior to January 1, 2006 for beneficiaries who do not opt for the new Medicare prescription drug plan; their Medigap policy will be modified to eliminate drug coverage and premiums will be adjusted. Beneficiaries with the new Medicare drug coverage can purchase Medigap policies that do not cover drugs.

VI. MEDICARE CANNOT NEGOTIATE DRUG DISCOUNTS.

The MMA prohibits the government from negotiating discounts on drugs purchases or otherwise interfering in drug pricing decisions.

VII. MEDICARE DOES NOT COVER PART D DRUGS.

Medicaid is prohibited from providing Part D drug benefits to dual eligible individuals.

VIII. PRESCRIPTION DRUG PLANS.

1. **Participation requires the beneficiary to take affirmative steps to enroll in a prescription drug plan**. In order for Medicare beneficiaries to take part in the Medicare Part D prescription drug program, it is incumbent upon them to enroll in a prescription drug plan. These plans are offered by insurance companies and other private companies and cover both generic and brand name drugs. Plans serving the fee-for-service Medicare population (original Medicare) are called prescription drug plans (PDPs), also known as stand-alone plans, and those serving Medicare Advantage enrollees are called Medicare Advantage prescription drug plans (MA-PDPs).

Rephrased, a PDP is a stand-alone plan that is defined as prescription drug coverage offered under an approved plan, contract or policy, by a PDP sponsor through a contract between CMS and the sponsor. An MA-PDP is offered through a Part C Medicare Advantage organization that offers comprehensive benefits, including outpatient prescription drug coverage.

2. **Exclusion of persons with end-stage renal disease (ESRD).** Persons with ESRD are excluded from taking part in the Medicare Part D prescription drug program. An individual who develops ESRD while enrolled in an MA plan may continue in that plan.

3. **PDP enrollees are locked-in.** Individuals who enroll in a PDP are locked-in to their plan for the remainder of the calendar year, even though the plan in which they enroll may change the formulary or cost-sharing arrangements during the year. Enrollees in PDPs must wait until the next annual enrollment period to switch plans, with enrollment in the new plan becoming effective on January 1 of the following year.

IX. ENROLLMENT -- ELIGIBILITY.

A. General.

A Medicare beneficiary who becomes entitled to Part B is not automatically enrolled in Part D. Enrollment in Part D requires the beneficiary to take affirmative steps to enroll and get Part D coverage. The beneficiary must first choose a drug plan from the options available in his/her area. Then, the beneficiary must enroll through the plan that he/she chooses. If the beneficiary may be eligible for the low-income subsidy, he/she must file a second affirmation.

The four (4) coverage enrollment periods are: (i) the initial enrollment period; (ii) open enrollment period; (iii) the annual coordinated election period; and (iv) special enrollment period.

In order to be eligible to enroll in a PDP plan, the individual must reside in the plan's service area and cannot be enrolled in a MA plan, (other than a Medicare Savings Account, or a private fee-for-service plan that does not provide qualified prescription drug coverage).

Individuals with the original Medicare plan, a Medicare fee-for-service plan that does not offer prescription drug coverage, a Medicare cost plan, or a Medical Savings Account plan, can join a Medicare prescription drug plan in their area. To obtain Medicare drug coverage, an individual must join a Medicare prescription drug plan if he/she is in the original Medicare plan, or the individual must join a Medicare Advantage plan that includes drug coverage.

If a Part D-eligible individual has prescription drug coverage from a former or current employer or union, he/she should contact his/her benefits administrator before making any changes to his/her coverage. If he/she joins a Medicare prescription drug plan or Medicare Advantage plan, such individual and his/her family may lose their employer or union coverage.

A Part D-eligible individual who is enrolled in a MA-PDP must obtain prescription drug coverage through that plan.

A PDP sponsor is not permitted to offer a prescription drug plan that provides enhanced or alternative coverage in a particular service area, unless it also offers a prescription drug plan that provides only basic prescription drug coverage.

An MA organization cannot offer a MA coordinated care plan in a service area unless that plan or another MA plan offered by the organization, includes either (i) basic prescription coverage, or (ii) enhanced alternative coverage, provided there is no MA monthly supplemental benefit premium applied under the MA-PDP Plan.

An MA organization may not offer prescription drug coverage (other than that required under Parts A and B of Medicare) to enrollees of a Medical Savings Account plan.

B. Enrollment Period.

There are four (4) enrollment periods as set forth below:

Initial Enrollment Period. The initial enrollment period for individuals who are first eligible to enroll in Part D, corresponds to the initial enrollment period for Part B, i.e., the seven- (7) month period running from three (3) months before the month the individual first becomes eligible and ending three (3) months after the first month of eligibility.

Open Enrollment Period. Beneficiaries who become eligible for Medicare may enroll in a Part D plan when they become eligible for Part A or Part B benefits. Open enrollment runs from October 15 through December 7, when original Medicare beneficiaries may switch from original Medicare to a Medicare Advantage plan or enroll in a stand-alone plan if they have not previously done so.

Rephrased: Beneficiaries may remain in original Medicare and receive prescription drug coverage through stand-alone prescription drug plans (drug only plan), or join a Medicare Advantage plan that offers comprehensive benefits, including outpatient prescription drugs.

Annual Coordinated Enrollment Period. The annual coordinated enrollment period corresponds to the annual coordinated enrollment period for Part C and runs from October15 through December 7.

Special Enrollment Periods. Individuals may be eligible for a special enrollment period, if:

> they did not enroll in Part D during their initial enrollment because they had other prescription drug coverage deemed to be creditable coverage, and they lose the creditable coverage;

> they were given incorrect information concerning the status of their other prescription drug coverage as creditable coverage;

> they were given incorrect information about enrollment by a Federal employee;

> they have Medicare and full Medicaid coverage or a Medical Savings Account program;

> they move out of a plan's service area;

> their PDP's contract with Medicare is terminated;

> they enrolled in a MA-PDPP during the first year of eligibility and want to return to traditional Medicare and a PDP; or,

> they move into or out of a nursing home.

5-Star Special Enrollment Period. Individuals can switch to a 5-star Medicare prescription drug plan at any time during the year. They can only switch to such a plan if one is available in their area. An individual can only use this period to switch to a 5-star plan one time each year.

C.   Effective Date of Enrollment.

Part D coverage becomes effective:

> the same month that Part A and/or Part B coverage becomes effective for individuals who enroll before their month of entitlement to Part A or enrollment in Part B;

the first day of the next calendar month after enrollment for individuals who enroll after the first month of entitlement for Part A or enrollment in Part B;

the following January 1, for individuals who enroll during the annual coordinated enrollment period; and

at the time specified by CMS for individuals who enroll during a special enrollment period.

D.   Involuntary Disenrollment.

An individual may be involuntarily disenrolled from a drug plan for reasons similar to the grounds for disenrollment from a Medicare Advantage plan. These include: no longer living in the plan's service area; loss of eligibility for Part D; death of the individual; termination of the PDP; failure to pay premiums on a timely basis; and, involvement in disruptive behavior that substantially impairs the ability of the plan to arrange for or provide services.

E.   Ability to Change Plan Mid-Year.

Changes during the Annual Coordinated Enrollment Period. All beneficiaries may switch plans once during the annual coordinated enrollment period, which runs from October 15 to December 7. Enrollment becomes effective on January 1 of the next year.

Changes during Open Enrollment Periods. Individuals enrolled in a Medicare Advantage (MA) plan also may change plans once during the open enrollment period, which extends for the first three (3) months of each year after. An enrollee in a MA-PDPP may use the open enrollment period (January through March) to change to another MA-PDP or to disenroll from the MA-PDP and return to traditional/original Medicare and a PDP. Someone who enrolls in a MA plan that does not offer prescription drug coverage may not change to an MA-PDP or to original Medicare and a PDP during the open enrollment period. The beneficiary must wait to change plans until the next annual election period.

Changes during Special Enrollment Periods. Beneficiaries are eligible to change plans mid-year if they qualify for a special enrollment period described above.

F.   Failure to Enroll on a Timely Basis.

A beneficiary who does not enroll in a Part D plan within sixty-three (63) days of his/her initial enrollment period, and who does not have other creditable prescription drug coverage, must pay a late penalty if he/she subsequently enrolls in a Part D plan. The penalty is assessed at one (1) percent of the national average premium for each month of delayed enrollment, for the remainder of the time in which the beneficiary is enrolled in a Part D plan. Thus, a beneficiary who first becomes eligible for Part D at age sixty-five (65), but who delays enrolling until age 70 may be assessed a sixty- (60) percent penalty on his/her premium (5 years x 12 months x 1%). Since the penalty is based on a percentage of the average premium each year, the dollar value of the penalty changes as the national average premium changes.

Late enrollment penalties will not be imposed if a beneficiary maintains creditable coverage (i.e., other coverage, equivalent to Medicare basic drug benefit, Veterans Administration coverage, Medigap coverage, and most employer (or union) sponsor retiree plans). Should a beneficiary's existing drug coverage end or change and thereby cease to be creditable, he/she has up to sixty-three (63) days to enroll in a Medicare drug plan.

G.   Automatic Enrollment for Individuals Who Are Full-Benefit Dual Eligible.

A full-benefit dual eligible individual under Part D means an individual who is determined eligible by the State for (i) medical assistance for full Medicaid benefits under Title XIX of the Social Security Act under any eligibility category covered under a state plan; or (ii) medical assistance under the Act authorized for the medical needy, or permitted by states that use more restrictive eligibility criteria than are used by the Supplemental Security Income (SSI) program. This definition is narrower than the definition of dual eligibles in other areas of the original Medicare program in that it excludes Specified Low-income Medicare Beneficiaries (SLMB), Low-income Qualified Individuals (QIs), and Qualified Disabled and Working Individuals (QDWI). (These individuals under MMA, however, are deemed full-benefit dual eligibles.)

Under the MMA there is a process of including automatic assignment into drug plans for individuals who are full-benefit dual eligibles, who are eligible for Medicare and Medicaid and who do not choose a PDP or MA-PDP during the initial enrollment period. Full-benefit dual eligibles at all times are automatically eligible for a special enrollment period.

Full-benefit dual eligibles cannot receive Medicaid drug coverage. They must join a MA-PDP or a Medicare stand-alone drug plan to obtain drug coverage. CMS must automatically enroll full-benefit dual eligible individuals who fail to enroll in a Part D plan into a PDP that offers basic prescription drug coverage in the area where the individual resides and that has a monthly beneficiary premium which does not exceed the low-income premium subsidy amount.

Full-benefit dual eligible individuals who are enrolled in an MA private fee-for-service (PFFS) plan or cost-basis HMO or competitive medical plan that does not offer qualified prescription drug coverage, or an MSA plan and who fail to enroll in a Part D plan must be automatically enrolled by CMS into a PDP plan.

Nothing prevents a full-benefit dual eligible individual from: (1) affirmatively declining enrollment in Part D; or (2) disenrolling from the Part D plan in which the individual is enrolled and electing to enroll in another Part D plan during the special enrollment period.

For individuals who are Medicaid eligible and subsequently become newly eligible for Part D, enrollment is effective on the first day of the month the individual is eligible for Part D. For individuals who are eligible for Part D and subsequently become eligible for Medicaid, enrollment is effective upon being identified by CMS as a full-benefit dual eligible individual.

X.   SUBSIDIES FOR LOW-INCOME INDIVIDUALS.

MMA provides for subsidies to meet all or some of the cost-sharing payments (deductibles and copayments) in the case of certain Medicare beneficiaries with incomes up to one-hundred fifty (150%) percent of the Federal poverty level. Subsidies differ depending on income, Medicaid status and institutional status. These beneficiaries are each a subsidy-eligible individual and according to income or status are (i) a full-subsidy-eligible individual, (ii) individuals treated (deemed) as full-subsidy eligibles, or (iii) individuals who are other low-income subsidy individuals.

A. Definitions.

A subsidy-eligible individual is a Part D-eligible individual who (i) is enrolled in or seeking to enroll in a Part D plan; (ii) has an income below one-hundred fifty (150%) percent of the Federal poverty level; and (iii) has resources at or below the thresholds set forth below.

There are two groups of subsidy-eligible low-income individuals. The first group is composed of persons who (i) either have incomes below one-hundred thirty-five (135%) percent of the Federal poverty level; have resources in 2012 no more than $8,440 for an individual and $13,410 for a couple (increased in future years by the percentage increase in the consumer price index (CPI); or (ii) are full-benefit dual eligibles, regardless of whether they meet eligibility standards.

The second group of subsidy-eligible individuals is persons meeting the same requirements, except that the income level is above one-hundred thirty-five (135%) percent but below one-hundred fifty (150%) percent of the Federal poverty level and an alternative resources standard (i.e., alternative to the resources standard in (i) above) may be used. The alternative standard in 2012 is $13,070 for an individual and $26,120 for a couple (increased in future years by the percentage increase in the CPI).

A full-subsidy eligible individual is a subsidy individual who has full Medicaid status (full-benefit dual eligible) and (i) income below one-hundred thirty-five (135%) percent of the Federal poverty level and (ii) has resources in 2012 not more than $8,440 (single person) or less than $13,410 (married couple); including $1,500 per person for burial expenses.

A subsidy individual treated (deemed) as a full-subsidy eligible is: (i) an individual enrolled in one of the following Medicare savings programs -- Qualified Medicare Beneficiary (QMB); Specified Low-income Medicare Beneficiary (SLMB); Qualifying Individual (QI) under a state's plan; or (ii) a recipient of SSI benefits without Medicaid.

All Medicaid full-benefit dual eligible individuals must be enrolled in Medicare Part D in order to receive drug benefits. Enrollment in Medicare Part D is a condition of eligibility for Medicaid. An individual will lose all Medicaid benefits for failure to enroll or remain enrolled in a plan. New applicants who are Part D eligible do not need to be enrolled in a Medicare prescription drug plan in order to open a Medicaid case. Once they have an open case, the state will send their name to CMS for automatic enrollment in a plan.

Full-benefit dual eligible individuals who reside in nursing homes are required to enroll in Medicare Part D.

Partial-subsidy individuals are those subsidy-eligible individuals who (i) have income above one-hundred thirty-five (135%) percent of the Federal poverty level, but income less than one-hundred fifty (150%) percent of the Federal poverty level, or (ii) have resources that do not exceed $13,070 (2012) if single, or $26,120 (including $1,500 for burial expenses) if married.

B.   Premium Subsidy Entitlements.
(See *also Premium/Medicare Part D Drug Coverage*.)

Full-subsidy eligible individuals (including those deemed full-subsidy eligible) are entitled to one-hundred (100%) percent of the premium subsidy amount.

Other low-income subsidy individuals (partial subsidy individuals) are entitled to a premium subsidy based on a sliding scale:

A premium subsidy equal to seventy-five (75%) percent of the subsidy for individuals with income greater than one-hundred thirty-five (135%) percent but at or below one-hundred forty (140%) percent of the Federal poverty level.

A premium subsidy equal to fifty (50%) percent of the subsidy for individuals with income greater than one-hundred forty (140%) percent but at or below one-hundred forty-five (145%) percent of the Federal poverty level.

A premium subsidy equal to twenty-five (25%) percent of the subsidy for individuals with income below one-hundred fifty (150%) percent of the Federal poverty level.

C.   Cost-Sharing Subsidies (Deductibles, Copayments).

The cost-sharing subsidies are set forth below.

Full-Subsidy Eligible. Full-benefit dual eligible beneficiaries who are recipients of Medicare and Medicaid will automatically, without the necessity of filing any application therefor, receive their prescription drug coverage through Medicare. Medicare Part D replaces Medicaid as the primary pharmacy coverage for dual eligible recipients. Generally, if a person has private health insurance that includes a drug benefit, in addition to Medicare Part D, the private insurance would be billed prior to billing Medicare Part D.

All full-subsidy individuals are entitled to a one-hundred (100%) percent subsidy for the low-income benchmark premium for a plan offering the standard Part D benefit.

The cost-sharing benefit for full-subsidy individuals includes:

No premiums;

No deductibles;

No doughnut hole (i.e., the amount of out-of-pocket drug costs that standard benefit beneficiaries are required to pay once their initial coverage limit of $2,930 (2012) is reached). Coverage continues through the doughnut hole; and

$1.10 copayment for generic drugs, or $3.30 for brand name drugs up to the out-of-pocket limit; thereafter all cost-sharing is eliminated for 2012.

Deemed Full-Subsidy Individuals. Individuals enrolled in one of the Medicare Savings Programs – Qualified Medicare Beneficiary (QMB), Specified Low-income Medicare Beneficiary (SLMB), or Qualified Individuals (QI) under a state plan program, and recipients of SSI benefits – are deemed eligible for low-income subsidy. They are treated the same as full-subsidy individuals.

Partial Subsidy-Eligible Individuals. Individuals who are not deemed eligible for the low-income subsidy may apply for the benefit. The following beneficiaries may apply for the low-income subsidy through SSA.

1. Medicare beneficiaries, who are not eligible for Medicaid, with resources less than $13,070 (for a single person in 2012) or less than $26,120 (for a married couple in 2012) and income below one-hundred thirty-five (135%) of the Federal poverty level will receive the following benefits:

No deductible;

Coinsurance of fifteen (15%) percent instead of the full twenty-five (25%) percent provided by the standard drug benefit (see *section III*), including coverage through the doughnut hole;

Copayments (2012) of $2.50 for each generic or preferred brand drug and $6.30 for each brand name drug, after an out-of-pocket limit is reached.

2. Beneficiaries with resources below $13,070 (for a single individual) in 2012 or $26,120 (for a married couple), and income between one-hundred thirty-five (135%) percent and one-hundred fifty (150%) percent of the Federal poverty level will receive the following benefits:

A $65 (2012) deductible;

Coinsurance of fifteen (15%) percent after the deductible up to the out-of-pocket limit, including continued coverage through the doughnut hole; and

Copayments (2012) of $2.60 for each generic or preferred brand drug or $6.50 for each brand name drug, after the out-of-pocket limit is reached.

Note: There is no cost-sharing for eligible individuals residing in a medical facility which is defined as a nursing home, psychiatric center, residential treatment center, development center, intermediate care facility. Individuals in other group residences such as assisted living programs, group homes and adult homes are subject to copayments.

(continued on next page)

Medicare Application
See also *Enrollment/Medicare.*

Enrollment in Medicare is automatic, without application, for persons who are age 65 or older, entitled to Social Security benefits and are actually receiving them. All other Medicare-eligible persons must file an application.

Medicare Cancellation

An individual's Medicare coverage will cease in the following instances:

> When a beneficiary's Medicare hospital insurance (Part A) is based on a spouse's work record, coverage will end if the beneficiary and his/her spouse are divorced during the first ten (10) years of their marriage. If the beneficiary is covered by Part A based on his/her own work record, coverage will continue as long as he/she lives.

> Medicare Part B coverage will be canceled if premiums are not paid. If a beneficiary cancels Part B and then later decides to re-enroll, he/she will have to wait for the general enrollment period from January 1 through March 31 of each year.

> If the beneficiary has purchased Medicare Part A by paying monthly premiums, he/she will lose it upon cancellation of Medicare Part B.

Medicare Catastrophic Coverage Act

This Federal law passed in 1988 was intended to broaden Medicaid and Medicare benefits, particularly in the area of Medicare outpatient prescription drugs and community-based long-term care. It was subsequently revised to repeal virtually all of the Medicare provisions, but many Medicaid provisions as amended were not repealed. Important amendments included additional income and recourse protection for the community spouse of a Medicaid nursing home resident, and the requirement for states to pay Medicaid cost-sharing for low-income Medicare beneficiaries.

Medicare Cost Contract/Managed Care
See also *Medicare HMO; Medicare Advantage.*

A contract between Medicare and a health plan under which the plan is paid by Medicare on the basis of reasonable costs to provide Medicare-covered services to plan participants.

Medicare Economic Index/Medicare
See also *Physician fee schedule/Medicare; Fee schedule charge/Medicare.*

An index by which Medicare calculates annual changes in the conversion factor in order to establish and adjust fee schedule charges for physician services and other procedures.

Medicare Eligibility of Persons Age 65 or Older
See also *Enrollment/Medicare.*

Entitlement to Medicare is based primarily on age and not on an applicant's financial status.

Part A. Generally, everyone age 65 and over who is entitled to <u>and</u> receiving Social Security retirement benefits and who has filed his/her application for these benefits is automatically enrolled in Medicare Part A. A dependent or survivor of a beneficiary entitled to Part A coverage, or a dependent of a beneficiary under age 65 who is entitled to Social Security retirement benefits, is likewise eligible for Part A if he/she is age 65 or older.

When a person age 65 or over is eligible for Medicare but does not receive Social Security benefits (for example, a person who has elected to defer retirement), he/she is entitled to Part A coverage. However, coverage is not automatic, and the person must make an application.

Part B. A person who is entitled to Part A coverage is entitled to Part B coverage but may elect to reject Part B coverage. Application for Part B coverage is voluntary. Should a person elect to receive Part B coverage, he/she will be required to pay a monthly premium, unlike the case of Part A coverage where no premium is required.

Medicare Health Insurance Card
See also *Enrollment/Medicare.*

Medicare-eligible persons receive a Medicare card in the mail following an application for Medicare or in certain cases automatically. The card shows that the beneficiary is entitled to receive Part A and/or Part B benefits and also indicates the beneficiary's Medicare claim number.

Medicare Health Plan

A Medicare health plan is a plan that is offered by a private company that contracts with Medicare to provide Part A and Part B benefits to people with Medicare who enroll in the plan. This includes all Medicare Advantage plans, Medicare cost plans, and Programs of All-Inclusive Care for the Elderly (PACE).

Medicare Part A Hospital Benefits

See also *Psychiatric Care/Medicare*.

Covered Services. With the exception of certain deductibles and copayments explained below, Medicare Part A will pay one-hundred (100%) percent of the following inpatient hospital services:

Bed and board in a semi-private room (two to four beds). Medicare will pay the cost of a private room only if it is required for medical reasons.

Nursing services provided by or under the supervision of licensed nursing personnel other than services of a private duty nurse or attendant.

Services of hospital medical social workers.

Use of regular hospital equipment, supplies and appliances, such as oxygen tents, wheelchairs, crutches, casts, surgical dressings and splints.

Drugs and biologicals ordinarily furnished by the hospital.

Diagnostic or therapeutic items and services ordinarily furnished by the hospital or by others, under arrangements made with the hospital.

Deductible and Copayments. For each benefit period or spell of illness requiring hospitalization, the beneficiary must pay a deductible equal to the first day's charges ($1,156 in 2012). For days 61-90 a copayment of $289 in 2012 per day is required, and during days 91-150 which are the non-renewable lifetime reserve days, a copayment of $578 in 2012 per day. Beneficiaries also must pay a deductible of the first three (3) pints of blood used each year.

Excluded Services. The following hospital services are not covered by Medicare:

Personal convenience items such as a telephone and television;

Private duty nurses or attendants unless the patient's condition requires such services and the nurse or attendant is a hospital employee; and

The first three (3) pints of blood.

Medicare Part B Benefits

See also *Medicare, section IV.B; Outpatient department hospital services/ Medicare; Drugs/Medicare.*

Covered Services.

Doctors' services which include the cost of house calls, office visits and doctors' services in a hospital or other institution. Also included are the fees of physicians, surgeons, pathologists, radiologists, anesthesiologists and osteopaths.

Services of clinical psychologists if they would otherwise be covered if furnished by a physician.

Services by chiropractors with respect to treatment of subluxation (i.e., partial dislocation) of the spine by means of manual manipulation.

Colorectal cancer screenings (see *Medicare, section IV.B* for more details.)

Fees of podiatrists, including the treatment of plantar warts, but not for routine foot care.

The costs of diagnosis and treatment of eye and ear ailments, including optometrist's treatment of aphakia.

Plastic surgery for repair of an accidental injury, an impaired limb or a malformed part of the body.

Radiological or pathological services furnished by a physician to a hospital inpatient.

The cost of blood-clotting factors and supplies necessary for the self-administration of the clotting factor.

Immunosuppressive drugs used in the first three (3) years after transplantation, plus an extension of up to eight (8) additional months.

Outpatient physical therapy and speech-language pathology services received as part of a patient's treatment in a doctor's office or as an outpatient in a participating hospital, skilled nursing facility, or through a home health agency, approved clinic, rehabilitative agency or public health agency, if the services are furnished under a plan established by a physician or physical therapist.

Services and supplies relating to a physician's services and hospital services rendered to outpatients; this includes drugs and biologicals which cannot be self-administered.

Dentist bills for jaw or facial bone surgery, whether required because of accident or disease. Also covered are hospital stays warranted by the severity of a non-covered dental procedure, and services provided by a dentist if they would otherwise be covered if provided by a physician.

The cost of psychiatric treatment outside a hospital for mental, psychoneurotic or personality disorders, but with forty- (40%) percent coinsurance instead of the usual twenty (20%). (By 2014 the copayment will decrease to twenty (20%) percent) The latter applies when services are provided on a hospital-outpatient basis if, in the absence of treatment outside a hospital, hospitalization would have been required. (For more details see *Medicare/Mental Health Services.*)

An unlimited number of home health services each calendar year, subject to the limitations as to the number of hours per day coverage and to the requirements of the Balanced Budget Act of 1997 (see *Part-time or intermittent/Medicare*). A doctor must certify as to an individual's need for these services each calendar year.

Radiation therapy with x-ray, radium or radioactive isotopes.

Surgical dressings, splints, casts and other devices for reduction of fractures and dislocations; rental or purchase of durable medical equipment, such as iron lungs, oxygen tents, hospital beds and wheelchairs for use in the patient's home; prosthetic devices, such as artificial heart valves or synthetic arteries, designed to replace part or all of an internal organ (but not false teeth, hearing aids or eyeglasses); braces, artificial limbs, artificial eyes (but not orthopedic shoes).

The cost of annual prostate cancer screening tests for men age 50 or over, including digital rectal exam and prostate-specific antigen (PSA) blood tests. Neither the Part B $140 (2012) annual deductible nor the twenty- (20%) percent coinsurance apply to the PSA test, but they do apply to the digital rectal exam.

Ambulance service to and from the hospital, nursing home and the patient's home if the patient's condition does not permit the use of other methods of transportation.

Comprehensive outpatient rehabilitation services performed by a doctor or other qualified professionals in a qualified facility.

The cost of training services in an ambulatory setting for diabetes outpatient self-management, if recommended by a physician. Also covered are a blood glucose lancet monitor and., every three (3) months, one-hundred (100) lancets plus one-hundred (100) test strips.

The cost of a flu shot each fall and one pneumonia shot per lifetime. Neither the annual deductible nor the twenty- (20%) percent coinsurance apply to the pneumonia shot.

The cost of hepatitis B vaccine for high- and intermediate-risk individuals when it is administered in a hospital or renal dialysis facility.

Screening pap smears for early detection of cervical cancer. Screening under normal circumstances is covered every three (3) years. The coverage is authorized on a yearly basis for women at high risk if developing cervical or vaginal cancer and for women of child bearing age who have had a negative test in the three (3) preceding years. The Part B annual deductible is waived for screening pap smears and pelvic exams, but the twenty- (20%) percent coinsurance must be paid by the beneficiary.

Screening mammography, which is defined as a radiologic procedure provided to a woman for the early detection of breast cancer, including a physician's interpretation of the results of the procedure. For women age 40 and over, screening under normal circumstances is covered every twelve (12) months. For woman age 30-39, Medicare will help pay for one baseline mammogram. The Part B annual deductible is waived, but not the twenty- (20%) percent coinsurance amount.

The cost of an injectable drug approved for the treatment of a bone fracture related to post-menopausal osteoporosis under the following conditions: the patient's attending physician certifies the patient is unable to learn the skills needed to self-administer, or is physically or mentally incapable of self-administering, the drug; and the patient meets the requirements for Medicare coverage of home health services.

Rental or purchase of durable medical equipment (See *Medicare/ Durable Medical Equipment).*

Costs relative to kidneys (for details see *Medicare, section IV.B)*

Depression screening, alcohol misuse counseling, and obesity screening and counseling (see *Medicare/Preventive Disease* for more details).

One pair of eyeglasses following cataract surgery.

The cost of bone mass measurements for women over age 65 who are at high risk for osteoporosis, and for beneficiaries with vertebral abnormalities and certain bone defects.

Deductibles and Copayments

For the covered services listed above unless otherwise indicated, Medicare beneficiaries are responsible for an annual Part B deductible of $140 (2012) and the twenty (20%) percent coinsurance. The number of services provided under Part B is limited by the general requirement that they must be reasonable and necessary.

Assignment and Balance Billing

There are two (2) billing methods for payment of benefits – assignment and balance billing.

When doctors provide services on assignment, they agree to charge no more than Medicare-approved charges for services. Patients assign their rights to collect benefits to their doctor, who in turn submits the assigned claims to Medicare and bills the beneficiaries for the twenty-(20%) percent coinsurance amount.

When doctors do not accept assignment, they are nevertheless responsible for handling the paper work of Medicare claims. They will bill and seek payment on the basis of an itemized bill. This method of billing is known as balance billing. Payment will be made by Medicare to the beneficiary for eighty (80%) percent of the Medicare-approved charge. The patient is responsible for paying the doctor's bill which cannot exceed one-hundred fifteen (115%) percent of the Medicare-approved charge. The capped charge is known as the limited charge. Several states by statute have prohibited balance billing and thus in effect have mandated assignment.

Excluded Services

Routine physical checkups and tests related to such examinations, except some Pap smears, mammograms and prostate cancer screening tests;

Eyeglasses (except after cataract surgery), hearing aids and vision and hearing examinations;

Drugs and medicines a patient buys with or without a doctor's prescription;

Immunizations, except pneumococcal pneumonia and hepatitis B vaccinations, flu shots and immunizations required because of an injury or immediate risk of infection;

Ordinary dental care and dentures;

Cosmetic plastic surgery;

Most routine foot care; and

Services required as a result of war.

*Medicare Savings Programs/Medicare

States have programs that pay Medicare premiums and, in some cases, may also pay Part A and Part B deductibles, coinsurance, and copayments. These programs help people with Medicare save money each year.

To qualify for a Medicare Savings Program, you must meet all of these conditions:

have Part A;

*have monthly income less than $1,239 and resources less than $6,600 –
single person; and*

*have monthly income less than $1,660 and resources less than $9,910 –
married and living together.*

*These amounts may change each year. Many states figure your income and
resources differently, so you may qualify in your state even if your income or
resources are higher. Resources include money in a checking or savings account,
stocks, and bonds. Resources don't include your home, car, burial plot, burial
expenses up to your state's limit, furniture, or other household items.*

Medicare Savings Programs

See also *Low-Income beneficiaries/Medicare Part D Drugs.*

Medicare savings programs (buy-in programs) will pay certain Medicare benefits
(deductibles, copayments, coinsurance, and/or premiums) for low-income
Medicare beneficiaries, as set forth below:

Qualified Medicare Beneficiary (QMB).

Federal law requires state Medicaid programs to buy-in Medicare
coverage for certain low-income Medicare beneficiaries. The buy-in
consists of payment of deductibles and coinsurance costs under
Medicare Part A and Part B, payment of premiums under Part B, and
payment of premiums under Part A for those not entitled to Part A by
virtue of receiving Social Security benefits. These beneficiaries are
known as Qualified Medicare Beneficiaries (QMB).

QMBs must:

> meet federally prescribed income and resource standards.
> Individuals must have incomes below one-hundred (100%) percent
> of the Federal poverty level, and their non-exempt resources cannot
> exceed twice the Supplemental Security Income resource standard
> ($4,000 for an individual and $6,000 for a family of two); and,

> be entitled to Part A hospitalization. If they otherwise would be
> eligible for QMB benefits but are not automatically eligible to
> Medicare Part A, the state must pay their Part A premiums to make
> them eligible for Part A.

Specified Low-income Medicare Beneficiary (SLMB).

An individual entitled to Medicare Part A benefits whose income is between one-hundred (100%) percent and one-hundred twenty (120%) percent of Federal poverty guidelines and whose non-exempt resources are $4,000 or less ($6,000 in the case of a couple) is eligible to have Medicaid pay his/her Medicare Part B premium. This individual is referred to as a SLMB. As with the Qualified Medicare Beneficiary program, the SLMB program is managed by the state agency that provides medical assistance under Medicaid.

Low-income Qualifying Individual (QI).

An individual is selected by the state as a qualified individual (QI). A QI is an individual who meets the QMB criteria, except that his/her income level is at least one hundred twenty (120%) percent but less than one-hundred thirty-five (135%) percent of the Federal poverty level for a family of the size involved and his/her non-exempt resources are $4,000 or less ($6,000 in the case of a couple). (There is no resource criterion in New York State and some other states.) The state Medicare program is required to pay the full amount of the Medicare Part B premiums of such a QI (but only for premiums payable during a statutorily prescribed period). However, the individual cannot be otherwise eligible for medical assistance under the state-approved plan.

Qualified Disabled and Working Individual (QDWI).

State Medicaid programs must pay Medicare Part A premiums for the individuals whose income is below two-hundred (200%) percent of the Federal poverty level who are entitled to Medicare on the basis of disability; who are in a trial work period and are entitled to continue Medicare coverage while they are in that work period; whose non-exempt resources do not exceed twice SSI resource levels ($4,000 for individuals, and $6,000 in the case of couples); and who are not otherwise eligible for Medicaid. They are not entitled to other Medicaid services.

Medicare Select /Medigap

Medicare Select is a type of Medigap policy. It began as a HCFA (now CMS) demonstration project authorized in fifteen (15) states and now is approved for sale throughout the country. Medicare Select policies are available to beneficiaries who agree to use providers within a network of providers. If a participant uses a non-network provider, other than for emergency services, the Medicare Select plan is not obligated to reimburse the participant's insured deductible or copayment.

The benefits covered under a Medicare Select policy are the same as those offered under one of the standardized Medigap plans. The advantage of Medicare Select policies to the enrollee is that premiums are likely to be lower than those charged for regular Medigap policies.

Medicare Summary Notice
See *Summary notice/Medicare.*

Medigap Insurance

Colloquial term for Medicare supplemental insurance.

(continued on next page)

MEDICARE SUPPLEMENTAL INSURANCE – MEDIGAP

Introduction

Medicare supplemental insurance is colloquially known as Medigap insurance. It is commercially sold to Medicare-eligibles and is specifically tailored to provide them supplemental coverage. Depending on the policy, Medigap policies pay some or all of Medicare deductibles and copayments and may also pay for some health services not covered by Medicare. Included among the items paid by some Medigap policies are: coinsurance for doctor bills; hospital deductible; coinsurance for hospital expenses after a sixty- (60) day stay; costs for the first three (3) pints of blood; annual doctor bill deductible; and skilled nursing home coinsurance after the Medicare benefit expires. The policies require, as does Medicare, that the services provided be medically necessary.

The history of changes to Medigap policies is set forth below.

   1. Until 1992, insurers designed their own Medigap policies. In 1992, Congress mandated that insurers could only issue ten (10) standard policies known as plans A-J.

   2. Starting in 2006 two (2) new policies (K and L) were added (see section I below). The premiums for the plans vary from insurer to insurer and from state to state.

   3. The Balanced Budget Act of 1997 added two other options: Plans F and J may be issued as a high-deductible insurance policy. The high-deductible features of these plans are described in section III below. Effective June 1, 2010, Plan J was no longer authorized for sale.

   4. Congress, in the MMA ("Act"), made changes to existing standard plans H, I and J. On or after June 1, 2006, plans H, I, and J cannot be sold, issued, or renewed to anyone with Medicare who was enrolled in or eligible for Medicare Part D. The Act created an exception for people with an H, I, or J policy that was issued before January 1, 2006. Those policies could be renewed for such individuals as long as the individuals are not enrolled in a Medicare Part D

prescription drug plan. Should an individual elect to keep a Medigap prescription drug plan, upon enrollment in a Medicare Part D drug plan, the Medigap plan's coverage will be modified to eliminate prescription drug coverage for expenses of prescription drugs incurred after the effective date of coverage under Part D. Premiums will also be adjusted to reflect the elimination of this coverage.

5.   Effective June 1, 2010, the Medicare Improvements for Patients and Providers Act (MIPPA) enacted the following Medigap changes:

i)   eliminated plans E, H, I, and J as they became duplicative of other plans after the implementation of the MMA;

ii)   the at-home recovery and preventive care benefits were eliminated as additional benefits Medigap plans could offer;

iii)   a new hospice benefit (which will cover all cost-sharing for Part A-eligible hospice care and respite care expenses) will be added as a core benefit eligible available with every Medigap plan offered for purchase; and

iv)   Plan G's eighty- (80%) percent excess charges benefit was increased to one-hundred (100%) percent.

6.   MIPPA added two high-deductible plans – M and N. These plans, which are described in section I.7(e) below, offer new options with higher beneficiary cost-sharing and lower anticipated premiums.

Medicare Select. Special Medigap policies known as Medicare Select are approved for sale in all states. Medicare Select is a managed care Medigap policy sold by private insurance companies or health maintenance organizations (HMO). It began as a Health Care Finance Administration (HCFA) (now known as Centers for Medicare and Medicaid Services (CMS)) demonstration project authorized in fifteen (15) states but now is approved for sale throughout the country. Medicare Select policies are available to beneficiaries who agree to use providers who participate in a preferred provider organization (PPO) or an HMO. If a participant uses a non-network provider, other than for emergency services, the Medicare Select plan is not obligated to reimburse the participant's incurred deductible or copayment. The benefits covered under a Medicare Select policy are the same as those offered by one of the standard Medigap plans depending on which plan is chosen to be offered for sale by the PPO or HMO and approved by the individual state. Premiums for Medicare Select policies are likely to be lower than those charged for standard Medigap policies.

I. CHARACTERISTICS OF MEDIGAP POLICIES.

Set below are the major characteristics of Medigap policies.

1. **Eligibility – Enrollment (Open Enrollment Period).** In order for an individual to purchase a Medigap policy, he/she must have Medicare Part A and Medicare Part B. The time to pick the policy is during the six- (6) month period (open enrollment period) that commences on the first day of the month in which the individual is both age 65 or older and enrolled in Medicare Part B.

2. **Free Look.** A period of time, usually thirty (30) days from the date an applicant receives a policy, in which the applicant can review a Medigap policy, or take a free look. If he/she is dissatisfied with the policy or changes his/her mind about wanting the coverage within this review period, the policy can be canceled, and the company must fully refund the premium paid.

3. **Pre-existing Conditions, Guaranteed Issue, Open Enrollment Period.** Under Federal rules, during the six (6) months (open enrollment period) after obtaining Medicare Part B medical coverage, an older person cannot be denied a Medigap policy for any medical reason. However, coverage for a pre-existing condition can be delayed for up to one-half year except for applicants who have creditable coverage. The term creditable coverage means coverage of an individual under one of the general medical health plans, such as a group health plan, Medicare Part A or Part B, or a state health benefit risk pool. In most states, except for certain individuals who are guaranteed issue of certain Medigap policies, Medigap coverage can be denied by insurers on medical grounds if the applicant misses the six- (6) month open enrollment window.

4. **Premiums**. Carriers use one of three methods to fix Medigap policy premiums:

> **Issue Age**. The premium is pegged to an applicant's age when he/she enrolls so that a consumer always pays the premium required of a person of the same age when the policy was issued. Thus, if an individual buys a policy at age 65, he/she will always pay the rate the company charges people who are age 65, regardless of his/her age.

Attained Age. Premiums increase as the beneficiary grows older.

Community Rating. Carriers charge all beneficiaries in a particular area the same amount; the rate is based on the demographics and health experience of the group.

5. **Availability of Policies**. With the exception of Plan A, not all of the standard Medigap policies are available in each state. However, in all states, except Minnesota, Massachusetts, and Wisconsin, insurers are required to sell Medigap policies that are one of the standard plans.

6. **Portability.** Some states restrict enrollees' movement (portability) from carrier to carrier or from one type of policy to another, particularly in the case of people with pre-existing conditions.

7. **Benefits of Standardized Plans.** With the exception of Minnesota, Massachusetts and Wisconsin, the benefits of the standardized plans are uniform throughout the United States. Because these three (3) states had alternative Medigap standardization programs in effect before the Federal legislation standardizing Medigap insurance was enacted, they were not required to change their plans.

The benefits of six (6) of the plans (A-D, F, and G) out of the ten (10) original standard plans (A-J) and the new K, L, M and N plans are summarized below.

(a) **Core or Basic Benefits (Plan A).** Plan A is the basic package, constituting the core or basic benefits contained in all other plans which have a mix of additional benefits (see (b) below). Plan A benefits are:

Medicare Part A hospital coinsurance for days 61-90 ($289 per day in 2012);

Medicare Part A hospital coinsurance for days 91-150 which count toward the non-renewable lifetime hospital inpatient reserve days ($578 per day in 2012);

All charges for a total of three-hundred sixty-five (365) lifetime reserve days of inpatient hospital treatment;

Part A deductible of the first three (3) pints of blood yearly; and

Medicare Part B's twenty (20%) percent coinsurance of Medicare-approved charges, including physician fees; fifty (50%) percent coinsurance of approved charges for outpatient mental health services after the $140 deductible (2012) is met.

Effective June 1, 2010, a new hospice benefit was added as a core benefit for all plans. It covers all cost-sharing for Part A-eligible hospice care and respite care expenses.

(b)   **Additional Benefits (Plans B, D, F and G)**. These plans include all core benefits plus various additional benefits.   The additional benefits are listed below with an indication of the plans that incorporate them.

Part A inpatient hospital deductible. Plans B, D, F and G pay Part A deductible ($1,156 in 2012).

Part A skilled nursing home coinsurance. Plans C, D, F and G pay the daily coinsurance for days 21-100 of skilled care in a nursing home per benefit period ($144.50 per day in 2012).

Part B annual deductible. Plans C and F pay the $140 (2012) annual deductible.

Part B excess doctor charges. Plans F and G pay one-hundred (100%) percent of excess doctor charges up to one-hundred fifteen (115%) percent of the Medicare-approved amount, and Plan G pays one-hundred (100%) percent.

Foreign travel emergency. Plans C, D, F and G cover eighty (80%) percent of medically necessary emergency care during the first two (2) months of each trip outside the USA. There is an annual $250 deductible and a lifetime maximum benefit of $50,000.

Hospice care. Effective June 1, 2010, a new hospice benefit was added as a core benefit for all plans. It covers all cost-sharing for Part A-eligible hospice care and respite care expenses.

(c)   **Plans K and L – Limited Benefits**. Starting on January 1, 2006, two (2) new Medigap plans (K and L) were authorized by Congress. (See the chart in section VI.)

Plan K offers fifty (50%) percent of cost-sharing under Medicare Parts A and B, except that the Part B deductible is not covered. One-hundred (100%) percent of cost-sharing is covered in addition fir the hospital coinsurance amount, and the three-hundred sixty-five (365) lifetime inpatient reserve days. The annual out-of-pocket amount under Parts A and B is limited to $4,640 in 2012 and thereafter is adjusted annually for inflation.

Plan L covers seventy-five (75%) percent of cost-sharing under Parts A and B, except for the Part B deductible. All hospital coinsurance is covered, in addition to the three-hundred sixty-five (365) lifetime inpatient reserve days. The annual out-of-pocket amount under Parts A and B are limited to $2,320 (2012) and thereafter is adjusted annually for inflation.

(d)   **Medigap Plan F High-Deductible Policy**   The Balanced Budget Act of 1997 allows Plans F and J, two (2) of the statutory standard Medigap plans, to offer an optional high-deductible insurance feature as part of the benefit package. Before the policy begins payment of benefits, a high-deductible insurance policy requires the beneficiary of the policy to pay annual out-of-pocket expenses, other than premiums, in the amount of a specified deductible, and requires the insurance company to pay one-hundred (100%) percent of the beneficiary's covered out-of-pocket expenses once the deductible has been satisfied in a year.

The Medigap Plan F high-deductible policy has a deductible amount at $2,070 (2012). In subsequent years, increases in the deductible amount will be tied to the consumer price index.

(e)   **Plans M and N.** Plan M offers the basic core benefits required of every Medigap plan and additionally covers fifty (50%) percent of the Medicare Part A deductible, skilled nursing facility copayments, and medically necessary emergency care in a foreign country.

Plan N offers the basic core benefits required of every Medigap plan and additionally covers one-hundred (100%) percent of the Medicare Part A deductible, skilled nursing facility copayments, and medically necessary emergency care in a foreign country. Plan N also includes copayments for covered services as follows: (1) the lesser of $20 or the Medicare Part B coinsurance or copayment for each covered health care provider office visit and (2) the lesser of $50 or the Medicare Part B coinsurance or copayment for each covered emergency room visit. However, this copayment for an emergency room visit will be waived if the insured is admitted to any hospital and the emergency visit is subsequently covered as a Part A expense.

II. MEDIGAP POLICIES MAY NOT COVER PRESCRIPTION DRUGS.

Starting in January 1, 2006, insurance companies may not sell existing Medigap policies that provide drug coverage to Medicare beneficiaries who are enrolled in or are eligible for Medicare out-patient prescription drug coverage. They are able, however, to renew the Medigap drug policies issued prior to January 1, 2006. The Medigap policies of beneficiaries with drug coverage who enroll in a new Medicare prescription drug plan will be modified to eliminate drug coverage, and premiums will be adjusted. Beneficiaries with the new Medicare drug coverage can purchase Medigap policies that do not cover drugs.

III. EXCLUSION (WAITING OR ELIMINATION) PERIOD.

Prior to enactment of the Balanced Budget Act of 1997 (Act), if a Medigap policy was purchased during the one-time six- (6) month open enrollment period permitted under the policy, an individual could not be turned down because of a pre-existing medical condition. However, the policy might impose a waiting (elimination) period (exclusion period), not exceeding six months, before coverage for the pre-existing condition will take effect.

Under the Act, if application for a Medigap policy is made during the initial six- (6) month open enrollment period, an exclusion or waiting (elimination) period for a pre-existing condition may not be imposed under certain circumstances. Commencing July 1, 1998, the exclusion may not be applied to any individual who, on the date of application for Medigap enrollment, has had at least six (6) months of creditable coverage (see *section I*). Persons having fewer than six (6) months of such coverage are entitled to have the period of any pre-existing condition exclusion reduced by the aggregate period of creditable coverage they have accumulated.

Creditable coverage, with respect to an individual, means coverage of the individual under any one of several medical health plans, such as a group health plan, Medicare Part A or Part B, or a state health benefit risk pool.

IV.   GUARANTEED ISSUE OF PLANS A, B, C, AND F.

If an individual seeks to purchase a Medigap policy after the six- (6) month open enrollment period, the applicant generally can be turned down due to a pre-existing medical condition. However, the Balanced Budget Act of 1997 created certain exceptions. Since July 1, 1998, certain individuals (see below) are guaranteed issue of certain of the Medigap policies despite a pre-existing medical condition and even if purchased after the six- (6) month open enrollment period.

Four (4) of the original standard Medigap policies — A, B, C, and F — are designated by the Act to provide such guaranty. It applies to individuals, specified below, continuously covered by a health policy. They may avail themselves of such guaranty, provided they enroll in one of the four (4) specified policies not later than sixty-three (63) days after termination of their prior coverage.

The following individuals are considered "continuously covered":

Individuals whose supplemental coverage under an employee welfare benefit plan terminates.

Individuals enrolled in a Medicare Advantage plan who disenroll for permissible reasons (e.g., termination of the plan's certification or a move out of the plan area) other than during an annual election period.

Individuals enrolled in risk or cost-basis HMOs or Medicare Select policies who disenroll for the permissible reasons explained above. With respect to Medicare Select policies, there must be no state law provision relating to continuation of coverage for this provision to apply.

Individuals whose enrollment in a Medigap policy ceases because of the bankruptcy or insolvency of the insurer issuing the policy, or because of other involuntary termination of coverage for which there is no state law provision relating to continuation of coverage.

Individuals previously enrolled under a Medigap policy who terminate such enrollment to participate, for the first time, in a Medicare Advantage plan, risk or cost-basis HMO, or Medicare Select policy, and who subsequently terminate their enrollment in such a plan during any permissible period within the first twelve (12) months of such enrollment.

Individuals who enroll in a Medicare Advantage plan upon first reaching Medicare eligibility at age 65 but disenroll from the plan within twelve (12) months.

In addition to the above, individuals who re-enroll in a Medigap plan, after the one-time test of a Medicare Advantage plan, risk or cost-basis HMO, or Medigap Select policy, may re-enroll in the same Medigap policy, if still available from the same issuer, as they had before trying a Medicare Advantage plan.

All Medigap plans must be offered without the pre-existing condition exclusion to persons who enroll in a Medicare Advantage plan upon first reaching eligibility at age 65, and disenroll from the plan within twelve (12) months.

V. MEDICARE SUPPLEMENTAL INSURANCE POLICIES FORBID MEDICARE PART D DRUG COVERAGE.

Since January 1, 2006, insurance companies have not been allowed to sell existing Medicare supplemental policies (Medigap) that provide drug coverage to Medicare beneficiaries who are enrolled in or eligible for Medicare outpatient prescription drug coverage. They are, however, able to renew the Medigap drug policies issued prior to January 1, 2006 for beneficiaries who do not opt for the new Medicare outpatient prescription drug coverage. For Medicare beneficiaries with Medigap drug policies who enroll in a new Medicare outpatient prescription drug plan, their Medigap policy will be modified to eliminate drug coverage, and premiums will be adjusted. Beneficiaries with the new Medicare drug coverage can purchase Medigap policies that do not cover drugs.

(continued on next page)

VI.   MEDIGAP BENEFITS SUMMARY CHART (see notes below chart).

BENEFITS	A	B	C	D	F*	G	K**	L**	M	N
CORE Plan pays 20% coinsurance for doctor's bills, copayment for hospital days 61-90 ($289/day), days 91-150 ($578/day) plus 365 lifetime hospital inpatient reserve days.	√	√	√	√	√	√	√	√	√	√
BLOOD (first 3 pints)	√	√	√	√	√	√	50%	75%	√	√
HOSPICE CARE coinsurance or copayments	√	√	√	√	√	√	√	√	√	√
HOSPITAL DEDUCTIBLE Plan pays the $1,156 for first day, not paid by Medicare.		√	√	√	√	√	50%	75%	50%	√
DOCTOR'S BILL DEDUCTIBLE Plan pays the annual $140 not paid by Medicare.			√							***
NURSING HOME COINSURANCE Plan pays $144.50/day for days 21-100.			√	√	√	√	50%	75%	√	√
DOCTOR'S CHARGES BEYOND MEDICARE LIMITS					√	√				
MEDICAL TREATMENT OUTSIDE THE U.S. Patient pays $250 deductible and 20% coinsurance. Plan pays $50,000 lifetime maximum.			√	√	√	√			√	√

NOTE: On June 1, 2010, Plans E, H, I, and J were eliminated from the ten original authorized Medigap plans and cannot be sold. Beneficiaries may keep their existing policies after June 1, 2010.

√   Means that the Medigap policy covers 100% of the described benefit.

*   Plans F offers a high-deductible option whereby the beneficiary pays the first $2,020 (2012) in Medigap-covered costs.

**   After the beneficiary meets the annual out-of-pocket limit $4,640 (2012) for Plan K and $2,320 (2012) for Plan L and the yearly Part B deductible, the plan pays 100% of covered services for the remainder of the calendar year.

***   Plan N includes copayments for covered services as follows: 1) the lesser of $20 or the Medicare Part B coinsurance for each covered health provider office visit and (2) the lesser of $50 or the Medicare Part B copayment for each covered emergency room visit. However, this copayment for an emergency room visit will be waived if the insured is admitted to any hospital and the emergency room visit is subsequently covered as a Part A expense.

Mental or Emotional Illness/LTCI

Most LTCI policies explicitly exclude payment of benefits for the treatment of mental or emotional illness, nor will they pay for substance abuse treatment. However, it is almost universally conceded that Alzheimer's disease is an organic condition of the brain, and therefore policy benefits cannot be refused under the mental illness exclusion if the benefit triggers are otherwise met.

*Mental Health Care/Medicare

To get help with mental health conditions such as depression or anxiety:, includes services generally given outside a hospital or in a hospital outpatient setting, including visits with a psychiatrist or other doctor, clinical psychologist, nurse practitioner, physician's assistant, clinical nurse specialist, or clinical social worker; substance abuse services; and lab tests. Certain limits and conditions apply.

What you pay will depend on whether you're being diagnosed and monitored or whether you're getting treatment.

*For visits to a doctor or other health care provider to **diagnose** your condition, you pay 20% of the Medicare-approved amount.*

*For outpatient **treatment** of your condition (such as counseling or psychotherapy), you pay 45% of the Medicare-approved amount in 2011. This coinsurance amount will continue to decrease over the next 3 years.*

The Part B deductible applies for both visits to diagnose or treat your condition.

Inpatient mental health care is covered under Part A hospital stays.

Methodology/Medicaid

The term is used to describe how a state counts an individual's income and resources to determine whether the individual meets its standard for Medicaid eligibility. For example, states may disregard, that is cannot count, payments for court-ordered support from an applicant's income. That disregard is part of the state's methodology. A methodology is distinguished from a standard, which is the dollar figure above which an individual is not eligible for the program.

Miller Trust/Medicaid

See also *Trust transfer penalty rules/Medicaid.*

One of three (3) types of trusts that is expressly exempted from the Medicaid trust transfer penalty rules. The Miller trust is named for the plaintiff in a lawsuit that first established its validity. It applies only in states without medically needy programs that have special eligibility categories for nursing facility care. In lieu of application of special Medicaid trust rules, income and resources of a Miller trust are governed by ordinary Medicaid eligibility principles.

Minimum Monthly Maintenance Needs Allowance/Medicaid

See also *Community spouse's income allowance/Medicaid.*

This term refers to an income allowance set by Federal law for the spouse of an institutionalized individual receiving Medicaid, and, at a state's option, an individual receiving home care services under a Medicaid waiver. The specific formula and exceptions to it are set forth below.

The basic allowance for the community spouse is equal to one-hundred fifty (150%) percent of the Federal poverty level for a two-person family, even though the community spouse is only one person. This amounts to a minimum monthly gross allowance of $1,838 (2012). The allowance is adjusted annually for inflation.

When the costs (e.g., rent, mortgage, taxes, maintenance charges on a co-op apartment or condominium, insurance and utilities) of maintaining the principal residence exceed thirty (30%) percent of the basic allowance, an excess shelter allowance is permitted. It is added to the basic allowance.

A cap of $2,841 (2012), as adjusted for inflation according to the Federal consumer price index, applies to the sum of the basic allowance and excess shelter allowance. In lieu of the allowance computed with the above two components (i.e., the basic allowance and the excess shelter allowance), a state may elect a flat monthly maintenance allowance, which may not exceed the two components together. California and New York have, for example, made this election. The flat monthly maintenance allowance is subject to the $2,841 cap.

The amount allowed for the community spouse is subject to increase if it can be shown at a fair hearing that there are exceptional circumstances causing him/her significant financial duress. A court may also grant the community spouse income from the institutionalized spouse in an amount higher than the income allowance. This additional income must be honored by the state in determining Medicaid eligibility.

If the community spouse's resource allowance is insufficient to generate income to bring his/her income up to the minimum monthly needs allowance, then the community spouse may resort to a fair hearing to increase his/her resource allowance to make up the income deficiency. However, the community spouse may not resort to the fair hearing process, to increase his/her resource allowance unless the institutionalized spouse has first made available to the community spouse, out of his/her income, an amount sufficient to make up the deficiency. (See also *Income first rule/Medicaid*.)

Modified Adjusted Gross Income (MAGI)
See also *Adjusted gross income*

Modified adjusted gross income is the taxpayer's adjusted gross income with the following add-backs to gross income and the following exclusion: interest exclusion that applied to savings bonds used to finance education; foreign earned income; foreign housing; U.S. possessions source income; amounts paid under an adoption assistance program of the employer; interest on qualified education loans; and all tax-exempt interest, such as tax-exempt interest received on municipal bonds which the taxpayer received or accrued during the tax year.

Monthly Income Allowance of Community Spouse/Medicaid
See *Minimum monthly maintenance needs allowance/Medicaid; Community spouse's income allowance/Medicaid.*

Moral Risk/LTCI
See *Induced demand/LTCI.*

(continued on next page)

N

Name-on-the-check rule/Medicaid

This rule assigns ownership of income to the individual whose name appears on the financial instrument, most often a check. Thus, the full amount of a check made out to John Jones will be attributed to Mr. Jones under this rule, regardless of whether a portion of the check is actually intended for Mr. Jones's spouse. This rule comes from the SSI program and is applied in certain circumstances to Medicaid income determinations, especially when states have not specified other rules or in states that do not use community property principles in determining Medicaid eligibility.

Naturally Occurring Retirement Community (NORC)

An apartment building, complex or community, in which, due to the longevity of the residents and their aging in place, the majority of the residents are 60 years of age or older. In such situations, an informal support system may develop where residents look out for one another. Currently, more formal comprehensive and accessible supportive services programs have become available to insure that residents do not "fall through the cracks" of public benefits and other private service systems.

Net Gift

A gift made upon the express condition that the recipient will pay the gift tax.

Network Model/Managed Care

This type of HMO enters into contract with one or more independent physician group practices. The physicians in the network may have individual and/or group practices. The physicians customarily work out of their own offices and provide care not only to HMO enrollees but also to non-HMO patients.

All entries preceded by an asterisk (*) are culled or copied from the official U.S. government **Medicare** handbook (*Medicare & You 2011*).

Network Pharmacy/Medicare Part D Drug Coverage

A licensed pharmacy that is under contract to a plan to provide Part D-covered drugs at negotiated prices to the plan's enrollees.

Neurologist

Neurology is the medical field that specializes in the study of the human nervous system. The nervous system encompasses the brain, spinal cord, nerves, and muscles. It can be affected by debilitating diseases, such as Parkinson's and Alzheimer's, as well as by mental disorders such as schizophrenia, depression, autism, and attention-deficit hyperactivity disorder (ADHD). The specialist doctors who treat patients suffering from these diseases and disorders are called neurologists.

Neurologists examine patients who have been referred to them by other physicians. There are many tests they can perform to diagnose a patient's illness. Depending on the symptoms, they may physically examine the nerves of the head and neck, or test the patient's balance, reflexes, muscle strength, and range of movement. They may also test the patient's cognitive abilities, including memory, speech and sensation.

Neurologists often have images made of parts of the nervous system through computed axial tomography (CAT) scans or magnetic resonance imaging (MRI). With these images they can usually diagnose the problem and prescribe a treatment plan.

No-payment Billing/Medicare
See also *Demand billing/Medicare.*

This term is synonymous with demand billing.

Non-covered Services (Exclusions)/Medicare, Medicaid
See also *Medicare, section IV.B.2; Medicaid, sections III and IV.*

Services not approved for Medicare or Medicaid reimbursement.

*Non-doctor Services/Medicare

Medicare covers services provided by certain non-doctors, such as physician assistants, nurse practitioners, social workers, physical therapists, and psychologists. Except for certain preventive services, you pay 20% of the Medicare- approved amount, and the Part B deductible applies.

Non-exempt Resources/Medicaid
See also *Exempt resources/Medicaid.*

A term used in SSI, Medicaid and other public benefits programs to describe those resources that are counted in determining eligibility. Generally speaking, these are bank accounts, certificates of deposits, stocks, bonds, personal goods and household possession over a certain value, automobiles over a certain value and real estate that is not the homestead.

Non-forfeiture Benefits/LTCI
See also *Long-term care insurance.*

A cash-value or other benefit in a LTCI policy which may be repaid by the insurer if the long-term care benefits are not used, or if the policy lapses. To be eligible for the tax advantages extended through the Health Insurance Portability and Accountability Act of 1996, policies sold after January 1, 1997 must offer an option to purchase non-forfeiture coverage.

Non-medical Home Care

Non-medical home care consists of home care services that require less training and skills than medical home health care and are performed by personal care aides (called attendants or home care workers). These services are often referred to as custodial care and consist of:

> **Personal care services** including help with bathing, dressing, eating, toileting, transferring (from chair to walker and from bed to wheelchair), turning and positioning; and

> **Homemaker/housekeeping services** including light house-work, preparing meals, shopping, laundry and cleaning, and management of money.

The foregoing services may be supplemented by other in-home services consisting of nutrition assistance, reassurance programs, day care, and other types of community-based services.

Non-participating Physician/Medicare

A physician who does not sign a participation agreement with Medicare and therefore is not obligated to accept assignment on Medicare claims.

Non-physician Practitioner

A health care professional who is not a physician, such as an advanced practice nurse and a physician's assistant.

Non-preferred Drug/Medicare Part D Drug Coverage.

A drug to which a plan discourages access. This is typically done by requiring a large co-pay.

Normal Retirement Age/Social Security

For purposes of Social Security, the normal retirement age historically has been 65 years of age for workers and spouses born in 1938 or before. After December 31, 1999, the normal retirement age was gradually increased to 67 years of age for those born in 1960 or later.

Notice by Hospital of Continued Stay Denial/Medicare
See also *Appeals (expedited) discharge of hospital patient/Medicare.*

This is a denial notice, also called a notice of non-coverage. It states that in the hospital's opinion and with the attending physician's concurrence, the beneficiary no longer requires inpatient hospital care. A patient's liability for hospital costs begins on the third day after his/her receipt of this notice from the hospital.

Notice of Non-coverage/Medicare
See *Notice by hospital of continued stay denial/Medicare.*

Nurse Practitioner (NP)/Medicare

An NP is a registered nurse licensed to practice nursing in the state in which services are performed, has acquired additional training beyond basic nursing education and provides primary care services. An NP is a broad term that includes a gerontological nurse, pediatric nurse, family nurse and obstetric-gynecologic nurse.

Historically, Medicare paid separately for an NP's services only when provided in collaboration with a physician and only in a nursing home or a rural area setting. Under the Balanced Budget Act of1997, NPs are eligible for separate Part B payments if they provide physician-type services in any setting and as long as Medicare does not pay the facility or provider for their services. They are paid at eighty (80%) percent of the lesser of either the actual charge or eighty-five (85%) percent of the Medicare physician fee schedule.

Nursing Facility/Medicaid

As defined by Medicaid, a nursing facility is an institution primarily engaged in providing skilled nursing and related services, rehabilitation services for injured, disabled or sick persons, or, on a regular basis, health-related care and services to individuals who because of their mental or physical condition require care and services (above the level of room and board) which can be made available to them only through institutional facilities.

Historically, Medicaid distinguished between skilled and intermediate nursing facilities. Since October 1990, all Medicaid-certified nursing homes have been simply called nursing facilities. The requirements of such nursing facilities to participate in Medicaid are virtually identical to those for skilled nursing facilities participating in Medicare. Medicaid retains the separate designation of intermediate care facility for the mentally retarded which applies to entirely different institutions.

Medicaid mandates that all states provide the categorically needy and optional categorically needy with nursing facility services. It is optional to states to provide such services under the medically needy program.

The major nursing facility services paid for by Medicaid include the following:

> Daily basic nursing care;
>
> Specialized rehabilitative services;
>
> Medically related social services;
>
> Board and lodging;
>
> Pharmacy and dietary services; and
>
> Emergency dental services for persons with mental illness or mental retardation.

Medicaid will also pay the Medicare Part B premiums for nursing facility residents who qualify for Medicaid.

Each Medicaid recipient must be under the care of a physician who is primarily responsible for that resident's care. Each recipient has the right to select a primary physician from among physicians who practice at the facility.

Access to nursing homes is limited to those Medicaid recipients or applicants who qualify medically for nursing facility care, according to an assessment procedure and criteria. The criteria are set forth in forms called a patient review instrument which is used to determine whether individuals need care in a nursing home or can be cared for in another setting such as their own home or other facility. Based on this assessment, an individual is assigned a resource utilization group (RUG), depending upon the person's medical condition, care needs and relative dependence or independence in performing activities of daily living. The RUG categories each indicate the amount a nursing facility will be reimbursed by Medicaid and the kind of care and staff time that will be needed.

The RUG is thus a method of scoring a resident's care needs upon which Medicaid reimbursement rates are based. A higher score results in higher Medicaid reimbursement.

The Nursing Home Reform law specifies when a Medicaid recipient in a nursing home may be involuntarily transferred or discharged. Such individual may be involuntarily transferred only for specified reasons. For details see *Nursing home reform law*.

Nursing Home Reform Law

Sometimes referred to as OBRA '87, this Federal law regulating aspects of nursing homes is contained in the Omnibus Budget Reconciliation Act of 1987. It sets Federal standards of care, including one stipulating that nursing homes may use physical and chemical restraints only in very specific circumstances and only after other interventions have been tried. The bill also establishes certain rights for patients and requires states and the Federal government to inspect nursing homes and to enforce standards through the use of a range of sanctions designed to promote compliance without forcing the relocation of residents due to the closing of facilities.

The resident's bill of rights, mandated in the nursing home reform law, includes a resident's rights to:

Admit and discharge oneself;

Control one's own medical care and be informed of all aspects of one's health;

Choose his/her own physician of own choice and refuse treatment;

Self-administer drugs;

Be free of restraints (physical or chemical);

See all his/her medical records;

Receive notice of any decision to transfer or discharge or change a roommate;

Manage own financial affairs;

Receive visitors of one's choice as well as refuse visitors; and

Have access to a private telephone.

Transfers or discharges are permitted only under three (3) situations:

If necessary for the resident's welfare and if her/his needs cannot be met in the facility;

If a resident's health has improved and he/she no longer needs care; or

If a resident's presence or non-payment of charges endangers the health and safety of other residents in the facility.

All residents, whether private pay or receiving Medicaid assistance or Medicare benefits, are entitled to due process, namely, a fair hearing. In this connection, the procedures for Medicaid fair hearings apply to nursing home transfers and discharges. The right to a pre-transfer hearing is mandated except for emergency transfers subject to a resident's right to a bedhold pending a post-transfer hearing.

The law requires every resident to undergo a process known as preadmission, screening, and annual resident review. Prior to admission there is to be a functional evaluation, and at the time of admission a comprehensive care plan must be developed. It must be prepared annually with a physician and nursing team.

The law contains a number of other significant requirements. Nursing homes may not require as a condition for admission or for continuing stay a guarantee of payment from a third party. They must provide coverage by a registered nurse, not less than eight (8) hours a day, seven (7) days a week. Aides must go through a training program and pass a nursing aide registry certification. States are required to create a nursing aide registry to train, certify and maintain a listing of all approved workers.

Nutrition Services

See *Older Americans Act; Meals on wheels.*

A variety of programs provide nutritional assistance to older persons. Nutrition services consist of meals provided to the elderly at home or as congregate meals at senior centers or adult day care programs.

Home-delivered meals consist of hot, nutritious meals, delivered once and sometimes twice a day, five (5) days a week to persons who are unable to cook for themselves.

Congregate meals are usually served in senior centers or adult day care programs.

Most nutrition programs are funded through the Federal Older Americans Act and are administered by local Offices for the Aging. There may be a sliding fee (or no fee), determined by the individual's ability to pay. Medicare will not pay for home-delivered meals (Meals on Wheels) or nutrition services at a senior center. Food stamps may be available to homebound Americans who are eligible for them because they meet the program's financial eligibility requirements. Food stamps consist of debit cards with pre-loaded amounts which can be used to purchase food in most supermarkets.

Nutrition Sites

Facilities such as adult day care centers, senior centers, churches, synagogues, schools or housing projects often serve as congregate settings where inexpensive, well-balanced meal programs are run.

*Nutrition Therapy Services/Medicare

Medicare may cover medical nutrition therapy and certain related services if you have diabetes or kidney disease, or you have had a kidney transplant in the last 36 months, and your doctor refers you for the services. Starting January 1, 2011, you pay nothing for these services if the doctor accepts assignment.

Nutritionist

A nutritionist may be requested by a home health nurse when a patient needs help planning a special diet or restricted eating plan. For example, persons with diabetes, heart conditions or high blood pressure must learn to eat fewer high fat foods, avoid sugar and/or restrict salt intake. The nutritionist prepares menus that are appetizing to the patient, free of harmful food and based upon the patient's food preferences.

(continued on next page)

O

Occupational Therapist

An occupational therapist may be needed by a patient who has suffered an illness or injury that has affected daily activities, movement or perceptual abilities. The occupational therapist evaluates the patient's ability to dress, wash, walk or perform other routine functions, and, when necessary, provides devices that add to the patient's comfort. Examples include using larger buttons on clothes to facilitate dressing, adding a board to the arm of a wheelchair to help support a patient's paralyzed arm and providing a leg or ankle splint to aid in walking.

*Occupational Therapy/Medicare

Evaluation and treatment to help you return to usual activities (such as dressing or bathing) after an illness or accident when your doctor certifies you need it. There may be limits on these services and exceptions to these limits. You pay 20% of the Medicare-approved amount, and the Part B deductible applies.

Occupational Therapy, Physical Therapy and Speech-Language Pathology, Home Care/Medicare

See also *Outpatient occupational therapy, physical therapy and speech-language pathology/Medicare; Qualifying skilled services/Medicare.*

Skilled therapy services may be furnished to a Medicare beneficiary as a "home health service" under Medicare Part A, or as "medical and other health services" under Medicare Part B, depending upon whether the patient satisfies prescribed home health requirements. While Medicare home health services, including skilled therapy, may be covered under Part A, if the beneficiary only has Part B, then the services will be covered under Part B if the individual qualifies for home health services.

All entries preceded by an asterisk (*) are culled or copied from the official U.S. government **Medicare** handbook (*Medicare & You 2011*).

The home health care service(s) of a physical therapist, speech-language pathologist or occupational therapist is considered skilled therapy if an inherent complexity of the service(s) is such that it can be performed safely and effectively only by or under the general supervision of a skilled therapist.

For skilled therapy services to be covered by Medicare as a home health service, the beneficiary must meet the following conditions:

> The skilled therapy services must be reasonable and necessary to the treatment of the patient's illness or injury or to the restoration or maintenance of function affected by the patient's illness or injury.

> The Medicare-eligible patient must meet certain home health eligibility requirements: he/she must be homebound, meet requirements for qualifying skilled services and obtain therapy services through a Medicare-certified home health agency according to a physician's plan of care.

A patient who satisfies the home health eligibility requirements set forth above may receive therapy services as an outpatient covered under Medicare Part B at a participating hospital, skilled nursing facility or rehabilitation center if and when required equipment is not readily available at the patient's residence. The hospital, skilled nursing facility or rehabilitation center must be Medicare-qualified providers of the service.

(continued on next page)

OLDER AMERICANS ACT (AREA AGENCY ON AGING)

INTRODUCTION

The Older Americans Act ("Act") is a Federal law enacted on July 14, 1965 to create a Federal program assisting state and area agencies and volunteer organizations to plan and develop services, research, and training programs.

The sections of the Act are the following:

Title I   -   Declaration of Objectives: Definitions

Title II   -   Administration on Aging

Title III   -   Grants for State and Community Programs on Aging

Title IV   -   Training, Research, and Discretionary Projects and Programs

Title V   -   Community Service Employment for Older Americans

Title VI   -   Grants for Native Americans

Title VII -   Elder Rights (Ombudsman)

Under Title III of the Act, the Federal government has developed a national aging network and distributes funds to state agencies (State Units of Aging), which utilize them for support of a wide range of home and community-based services. The statewide programs are operated at the local level by Area Agencies on Aging (AAA).

I. INFRASTRUCTURE.

The Act is structurally administered in three tiers. (i) On the Federal level is the Administration on Aging (AoA), part of the Department of Health and Human Services and consisting of ten (10) regional offices; AoA is the administrative point of the national aging network. (ii) Each state has a State Unit on Aging, which oversees statewide programs and distributes funds to localities in the states;

(iii) Area Agencies on Aging, of which there are over six-hundred (600) nationwide, operate at the local level. They are non-profit, public and private organizations, or units of a local government, designated by the state and responsible for a given geographical area to develop and advance plans to advocate on behalf of elderly persons with the greatest economic and social need.

II.   ELIGIBILITY.

Persons age 60 and older are eligible for Act services. Generally, while eligibility does not depend on income, the states and AAAs must give priority to those elderly persons with the greatest economic and social need who are frail, homebound by reason of illness or disability, or isolated. The term "frail" is defined as having a physical or mental disability, Alzheimer's disease or a related disorder, or neurological or organic brain dysfunction that restricts a person's ability to perform normal daily tasks or that threatens an individual's capacity to live independently. Services under the Act are free of charge although voluntary contributions may be sought. In the case of nutrition services, a fee may be charged determined by an individual's ability to pay.

III.   SERVICES.

The Older Americans Act is best known as a source of funding of the following services:

In-home services.

homemaker and home health aides;

personal care services;

visiting and telephone reassurance;

chore maintenance;

in-home respite care for families, and adult day care as a respite service for families; and

minor modification of homes that is necessary to facilitate the ability of older individuals to remain at home, that is not available under other programs, and that does not exceed $150 per client for such modification.

Nutrition services.

The Act funds two types of food services:

Home-delivered Meals Program. Popularly known as meals on wheels, this program provides a hot, nutritious, home-delivered meal, once and sometimes twice a day, five (5) days a week, to persons at home who are unable to cook for themselves. Usually a sliding fee (or no fee) is charged, based upon the individual's ability to pay.

Congregate Meals Program. This program provides for the serving (with the same frequency as home-delivered meals) of congregate meals in settings such as senior or adult day care centers.

Senior Centers.

Senior centers provide the site and the opportunity for social contact, recreational activities and information and referral for the elderly. They also offer health screening and education programs. Many serve meals on weekdays, and some have extensive health and social service programs, including adult thy care. Senior centers are an important facility for coordinating and delivering community-based services. The centers in addition to being funded by the Act are supported by local governments, philanthropic organizations, participant contributions and senior volunteers.

IV. OMBUDSMAN.

Under the Older Americans Act, the State Unit on Aging is required to have a state long-term care ombudsman office. The ombudsman, as an impartial mediator, receives, investigates and settles complaints from long-term care residents, families or facilities. The state may operate the ombudsman program directly, or it may contract with a local government agency or a private non-profit organization for this purpose. The ombudsman maintains a staff of volunteers who visit long-term care facilities on a regular basis and work with staff to improve the quality of residents' care.

V. MISCELLANEOUS SERVICES.

Services and activities furnished by the Act also include transportation, information and referral, legal assistance, senior employment opportunities, elder abuse protection, and volunteer service for other seniors in the community at large.

(continued on next page)

Ombudsman

See also *Older Americans Act (Area Agency on Aging), section IV.*

Under the Older Americans Act, the State Unit on Aging is required to have a state long-term care ombudsman office. The ombudsman, as an impartial mediator, receives, investigates and settles complaints from long-term care residents, families or facilities. More specifically, the Ombudsman's responsibilities include: 1) responding to complaints, grievances and inquiries concerning any aspect of the Medicare program; 2) assisting beneficiaries in collecting information needed to more appeals; 3) helping beneficiaries with enrollment and disenrollment problems; 4) assisting beneficiaries with issues related to premiums; and 5) working with the aging and disability communities to improve beneficiaries' understanding of their rights and protections within the program.

The state may operate the ombudsman program directly, or it may contract with a local government agency or a private non-profit organization for this purpose. The ombudsman maintains a staff of volunteers who visit long-term care facilities on a regular basis and work with staff to improve the quality of residents' care.

Omnibus Budget Reconciliation Act (OBRA '87)

Passed almost every year since 1980, OBRA in one piece of legislation mandates changes in Federal programs in order to reconcile the budget to existing legislation. In the context of elder rights issues, OBRA '87 contains the Nursing Home Reform Law of 1987.

Open Enrollment Period/Medicare Advantage

In addition to initial enrollment period, beneficiaries are able to enroll on an annual basis in a Medicare Advantage plan in an annual coordinated election period. They are also able to switch between original Medicare and Medicare Advantage or enroll in an MSA plan during an open enrollment period once every year. The open enrollment period is between October 15 and December 7.

An election made during an open enrollment period will become effective on January 1.

A Medicare Advantage organization must accept eligible beneficiaries who elect that organization's plan during an open enrollment period without restrictions, waiting period, or pre-existing medical exclusion.

A beneficiary can elect an MSA plan only during the initial enrollment period or the annual coordinated election period.

Open Enrollment Period/Medicare Part D Drug Coverage

Beneficiaries who become eligible for Medicare may enroll in a Part D plan when they become eligible for Part A or Part B benefits. In addition, they may elect to enroll during an open enrollment period. Open enrollment runs from October 15 through December 7, when original Medicare beneficiaries may switch from Original Medicare to a Medicare Advantage plan or enroll in a stand-alone plan if they have not previously done so. Rephrased: Beneficiaries may elect during an open enrollment period to remain in original Medicare and receive prescription drug coverage through stand-alone prescription drug plans (drug only plan), or join a Medicare Advantage plan that offers comprehensive benefits, including outpatient prescription drugs.

Open Enrollment Period/Medigap

See also *Pre-existing condition, waiting period/Medigap*.

The open enrollment period for Medigap insurance lasts six (6) months, beginning in the first month in which a person age 65 or older enrolls for Medicare Part B benefits. (Enrollment in Part B typically occurs at age 65 or upon retirement after age 65.) Persons purchasing Medigap insurance during the open enrollment period cannot be denied the insurance for any reason, although there may be a waiting or exclusion period of up to six (6) months for coverage of preexisting conditions. However, this waiting or exclusion period may not be imposed under certain circumstances; (see *Preexisting condition, guaranteed issue/Medigap*).

Open Panel Model/Managed Care

See *Managed Care*.

Optional Categorically Needy/Medicaid

See also *Income cap states/Medicaid; Spend down/Medicaid*

This is one of the three (3) main groups of individuals eligible for Medicaid assistance – categorically needy, medically needy and optional categorically needy. For older people, probably the most significant subcategory within the larger rubric of optional categorically needy is the so-called three-hundred (300%) percent program. It provides nursing home care to people who are in a medical institution for at least thirty (30) days and whose gross income does not exceed more than three-hundred (300%) percent of the SSI benefit for an individual. Unlike the medically needy, the optional categorically needy are not permitted to spend down and will not qualify if they have even one dollar of income above the three-hundred (300%) percent level. The program permits states to cover nursing home care for people above the SSI level without having a full medically needy program for nursing home care.

States with a three-hundred (300%) percent program are sometimes referred to as income cap states. They are Alabama, Alaska, Colorado, Delaware, Idaho, Mississippi, Nevada, New Mexico, South Carolina, South Dakota and Wyoming. A second group of states – Arizona, Arkansas, Florida, Iowa, Louisiana (subject to the availability of state funds for individuals above the income cap), Oklahoma and Oregon plus Texas which does not cover the elderly – as a practical matter operate like income cap states. Although they have a medically needy program, these states do not permit nursing home expenses to be counted in calculating spend down expenses.

Optional Services/Medicaid
See also *Mandated Benefits/Medicaid*.

Medicaid will pay for certain specific services, in addition to those that may be designated by the Secretary of Health and Human Services. Of these, several are mandated; that is, states must provide them to categorically needy persons.

Optometrist Services/Medicare

Medicare pays only for very limited services by an optometrist licensed by the state in which he/she performs them. Routine eye exams and eyeglasses are not covered, except for one pair of glasses after a cataract operation.

Organization Determination/Medicare Advantage
See *Appeals/Medicare Advantage, section I*.

Original Medicare

This term refers to the health insurance available under Medicare Part A and Part B through the traditional fee-for-service payment system.

*Orthotic Items/Medicare

Includes arm, leg, back and neck braces; artificial eyes; artificial limbs (and their replacement parts); some types of breast prostheses (after mastectomy); and prosthetic devices needed to replace an internal body part or function (including ostomy supplies, and parenteral and enteral nutrition therapy) when your doctor orders it. For Medicare to cover your prosthetic or orthotic, you must go to a supplier that is enrolled in Medicare. You pay 20% of the Medicare-approved amount, and the Part B deductible applies.

Out-of-Network Pharmacy/Medicare Part D Drug Coverage

A licensed pharmacy that is not under contract with a Part D sponsor to provide negotiated prices to Part D plan enrollees.

Out-of-Pocket Spending/Medicare Part D Drug Coverage

See also *Out-of-Pocket threshold/Medicare Part D Drug Coverage; Catastrophic coverage/Medicare Part D Drug Coverage; Doughnut hole/Medicare Part D Coverage.*

The amount a beneficiary must pay on Part D-covered drugs to reach catastrophic coverage. An individual's payment of the deductible, coinsurance and/or copayments, and drug costs during the doughnut hole period counts towards out-of- pocket spending.

Out-of-Pocket Threshold/Medicare Part D Drug Coverage

See also *Out-of-Pocket spending/Medicare Part D Drug Coverage; Doughnut hole/Medicare Part D Coverage.*

This also is an official name for the drug costs Part D-eligibles must pay under Medicare Part D for deductibles, copayments and/or coinsurance, and drug costs during the doughnut hole period.

Outcome and Assessment Information Set (OASIS)/Home Care/Medicare

This form prescribed by the Secretary of HHS sets forth data concerning a patient's condition and is a significant part of the comprehensive assessment that a certified home health agency is required to make of each patient in determining his/her eligibility for Medicare home health benefits. The OASIS must be updated and revised as the patient's condition warrants.

Outpatient

A patient who receives services at a hospital, skilled nursing facility, clinic, rehabilitation facility, public health agency, or through a home health agency but does not stay overnight.

Outpatient Department Hospital Services/Medicare

Medicare Part B helps pay for the following outpatient department services:

> Blood transfusions furnished to a person as an outpatient;
>
> Drugs and biologicals that cannot be self-administered;
>
> Laboratory tests billed by the hospital;
>
> Mental health care if a physician certifies that inpatient treatment would be required without it;
>
> Medical supplies such as splints and casts;
>
> Services in an emergency room or outpatient clinic; including same day surgery; and
>
> X-rays and other radiology services billed by a hospital.

If an individual receives outpatient department (OPD) services at a hospital, other than for mental health, he/she is responsible for paying twenty (20%) percent of whatever the hospital charges not to exceed the standard Medicare hospital inpatient deductible – not merely the customary and lesser twenty (20%) percent of the Medicare-approved amount for Part B services rendered in other settings. According to CMS rules issued as a result of the Balanced Budget Act of 1997, this disparity in the amount of coinsurance for OPD services is scheduled to diminish generally and become the same as the standard copayment. Under these rules, the copayment for hospital OPD services is subject to a cap equal to the hospital inpatient deductible. If an individual receives outpatient mental health services, his/her coinsurance share is fifty (50%) percent of the Medicare-approved amount. (See also *Prospective payment system/Medicare.*)

Medicare Part B does not pay for a number of services, some of the most important being dental care and prescription drugs.

Outpatient Home Care/Medicare

See also *Outpatient services/Medicare.*

Outpatient services include any items of services covered by Medicare that are provided on an outpatient basis at a hospital, skilled nursing facility (SNF) or rehabilitation center and that require equipment not readily available at the patient's place of residence. The hospital, SNF, or rehabilitation center must be qualified providers of services.

*Outpatient Hospital Services/Medicare

You pay a coinsurance (for doctor services) or a copayment amount for most outpatient hospital services. The copayment for a single service can't be more than the amount of the inpatient hospital deductible.

For approved procedures (like x-rays, a cast, or stitches), you pay the doctor 20% of the Medicare-approved amount for the doctor's services. You also pay the hospital a copayment for each service you get in a hospital outpatient setting. For each service, the copayment can't be more than the Part A hospital stay deductible. The Part B deductible applies, and you pay all charges for items or services that Medicare doesn't cover.

Outpatient Mental Health Services/Medicare

See *Psychiatric care/Medicare.*

Outpatient Occupational Therapy, Physical Therapy and Speech-Language Pathology/Medicare

Skilled therapy services may be furnished to a Medicare beneficiary, whether or not homebound, on an outpatient basis by a participating hospital, skilled nursing facility, clinic, rehabilitation center, comprehensive outpatient rehabilitation facility, public health agency, or also, if the beneficiary is not homebound, by a home health agency. The provided services are covered as one of the "medical and other health services," as distinguished from "home health services," under Medicare Part B.

Outpatient therapy services are required to be reasonable and necessary. To be considered such, the services must provide a specific, safe and effective treatment for the beneficiary's condition. The required services must be sufficiently complex or the condition of the beneficiary such that the services can be performed only by a qualified therapist. There also must be an expectation that the beneficiary's condition will improve materially in a reasonably predictable period of time or that such services are necessary to establish a safe maintenance program.

Medicare will not make payment for outpatient occupational therapy services or outpatient physical therapy, furnished as an incident to a physician's professional services, which do not meet the standards applicable to a therapist furnishing such services in a clinic, rehabilitation agency or public health agency.

In addition to being reasonable and necessary, outpatient therapy services must meet the following conditions:

The outpatient must be under the care of a physician.

Services must be furnished and related directly to and specifically under a written plan of treatment established by a physician or the therapist who will provide the therapy services. The plan must be established before the treatment is begun and reviewed by the attending physician in consultation with the therapist at least every thirty (30) days.

The physician must certify at intervals of at least every thirty (30) days that a continuing need exists for such services and should estimate how long the services will be needed.

Recertification should be obtained at the time the plan of treatment is reviewed.

The provider of therapy services, other than a hospital outpatient department, may charge the patient any part of the Medicare Part B annual deductible not met, and the twenty- (20%) percent copayment of the Medicare-approved charge. However, if an individual receives outpatient services at a hospital outpatient department, as opposed to the other settings, his/her copayment is twenty (20%) percent of the hospital bill – a much higher amount than the standard copayment of twenty (20%) percent. However, this disparity gradually will diminish so that the copayment in time will equal the standard copayment.

An annual limit of $1,500 applies to all outpatient physical therapy services, including speech language pathology. A separate $1,500 applies to occupational therapy services. However, a hospital outpatient is not and will not be subject to any cap.

Instead of obtaining skilled therapy services from a participating Medicare facility, patients can receive services directly from private practicing, Medicare-approved therapists performing such services in their office or in the patient's home, if a doctor prescribes such treatment.

Medicare reimbursements to all providers of therapy services are made on a prospective basis and are based upon eighty (80%) percent of the lesser of the actual charge for the services, or the amount payable under the Medicare physician fee schedule.

Outpatient Services/Medicare

Medicare beneficiaries, including homebound patients who qualify for and receive home health care, are eligible to receive any services provided on an outpatient basis at a hospital, skilled nursing facility or rehabilitation center and that require equipment that is not readily available at the patient's place of residence or is furnished while the patient receives services at the facility.

Over-Resourced/Medicaid
See also *Spend down/Medicaid.*

Possessing non-exempt resources higher than the level permitted under a state's Medicaid plan to be eligible for Medicaid assistance.

Oxygen/Medicare
See also *Durable medical equipment/Medicare.*

Covered by Medicare.

(continued on next page)

P

Palliative Care

This is care provided to a terminally ill patient, often through a hospice program. It is intended to ease suffering and promote physical and emotional comfort but not to cure illness or prolong life.

*Pap Test/Medicare

Checks for cervical, vaginal and breast cancers. Medicare covers these screening tests once every 24 months, or once every 12 months for women at high risk, and for women who have Medicare and are of childbearing age who have had an exam that indicated cancer or other abnormalities in the past 3 years. You pay nothing for the Pap lab test. Starting January 1, 2011, you also pay nothing for Pap test specimen collection, and pelvic and breast exams if the doctor accepts assignment.

Pap Smear Screening and Pelvic Exam/Medicare

For beneficiaries at average risk, Medicare Part B helps pay for Pap smear screenings and pelvic exams every three (3) years. This coverage is authorized on a yearly basis for women at high risk of developing cervical or vaginal cancer and for those of childbearing age who have not had a negative test in each of the preceding three (3) years. Although the Medicare Part B deductible is waived for Pap smear screenings and pelvic exams, the twenty- (20%) percent copayment is not.

Parent Survivor Benefits/Social Security
See Social Security Program (Title II), section VII.C; Dependent benefits/Social Security.

All entries preceded by an asterisk (*) are culled or copied from the official U.S. government **Medicare** handbook (*Medicare & You 2011*).

Part A/Medicare

See also Medicare Part A hospital benefits.

The part of Medicare that covers inpatient hospital care, care in a skilled nursing facility, hospice care and limited home health care. Generally people age 65 and over can get premium-free Medicare Part A benefits based on their own or their spouse's employment. Such is the case if a person age 65 or over is entitled to receive retirement benefits under Social Security, or if a person under age 65 is a disabled beneficiary under Social Security or has end-stage renal disease.

Part B/Medicare

See also Medicare Part B benefits.

This part of Medicare covers doctor's services, limited home care, hospice, outpatient hospital care, lab tests, x-rays, ambulances and durable medical equipment. Any person who is entitled to premium-free Medicare Part A benefits can enroll for Part B, by paying the monthly Part B premium, which is deducted from a patient's Social Security check.

Part C/Medicare

The part of Medicare created by the Balanced Budget Act of 1997 replacing Medicare risk contracts with contracts under Medicare+Choice, now known as Medicare Advantage program. The program expanded the HMOs into a variety of private managed-care plan options for Medicare beneficiaries.

Part D/Medicare

The part of Medicare created by the Medicare Prescription Drug Improvement and Modernization Act of 2003 (i) establishing a voluntary prescription drug benefit program for Medicare beneficiaries entitled to Part A; (ii) authorizing, among other matters, changes to the Medicare+Choice program and replaced the term Medicare+Choice (phased out in 2005-2006) by the term Medicare Advantage (MA); and (iii) expanding the array of private managed plans available to Medicare enrollees, as alternatives to original Medicare. An individual is eligible for the Medicare prescription drug program if he or she is entitled to Medicare Part A or is enrolled in Part B. These beneficiaries are able to obtain prescription drugs with either (i) a stand-alone prescription drug program available to enrollees in original Medicare or (ii) a Medicare Advantage plan.

Part D Drugs/Medicare Part D Drug Coverage

Covered Part D drugs are drugs dispensable by prescription, biological products or insulin and corresponding medical supplies or vaccines. Certain drugs are not included. Plans may use formularies. If a drug is otherwise covered under Part D, but paid for under Part A or B, then the drug is not be considered for Part D payment. Part D drugs also may not be covered under the general exclusions from Medicare coverage, or if not prescribed according to the plan or statute.

Part D-eligible Individuals/Medicare Part D Drug Coverage

Individuals who are entitled to Part D benefits under Medicare Part A or enrolled in Medicare Part B.

Partial Subsidy Eligibles/Medicare Part D Drug Coverage

Individuals are eligible for the following partial subsidies if they have income up to one-hundred fifty (150%) percent of Federal poverty level and resources of not more than $13,070 per individual, and $26,120 (2012) per couple.

Premium Subsidy

Partial subsidy individuals are entitled to a premium subsidy based on a sliding scale as follows:

> A premium subsidy equal to seventy-five (75%) percent of the subsidy for individuals with income greater than one-hundred thirty-five (135%) percent but at or below one-hundred forty (140%) percent of the Federal poverty level.

> A premium subsidy equal to fifty (50%) percent of the subsidy for individuals with income greater than one-hundred forty (140%) percent but at or below one-hundred forty-five (145%) percent of the Federal poverty level.

> A premium subsidy equal to twenty-five (25%) percent of the subsidy for individuals with income below one-hundred fifty (150%) percent of the Federal poverty level.

Cost-sharing Subsidy

Partial subsidy individuals are entitled to cost-sharing subsidies (deductibles, copayments, and coinsurance) as follows:

Individuals with resources less than $13,070 (for a single person in 2012) or less than $26,120 (for a married couple in 2012) and income below one-hundred thirty-five (135%) percent t of the Federal poverty level will receive the following benefits:

No deductible;

Coinsurance of fifteen (15%) percent instead of the full twenty-five (25%) percent provided by the standard drug benefit, including coverage through the doughnut hole;

Copayments of $2.60 for each generic or preferred brand drug and $6.50 (2012) for each brand name drug, after an out-of-pocket limit is reached.

Individuals with resources below $13,070 (for a single individual) in 2012 or $26,120 (for a married couple, 2012), and income between one-hundred thirty-five (135%) percent and one-hundred fifty (150%) percent of the Federal poverty level will receive the following cost-sharing benefits:

A $65 (2012) deductible;

Coinsurance of fifteen (15%) percent after the deductible up to the out-of-pocket limit ($4,700, 2012), including continued coverage through the doughnut hole; and

Copayments of $2.60 for each generic or preferred brand drug or $6.50 for each brand name drug, after the out-of-pocket limit is reached.

Note: There is no cost-sharing for eligible individuals residing in a medical facility. (A medical facility is defined as a nursing home, psychiatric center, residential treatment center, development center, or intermediate care facility. Individuals living in the group residences such as assisted living programs, group homes and adult homes are subject to copayments.)

Participating Physician or Supplier/Medicare

A physician or supplier who agrees to accept assignment on all Medicare claims. Physicians who are not participating providers can still agree to accept assignment for any individual patient.

Partnership Program for LTCI
See *Robert Wood Johnson Program/LTCI.*

Part-time Care/Medicare
See also *Intermittent care/Medicare; Part-time or intermittent care/Medicare.*

Part-time is not a separately defined term in legislation or elsewhere. However, it is included by the Balanced Budget Act of 1997 within the term "part-time or intermediate" as a coverage limitation describing the period of time that home health aide services combined with skilled nursing services or provided separately will be covered by Medicare.

Part-time or Intermittent Care/Medicare
See also *Intermittent care/Medicare; Part-time care/Medicare.*

The Balanced Budget Act of 1997 (Act) defines intermittent as an eligibility factor. However, for purposes of determining the extent of coverage of home health care, as contrasted with eligibility for such care, the Act does not define intermittent separately. Instead, it refers to the statutory term "part-time or intermittent nursing care" or "part-time or intermittent services of a home health aide." In this context as a coverage limitation, part-time or intermittent services are defined to mean skilled nursing and home health aide services (combined) furnished any number of days per week so long as they are provided: less than eight (8) hours a day and twenty-eight (28) or fewer hours per week; or, on a case-by-case basis, subject to review as to the need for care, less than eight (8) hours a day and thirty-five (35) or fewer hours per week. The Secretary of HHS is authorized under the Act to establish normative guidelines for the frequency and duration of these and other home health services.

Patient Bill of Rights

A list of policies and procedures to be followed to ensure that patients receiving health care services are treated with dignity and participate fully in decisions relevant to their health care.

Patient Dumping

The transfer to other institutions of a patient unable to pay enough to cover his/her costs.

Patient Review Instrument/Medicaid

This form is used to determine the level of medical care and services a patient requires prior to placement in a nursing home, and to determine Medicaid reimbursement to nursing homes for services provided to resident patients.

Payer

An organization, such as Medicare or a commercial insurance company, that furnishes money to pay for health care services.

Payments for Part A Services/Medicare

Generally, Medicare will directly pay the service provider (e.g., a hospital) when the patient requests it to submit his/her claim to Medicare. Payment is prospectively based upon a Medicare-approved cost for the diagnosis-related group associated with the patient's illness or injury.

Payments for Part B Services/Medicare

In the case of services rendered under Part B by institutional providers (hospitals, skilled nursing facilities, home health agencies, hospices) – payments are made by Medicare directly to the provider. The provider in turn may then charge the beneficiary for applicable deductibles and coinsurance payments.

In the case of services rendered under Part B by physicians, practitioners, durable equipment suppliers – payment may be made by Medicare to the physician or other providers only if the right to payment is assigned to them by the beneficiary, and they agree to be paid according to the rules of assignment (see *Assignment/Medicare*).

Peer Review Organization (PRO)/Medicare
See *Quality Improvement Organization/Medicare*.

*Penalty (Late Enrollment)/Medicare

Part A – *If you aren't eligible for premium-free Part A, and you don't buy it when you're first eligible, your monthly premium may go up 10%. You will have to pay the higher premium for twice the number of years you have had Part A, but didn't sign up. For example, if you were eligible for Part A for 2 years but didn't sign up, you will have to pay the higher premium for 4 years. Usually, you don't have to pay a penalty if you meet certain conditions that allow you to sign up for Part A during a Special Enrollment Period.*

__Part B__ – If you don't sign up for Part B when you're first eligible, you may have to pay a late enrollment penalty for as long as you have Medicare.

Your monthly premium for Part B may go up 10% for each full 12-month period that you could have had Part B, but didn't sign up for it. Usually, you don't pay a late enrollment penalty if you meet certain conditions that allow you to sign up for Part B during a special enrollment period.

__Part D__ – The late enrollment penalty is an amount that is added to your Part D premium. __You may owe a late enrollment penalty if one of the following is true__:

You didn't join a Medicare drug plan when you were first eligible for Medicare, and you didn't have other creditable prescription drug coverage.

You didn't have Medicare prescription drug coverage or other creditable prescription drug coverage for 63 days or more in a row.

Pension Benefit Guaranty Corporation (PBGC)

A Federal agency that collects premiums from employers under an insurance scheme designed to guarantee payment of benefits under defined benefit pension plans, but not defined contribution plans.

Pension Plan
See *Defined benefit plan; Defined contribution plan; Private pension.*

Per Diem Hospital Cost

The inpatient hospital costs for a day of care. Per diem costs are an average and do not reflect the true cost for each patient.

Percent of Federal Poverty Level/Medicaid
See also *Federal poverty level.*

Several determinations under Medicaid are linked to percentages of the Federal poverty level (FPL). Eligibility as a qualified Medicare beneficiary (QMB) is open to people with incomes at or below one-hundred (100%) percent of the FPL for a family of the size involved. Medicaid determination of a minimum monthly needs allowance for a community spouse of a nursing facility resident is based upon one-hundred fifty (150%) percent of the FPL for two people, on the theory that when spouses cease living together, the expenses of the spouse remaining at home are not cut in half. The respective amounts based on the FPL are set forth in guidelines published the U.S. Department of Health and Human Services each year, usually in February.

Period of Ineligibility/Medicaid

See also *Transfer penalty (civil)/Medicaid.*

This is the period, stated as a number of months, that an individual who has made a transfer of assets for less than fair market value within the look-back period (as defined in *Transfer Penalty (civil) Medicaid*) shall remain ineligible for certain Medicaid services.

For an institutionalized person, the period ineligibility equals, and for a non-institutionalized person is not greater than, the number of months calculated by dividing the total uncompensated value of all assets an individual disposed of during the look-back period by a private patient's average cost of nursing facility care per month. The ineligibility period, except when multiple transfers are made, begins on the first day of the first month when the transfer of assets took place, or, at a state's option, on the first day of the following month.

When multiple transfers are made during the look-back period, they are treated as follows:

> For multiple transfers during the look-back period when assets have been transferred in amounts or in frequency that would make the calculated periods overlap, the transfers must be added together and then divided by the average monthly payment for nursing facilities within a state, or, at the option of the state, within a designated region of the state. The period of ineligibility will be determined on the basis of the total amount transferred. The period of ineligibility begins with the first day of the month following the month in which the first transfer is made.

> When multiple transfers are made in such a way that the penalties for each do not overlap, each transfer is treated as a separate event, with its own penalty period.

Permitted Deductions/Medicaid

An institutionalized spouse is required to apply all of his/her income to the cost of institutional care after certain permitted deductions. These deductions pertain to income that is deducted or exempted from either the eligibility or post-eligibility process of determining income for Medicaid purposes. In determining eligibility, for example, $20 per month of unearned income is deducted or exempted. In the post-eligibility process, different deductions are permitted from a Medicaid recipient's income to determine how much of that income an individual must pay to the Medicaid system. Included as permitted deductions are: a personal needs allowance of at least $30 per month per institutionalized individual; the community spouse's monthly income allowance; a family allowance; and amounts incurred for medical or remedial care expenses. Under current law, states cannot choose which or how much to allow for these deductions since the applicant/recipient is entitled to them by Federal law.

Personal Care
See *Custodial care*.

Personal Care/Medicaid
See also *Personal care services/Home Care*.

Non-medically oriented services provided to a Medicaid-eligible individual in the home or other location are optional to states. Personal care provided by Medicaid comprises some or total assistance with personal hygiene, dressing, feeding, nutritional and environmental support functions and health related tasks. These services do not necessarily have to be in support of a skilled service. States are authorized to provide personal care services either through Medicaid home and community-based waivers, or through the personal care services option specified in statute as a separate Medicaid services. The following requirements must be met:

> The services must be according to a physician's written plan of care – or at the state's option, in accordance with a service plan approved by the state – and may not be provided by a family member.

> The plan of care must be reviewed by the physician every sixty (60) days.

> Under CMS regulations, the services need not be supervised by a registered nurse.

The services must be provided at home, or at a state's option in another location. Medicaid coverage of personal care is not available to an individual who is an inpatient at a hospital facility, nursing facility, intermediate care facility for the mentally retarded or an institution for mental diseases.

The services must be medically necessary as determined by the physician.

The client's health and safety must be able to be maintained in the home.

Applications for personal care are based upon a physician's order submitted to a state-prescribed Medicaid office. The application process includes one or more of several assessments:

Nursing. This assessment focuses on such matters as the recommended hours per day and days per week.

Social. Usually a case manager will complete a social assessment form covering such matters as the availability of informal caregivers to help care for the patient and thus reduce the need for personal care services.

Fiscal. Determination whether institutional placement would be more cost effective.

Efficiency. This analysis is made to ensure that the most cost effective services are used.

Personal Care Home
See *Assisted living facility.*

Personal Care Services/Home Care

Personal care services are hands-on, unskilled services that assist the patient with such activities as eating, bathing, dressing, transferring from chair to walker or from bed to wheelchair, toileting and turning and positioning. The services sometimes include housekeeper/chore services.

Personal care is one of the three basic categories of home care services. The other two are medical home health services and non-medical services.

Medicare will not cover personal care services as a separate service. Hence, if a beneficiary needs only personal care services, a source other than Medicare coverage must be obtained. However, Medicare may cover personal care service if it is incidental to qualified skilled services provided to a homebound patient eligible for home health care. In order to obtain Medicare coverage, personal care service must be prescribed by a physician and furnished by a qualified home health aide through a certified home health agency.

Home health long-term care insurance policies covering personal care are obtainable by individuals who can afford the premiums. These policies may provide for medical and non-medical services that are incidental to home care, including not only nursing and home health aide services but also personal care services.

Personal Care Services Option/Medicaid
See *Personal care/Medicaid.*

Personal Emergency Response System (PERS)

Equipment that monitors the safety of older people in their homes through signals electronically transmitted over the telephone to a twenty-four- (24) hour emergency monitoring center. A PERS is a small device worn around the neck or wrist that allows the wearer to signal for help by pressing a button that activates the system. Consumers can purchase, lease or rent this equipment.

Personal Needs Allowance/Medicaid
See also *Permitted deductions/Medicaid.*

This is an amount of money required to be set aside for an institutionalized individual receiving nursing facility services paid by Medicaid in order to pay for personal needs such as clothing, reading material and stationery, snacks not required to be provided by the facility, and activities not required to be provided by the facility. At a minimum, the allowance must be $30 per month. It is not indexed annually according to changes in the consumer price index. States can increase the personal needs allowance above the minimum.

Physical Examination/Medicare

Medicare Part B does not cover a routine physical examination or tests directly related to it.

Physical Therapist
See also *Occupational therapist.*

Physical therapy is frequently needed by a patient whose limbs or muscles are impaired because of an illness or accident. After reviewing a physician's medical diagnosis and treatment plan, a physical therapist may visit the patient at home, as required under a plan of care. The therapist generally prepares a treatment schedule and visits the patient on a routine basis until determining, after consultation with the physician, that therapy is no longer necessary or advisable.

*Physical Therapy/Medicare

Evaluation and treatment for injuries and diseases that change your ability to function when your doctor certifies your need for it. There may be limits on these services and exceptions to these limits. You pay 20% of the Medicare-approved amount, and the Part B deductible applies.

Physical Therapy/Medicare

See also *Qualifying skilled services/Medicare; Occupational therapy, physical therapy and speech-language pathology, Home Care/Medicare; Outpatient occupational therapy, physical therapy and speech-language pathology/ Medicare.*

Treatment of injury and disease by additional means, such as heat, light exercise and massage. Physical therapy is characterized by Medicare as one of the qualifying skilled services. The need for a qualifying skilled service is one of the Medicare requirements for obtaining home health coverage.

Physician Assistant (PA)/Medicare

A physician assistant is a health professional qualified by training and licensure to provide health care services under the supervision and direction of a physician. The PA's functions include assisting the physician in performing diagnostic, therapeutic, preventive and health maintenance services in the setting in which the physician renders such care.

PAs are eligible for Part B payment if they render physician-type services in any setting as long as Medicare does not pay the facility or provider for their services.

PAs are paid eighty (80%) percent of the lesser of either the actual charge or eighty-five (85%) percent of the Medicare physician fee schedule. When they serve as assistants at surgery, payment to PAs is eighty (80%) percent of the lesser of either the actual charge or eighty-five (85%) percent of the physician fee schedule for assistance at surgery. A PA may be an independent contractor of the physician. However, the requirement of physician supervision continues.

584

Physician Charges/Medicare
See *Fee schedule charge/Medicare.*

Physician Fee Schedule/Medicare
See also *Fee schedule charge/Medicare; Resource-based relative value scale (RBRVS)/Medicare.*

Medicare Part B reimburses physicians for Medicare-covered services based on a fee schedule, also known as the resources-based relative value scale. The factors that enter into calculating the payment for each medical service under the physician fee schedule are:

> A nationally uniform relative value for the services;
>
> A geographic adjustment factor for the area where a physician practices; and
>
> A uniform conversion factor for the services.
>
> The particular relative value, in turn, is based on the following resources needed to furnish the services:
>
>> value of the physician services;
>>
>> physician costs or practice expenses; and
>>
>> cost of malpractice.

The fee schedule amount for a particular service is determined by multiplying the relative value for the service by the geographic adjustment factor and the conversion factor. This results in a specific dollar amount for the service.

Physician Hospital Organization (PHO)
See *Managed care.*

Physician Practice and Malpractice Expenses/Medicare
See *Physician fee schedule/Medicare.*

Pickle People/Medicaid

Former SSI recipients who would have lost categorical Medicaid eligibility due to increased income resulting from Social Security cost-of-living increases, if it were not for the "Pickle amendment" sponsored by Congressman Pickle in 1976.

Plan of Care/Medicare

The need for a home health qualifying skilled service must be provided and certified as necessary under a plan of care established by a qualified physician. The care plan must be reviewed by the physician at least every sixty (60) days. In some circumstances, verbal orders can later be incorporated into a plan.

Plan Sponsor/Medicare Part D Drug Coverage

Any private insurance company that is certified by Medicare to provide Medicare prescription drug coverage. It can be a stand-alone prescription drug plan that one chooses along with traditional Medicare or Medicare Advantage plans that offers Part D coverage.

Plenary Guardian
See *Adult guardian.*

*Pneumococcal Shot/Medicare

Helps prevent pneumococcal infections (like certain types of pneumonia). Most people only need this shot once in their lifetime. You pay nothing if the doctor or supplier accepts assignment for giving the shot.

Pneumococcal Pneumonia Vaccine/Medicare

Medicare Part B pays the full, approved charges for pneumococcal pneumonia vaccine and its administration once during a beneficiary's lifetime. Neither the annual deductible nor the twenty- (20%) percent coinsurance apply to this service.

Podiatrist Services/Medicare

Medicare Part B helps pay for any covered services of a licensed podiatrist to treat injuries and diseases of the foot. Examples of common problems include ingrown toenails, hammertoe deformities, bunion deformities and heel spurs. Medicare generally does not pay for routine foot care, such as cutting or removal of corns and calluses, trimming of nails and other hygienic care.

Point of Service (POS)/Medicare Advantage
See also *Medicare HMO*.

A form of managed care offered by organizations such as HMOs. POS organizations feature a network of doctors, hospitals and other health care providers. Participants have a choice of using the network or any other provider each time they seek medical care. This is a point of service choice. The network coverage is broadly comprehensive using preventative care as well as major medical and hospital coverage. Should a participant choose care outside the network, he/she is subject to paying copayments and deductibles which are usually higher than in a typical HMO. As with a preferred provider organization, the participant has a choice of providers and is not locked in.

Pool of Funds Policy/LTCI
See *Long-term care insurance*.

Pooled Trust/Medicaid
See also *Trusts, Medicaid eligibility rules; Trust transfer penalty rules/Medicaid*.

A pooled trust is created for a disabled individual, regardless of age, with the assets of that individual. They are pooled together with assets of others, but kept in a separate account and managed by a trustee that must be a non-profit association.

Upon the death of the disabled person, the trust is required to pay back Medicaid out of any funds remaining in the trust.

Post-Institutional Home Health Care Services/Medicare
See *Home Care, section V; Medicare/Home Health Care, section III*.

Pourover Will

The testator provides in his/her will that designated assets will be paid over and distributed to a previously established trust.

Power of Appointment Trust
See also *Terminable interest property*.

The transfer of terminable interest property does not qualify for a marital deduction, subject to certain exceptions, one of which is a power of appointment trust. This is a testamentary trust created by a decedent spouse. It passes to the surviving spouse in the form of a trust or a life estate in the decedent's property with the income payable to the surviving spouse for life. This trust vests in the surviving spouse a general power of appointment over the remainder of the property. The power of appointment must be exercisable by the surviving spouse either by will or during life. Such a trust qualifies for a marital deduction.

As an alternative, the terminable interest property need not be transferred in the form of a trust. The surviving spouse may be given a legal life estate by the decedent spouse with a general power of appointment as to the remainder.

Power of Attorney
See also *Durable power of attorney; Springing power of attorney.*

A legal document signed by a person, known as a principal, giving another person, known as an attorney-in-fact or agent, authority, which the principal may revoke at any time, over all the principal's financial transactions or personal actions, or only over those transactions and actions specifically set out in the document. If not revoked by the principal, the power of attorney continues indefinitely during the lifetime of the principal so long as he/she is competent. If the principal becomes non-cognitive or dies, the power of attorney automatically expires.

Pre-Demise Payment/Life Insurance Policies
See also *Accelerated benefits.*

An increasing trend among insurers is to permit life insurance policies to be tapped during the lifetime of the insured person based on a diagnosis of a terminal illness or a need for long-term care. Some policies also make benefits available for home care as well as institutionalization. These "living benefits" permit the insured person, usually on consent of the beneficiary, to access a percentage of the policy's death benefit during the insured's life.

Preexisting Condition/LTCI

The typical older LTCI policy may not cover treatment of a preexisting condition that is an injury, disease or a physical condition known to exist prior to the issuance of the policy. Newer LTCI policies will cover such conditions that are disclosed on the application. The National Association of Insurance

Commissioners model LTCI policy and state law usually limit the definition of preexisting condition, generally forbidding any definition more restrictive than a condition that was not admitted on the application, for which medical advice was or should have been sought during the six (6) months before the policy became effective date. The Health Insurance Portability and Accountability Act of 1996 requires that if replacement LTCI insurance policies are to be tax-qualified they can have no limitation for preexisting conditions.

Preexisting Condition Exclusion

A practice of some health insurers under private insurance policies to deny coverage to individuals for a certain period for health conditions that existed when coverage was obtained.

Preexisting Condition, Guaranteed Issue/Medigap
See also *Medicare Supplemental Insurance-Medigap, section V.*

During the first six (6) months after obtaining Medicare coverage, known as the open enrollment period, an applicant for a Medigap policy cannot be denied a policy because of a medical condition, preexisting or otherwise. If the applicant should miss the six- (6) month open enrollment window, in most states Medigap insurance can be denied on Medical grounds. The Balanced Budget Act of 1997, however, exempted several classes of applicants (see below) from this ban and guaranteed them issuance of a Medigap policy despite the existence of a preexisting medical condition, and even if purchased after the six-month open enrollment period.

An applicant may enroll in any of four (4) standard Medigap policies A, B, C or F if he/she is provided with such insurance and has had continuous coverage, as defined below, in an existing health policy and enrolls in one of the four (4) policies no later than six (6) days after the determination of prior coverage. Continuously covered applicants are:

> Individuals whose supplemental coverage under an employee welfare benefit plan terminates;
>
> Individuals enrolled in a Medicare Advantage plan who disenroll for permissible reasons (e.g., termination of the plan's certification or move out of the plan area) other than during an annual election period;

Persons enrolled in cost-based HMOs or Medicare Select policies who disenroll under the same circumstances described in the section about Medicare Advantage enrollees. With respect to Medicare Select policies, there must be no state law relating to continuation of coverage for this provision to apply;

Individuals whose enrollment in a Medigap policy ceases because of the bankruptcy or insolvency of the insurer issuing the policy, or because of other involuntary termination of coverage for which there is no state law relating to continuation of coverage;

Individuals previously enrolled under a Medigap policy who terminate such enrollment in order to participate, for the first time, in a Medicare Advantage plan, cost-based HMO, or Medicare Select policy and who subsequently terminate their enrollment in such a plan within the first twelve (12) months of enrollment; and

Persons who enroll in a Medicare Advantage plan upon first reaching Medicare eligibility at age 65 but disenroll from the plan within twelve (12) months of enrollment.

Applicants who were previously enrolled under a Medigap policy, after a one-time test of a Medicare Advantage, may enroll in the same Medigap policy, if still available from the same issuer, that they had before trying a Medicare Advantage Plan.

Applicants, who upon first reaching Medicare eligibility at age 65 enroll in a Medicare Advantage plan, may disenroll from that plan within twelve (12) months and enroll in any Medigap plan.

Preexisting Condition, Waiting Period/Medigap
See also *Open enrollment period/Medigap.*

Prior to the Balanced Budget Act of 1997 (Act), even though an applicant with a preexisting medical condition purchased a Medigap policy during the one-time, six-(6) month open enrollment period, he/she could be required to wait up to six (6) months before coverage of the condition became effective. The Act eliminated this waiting period for any applicant who on the date of application for Medigap enrollment has had at least six (6) months of creditable coverage. Persons having fewer than six (6) months of such coverage are entitled to have the period of any preexisting condition exclusion reduced by the length of time they had such coverage. The term creditable coverage means coverage of the applicant under any one of several medical health plans such as a group health plan, Medicare Part D or Part B, or a state health benefit risk pool.

Preferred Drug/Medicare Part D Drug Coverage

A drug that a plan encourages physicians and patients to choose. This drug is typically included on a formulary and requires lower cost-sharing than that of a non-preferred drug.

*Preferred Provider Organization (PPO) Plan/Medicare

There are two types of PPOs: Regional PPOs and Local PPOs. Regional PPOs serve one of 26 regions set by Medicare. Local PPOs serve the counties the PPO Plan chooses to include in its service area. You do not need to select a primary care doctor and you don't need a referral to see a specialist. In most cases, prescription drugs are covered. Ask your plan. If you want drug coverage, you must join a PPO Plan that offers it. You can also receive your health care from any doctor or hospital. PPOs have network doctors and hospitals, but you can also use out-of network providers for covered services, usually for a higher cost.

Preferred Provider Organization (PPO)/Medicare Advantage

An arrangement between an employer or insurance company and a network of health providers whereby the providers, called preferred providers, furnish health services in return for the guaranty of a certain volume of patients. As part of the arrangement, the insurance company or employer negotiates discounted fees with the PPO so that the insured enrollees receive services from the providers on a lower than the customary fee-for-service basis. A variant of the classic HMO, the PPO uses a primary care physician who acts as a gatekeeper. The insured individual can use doctors, hospitals and providers that belong to the network and they may obtain services outside the PPO but must pay higher copayments or deductibles for such services.

Medicare Advantage PPO is one type of a Medicare Advantage coordinated care plan. Any coordinated care organization may offer a PPO plan if the PPO meets the requirements of a Medicare Advantage coordinated care plan.

The conditions set forth in the entries *Medicare Advantage plans (MAP)*; *Medicare Advantage (MA) coordinated care plans – Common Features* (except where noted) apply to a Medicare Advantage PPO.

Premium/LTCI

The premium for a LTCI policy depends on actuarial factors such as the age and predicted need for care of the class of insured, adjusted in light of the policy's lapse rate. It also depends on the coverage chosen by the insured. The more risk the insured person is willing to accept, and the more private payment he/she is willing to assume before insurance benefits are available, the lower the premium will be. Conversely, the more risk the insurer must assume, the higher the premium will be.

LTCI policies are usually level premium policies. The premium is set based on the insured person's entry age, that is, the age at which a person first purchases coverage. Thus, premiums are low for an early entry age but increase dramatically the older a purchaser is. However, insurers can raise the level premium only on a class-wide basis for all policyholders with the same class of policy. So the premium for a level premium policy probably will increase over time.

Premium/Medicare
See also *Medicare section V.C.*

Part A

Individuals age 65 or over who are entitled to Social Security or Railroad Retirement benefits generally are entitled to Medicare Part A benefits without payment of a premium.

Persons (called voluntary enrollees) not entitled to Part A benefits may be able to purchase them by paying the following premiums:

$451.00/month (2012) if individual has twenty-nine (29) or fewer quarters of Social Security coverage; and

$248.00/month (2012) if individual has thirty (30) to thirty-nine (39) quarters of Social Security coverage.

Part B

All beneficiaries enrolled in Medicare Part B must pay a premium which CMS annually establishes ($99.90/month in 2012) together with a surcharge (monthly adjustment amount) for higher income beneficiaries. The premium has been income-related for individuals with higher incomes since 2007. In 2012, individuals with incomes of $85,000 or more and couples with incomes of $170,000 or more will pay higher Part B premiums than those below these income levels. The income levels for determining the Part B premium are adjusted each year based on the Consumer Price Index for urban consumers.

Income is the adjusted gross income of the individual plus certain types of additional income such as tax-exempt interest and capital gains. The adjusted gross income combined with these additional types of income is called modified adjusted gross income (MAGI). The MAGI is separated into ranges or thresholds (levels) (e.g. below $85,000 or above $85,000).

Medicare then prescribes certain monthly adjustment amounts (surcharges) associated respectively with the different levels of related income. (See Part B premium table below.)

Payment of the premium is made either by deductions by the government from Social Security benefits payable monthly to the beneficiary or by direct remittance by the beneficiary.

Part B Premium

The MAGI Range			
Individual Tax Return ($)	Joint Tax Return ($)	Married but File a Separate Tax Return	Monthly Premium (2012)
85,000 or below	170,000 or below		$99.90
85,001 - 107,000	170,001 -214,000		139.90
107,001 - 160,000	214,001- 320,000		199.80
160,001 - 214,000	320,001- 428,000	Greater than $85,000 but less than or equal to $128,000	259.70
Above 214,000	Above 428,000	Greater than $128,000	319.70

Premium/Medicare Part D Drug Coverage

The MMA does not mandate a set Part D drug monthly premium amount. Premiums are determined by a bidding process and vary from plan to plan and from region to region. Private insurance companies must submit new bids each year.

The premium is defined as the base beneficiary premium. The amount of the premium is equal to the product of the beneficiary premium percentage (see below) and the national average monthly bid amount (see below) for the month.

Base Beneficiary Premium. The beneficiary premium percentage is equal to twenty-five and one-half (25½%) percent divided by one-hundred (100%) percent, minus a percentage equal to the total reinsurance payments for the coverage year, divided by the sum of the reinsurance payments and the total payments the Secretary estimates will be paid to PDPs and MA-PD plans that are attributable to the standardized bid amount (see below) for the year. For a PDP that provides basic prescription drug coverage, the standardized bid amount is the PDP-approved bid. For a PDP that provides supplemental prescription drug coverage, the standardized bid amount is the portion of the PDP-approved bid that is attributable to basic prescription drug coverage. The PDP approved bid is the bid amount approved for the plan. For MA-PD plans, the standardized bid amount is the portion of the accepted bid amount that is attributable to the basic prescription drug coverage.

If for a month the standardized bid amount exceeds the national average monthly bid amount, the base beneficiary premium for the month is adjusted by the excess. If for a month, the national average monthly bid amount exceeds the standardized bid amount, the base beneficiary premium for the month will be decreased by the amount of the excess. The base beneficiary premium will be increased by the portion of the PDP-approved bid that is attributable to supplemental prescription drug benefits.

For each year beginning in 2006, the Secretary must compute a national average monthly bid amount equal to the average of the standardized bid amounts.

Premium/Medicare Supplemental Insurance (Medigap)

Carriers use one of three (3) methods to fix Medigap policy premiums:

Issue Age. The premium is pegged to an applicant's age when he/she enrolls so that a consumer always pays the premium required of a person of the same age when the policy was issued. Thus, if an individual buys a policy at age 65, he/she will always pay the rate the company charges people who are age 65, regardless of his/her age.

Attained Age. Premiums increase, as the beneficiary grows older.

Community Rating. Carriers charge all beneficiaries in a particular area the same amount; the rate is based on the demographics and health experience of the group.

Prepaid Health Plan (PHP)/Managed Care

A type of managed care organization. In certain health centers located in medically underserved areas, PHPs contract with a state Medicaid agency for a less-than-comprehensive list of services or on a non-risk basis and are statutorily exempt from HMO requirements.

*Prescription Drugs/Medicare

Includes a limited number of drugs such as injections you get in a doctor's office, certain oral cancer drugs, drugs used with some types of durable medical equipment (like a nebulizer or external infusion pump) and under very limited circumstances, certain drugs you get in a hospital outpatient setting. You pay 20% of the Medicare-approved amount for these covered drugs.

If the covered drugs you get in a hospital outpatient setting are part of your outpatient services, you pay the copayment for the services. However, if you get other types of drugs in a hospital outpatient setting (sometimes called "self-administered drugs" or drugs you would normally take on your own), what you pay depends on whether you have Part D or other prescription drug coverage, whether your drug plan covers the drug, and whether the hospital's pharmacy is in your drug plan's network. Contact your prescription drug plan to find out what you pay for drugs you get in a hospital outpatient setting that aren't covered under Part B.

Other than the examples above, you pay 100% for most prescription drugs, unless you have Part D or other drug coverage.

Prescription Drug Plan (PDP)/Medicare Part D Drug Coverage

A plan that offers the outpatient prescription drug benefit to beneficiaries who choose to be enrolled in the original Medicare program, distinct from the comprehensive managed care drug plan (MA-PDP). The PDP is called the stand-alone drug plan.

Prescription Drugs/Medicare
See *Drugs/Medicare*.

Present Value Calculation

A calculation that shows the current worth of money to be paid in the future.

Prevailing Charge/Medicare

See also *Fee schedule charge/Medicare.*

Now supplanted by the fee schedule charge, a prevailing charge was customarily used by Medicare in the context of establishing the reasonable charge. Under the former system, a prevailing charge was within the range of charges used in a locality for a particular medical service or procedure and was distinguished from the Medicare reasonable charge which was the lower of the actual charge, customary charge or prevailing charge.

*Preventive Services/Medicare

Health care to prevent illness or detect illness at any early stage, when treatment is likely to work best (for example, preventative services include Pap tests, flu shots, and screening mammograms).

Preventive Services

Health care to prevent illness or detect illness at an early stage. Preventive services include Pap tests, flu shots, and screening mammograms.

*Primary Care Doctor/Medicare

Your primary care doctor is the doctor you see first for most health problems. He or she makes sure you get the care you need to keep you healthy. He or she also may talk with other doctors and health care providers about your care and refer you to them. In many Medicare Advantage Plans, you must see your primary care doctor before you see any other health care provider.

Primary Care/Managed Care

As a means to control health care delivery, managed care systems emphasize the initial or primary care level at which a patient first seeks treatment. This initial contact is with a primary care physician – a general practitioner or internist – who arranges routine health care needs. Care requiring more specialized knowledge or skill is referred to a specialist by the primary care practitioner.

Primary Care Case Management/Medicaid

One type of arrangement under which Medicaid provides managed care is called primary care case management (PCCM). Under PCCM arrangements, a primary care physician coordinates and approves an array of services in addition to providing primary care services. In most PCCM systems, physicians are paid case management fees in addition to their regular fee-for-service payments for the primary care services they provide. In a few PCCM systems, physicians are placed at financial risk for some services, usually ambulatory care. They may determine the level of their Medicaid caseloads, up to a state-specified limit.

Primary Care Physician
See also *Gatekeeper*.

The physician in a managed care system whom a patient consults first when a health problem occurs and on whom the patient relies for advice, referrals and on-going care.

Primary Caregiver
See also *Caregiver*.

The individual who has the main responsibility for helping an older person and who is usually the one making decisions and organizing care and services.

Primary Insurance Amount (PIA)/Social Security

The PIA is the figure from which almost all Social Security cash benefit amounts are derived, including monthly benefits for workers, their dependents and their survivors. The PIA is based on a formula which takes various percentages at successive earning levels called bend points of an individual's taxable earnings averaged over his/her working lifetime. Numerous PIA formulas may apply depending on the year of birth and earnings record of the individual. The most common formula today is based on the average indexed monthly earnings (AIME). Up to the first bend point, Social Security replaces ninety (90%) percent of AIME. Between the first and second bend points, Social Security replaces thirty-two (32%) percent of AIME.

Above the second bend point, Social Security replaces fifteen (15%) percent of the AIME. The PIA is then the sum of these three (3) calculations. The mentioned percentages are termed replacement rates and specify the proportion of a worker's earnings prior to retirement that is replaced by the Social Security pension benefits he/she receives.

Primary Payer/Medicare

If an employee or an individual is covered by a health plan, then that plan must be the primary payer. Medicare is the secondary payer for these individuals and will not pay for items of care covered by another other health plan.

Principal

When an individual creates a trust during his/her life or by will, the assets that are placed in the trust are known as principal or corpus of the trust.

Prior Hospitalization/LTCI

A requirement, now forbidden by several states and largely absent from newer policies, that a person be discharged from a hospital shortly before receiving long-term care that is covered by the policy. To be considered qualified for Federal income tax benefits, policies issued after January 1, 1997 may not have a prior hospitalization requirement.

Prior Hospitalization/Medicare

Before Medicare will provide coverage in a skilled nursing facility, the beneficiary must have been first hospitalized at least three (3) consecutive days, not counting the day of discharge, before entering the nursing facility. However, in the case of home health care services covered by Medicare Part B, prior hospitalization is not a prerequisite for coverage of such services.

Private Annuity

A person may transfer property to another individual or organization in return for the transferee's promise to make annual payments to the transferor for a term of years or for his/her life. This plan is known as a private annuity.

*Private Contract/Medicare

A "private contract" is a written agreement between you and a doctor or other health care provider who has decided not to provide services to anyone through Medicare. The private contract only applies to the services provided by the doctor or other provider who asked you to sign it. You don't have to sign a private contract. You can always go to another provider who gives services through Medicare. If you sign a private contract with your doctor or other provider, the following rules apply:

Medicare won't pay any amount for the services you get from this doctor or provider.

You will have to pay the full amount of whatever this provider charges you for the services you get.

If you have a Medigap (Medicare Supplement Insurance) policy, it won't pay anything for the services you get. Call your Medigap insurance company before you get the service if you have questions.

Your provider must tell you if Medicare would pay for the service if you got it from another provider who accepts Medicare.

Your provider must tell you if he or she has been excluded from Medicare.

Private Contract/Medicare
See *Medicare/Private Contracts.*

Private Duty Nursing

Shift or private duty nursing obtained by a patient on a private-paying basis provides nursing in a patient's home or hospital facility. These services, in the limited instances when provided by the government, are most commonly funded by Medicaid under either the private duty nursing option or through Medicaid waivers available to states by application to CMS. Skilled nursing, other than private duty, may be covered by Medicare as part of home health care services, subject to the limitation that in duration it is part-time or intermittent.

*Private-Fee-For-Service (PFFS) Plans/Medicare Advantage

PFFS Plans aren't the same as Original Medicare or Medigap. The plan decides how much you pay for services. Some PFFS Plans contract with a network of providers who agree to always treat you even if you've never seen them before. If you join a PFFS Plan that has a network, you may pay more if you choose an out-of-network doctor, hospital or other provider.

Out-of-network doctors, hospitals, and other providers may decide not to treat you even if you've seen them before. In an emergency, doctors, hospitals, and other providers must treat you.

In some cases you can receive your health care from any doctor or hospital. You can go to any Medicare-approved doctor or hospital that accepts the plan's payment terms and agrees to treat you. Not all providers will. If you join a PFFS Plan that has a network, you can also see any of the network providers who have agreed to always treat plan members.

Under certain circumstances, prescription drugs are covered. If your PFFS Plan doesn't offer drug coverage, you can join a Medicare Prescription Drug Plan (Part D) to get coverage.

You do not need to choose a primary care doctor nor do you need to get a referral to see a specialist.

Private Fee-For-Service Plan/Medicare Advantage (MA)
See also *Medicare Advantage/Private Fee-For-Service (PFFS) Plans.*

Beneficiaries entitled to Medicare Part A and enrolled in Part B are eligible to enroll in a MA private fee-for-service (PFFS) plan that serves the geographic area where they reside. Beneficiaries with end-stage renal disease (ESRD) are not eligible; however, beneficiaries who develop ESRD while enrolled in a plan may remain in it.

A PPFS plan is a plan that:

> reimburses hospitals, physicians and other providers at a rate determined by the plan on a fee-for-service basis without placing the providers at financial risk;

> does not vary its rates for such providers based on utilization of the PFFS plan by the providers;

> does not restrict the selection of providers by enrollees to only those who provide the services and agree to accept the terms and conditions of payment established by the plan;

> provides access to any Medicare-approved doctor or hospital that accepts the plan's payment; the plan rather than the Medicare program determines how much it will pay and what the beneficiary pays for the services he/she is rendered;

may provide supplemental benefits (i.e., benefits in addition to items and services available under Parts A and B) and coverage of additional services that the plan finds to be medically necessary; and unlike all other plans, except MSAs, may provide for payment by enrollees of an extra premium for Medicare basic benefits in addition to the regular Medicare premiums. Beneficiaries are liable for the full amount of any premium that the plan may charge.

The conditions set forth in the entry Medicare Advantage Plans (MAP)/Common Features, except where noted, apply to the Medicare Advantage PFFS plan.

Private Pension

See also *Cash balance pension plan; Defined benefit plan; Defined contribution plan.*

The law does not obligate employers to provide employees with a pension plan. When companies do maintain pension plans, there are basically two (2) kinds: defined contribution plans and defined benefit plans. Plans that satisfy the requirements of the Internal Revenue Code are referred to as qualified plans. Eligibility to participate in a pension plan may depend on a variety of factors such as a minimum age or a minimum number of years of employment with the plan sponsor.

Depending on the terms of the plan, pension participants usually have a right to retain some portion of their benefits when they terminate employment with the plan sponsor. This is called vesting and is generally determined by the length of an employee's service.

Several salient income tax regulations are pertinent to private pensions.

The employer's contributions are tax deductible by the employer within specified limits.

The compensation paid into the plan is deferred compensation, and taxation upon the employee is generally deferred until the employee draws benefits from the plan.

Should an employee withdraw pension benefits prior to age 59½ (premature withdrawal), the Internal Revenue Code imposes as ten- (10%) percent penalty excise tax. However if an employee's employment ends before he/she attains the age of 55, a tax penalty will not be imposed if: the employee receives distribution in a series of substantially equal payments over his/her life or life expectancy; of if an employee rolls over the benefit distribution into an IRA or into a new employer's qualified plan. An employee who separates from his employer after age 55 is not subject to a penalty tax upon benefits received.

Pension distributions under qualified plans (other than distributions to five- (5%) percent employer-employee owners) must be made by April 1 of the year after a participant attains the age of 70½ but, if a participant continues working, may be delayed, at the employer's option, until the participant's actual retirement.

To project a surviving spouse of an employee, pension plans for married participants commonly provide for joint and survivor annuity payments; that is, an annuity for the life of the participant with a survivor annuity for the life of a spouse. Should a married employee decide on a payment other than that of a joint survivor annuity, the spouse must express his/her written consent. Customarily periodic payments will continue until both the worker and the worker's spouse have died, subject to a reduction in the amount of each payment after the first death.

(continued on next page)

PROGRAM FOR ALL-INCLUSIVE CARE FOR THE ELDERLY (PACE)

INTRODUCTION

*Programs of All-Inclusive Care for the Elderly (PACE)/Medicare

PACE is a Medicare and Medicaid program offered in many states that allows people who otherwise need a nursing home–level of care to remain in the community.

To qualify for PACE, you must meet the following conditions:

> *You're 55 or older.*

> *You live in the service area of a PACE organization.*

> *You're certified by your state as needing a nursing home-level of care.*

> *At the time you join, you're able to live safely in the community with the help of PACE services.*

PACE provides coverage for prescription drugs, doctor visits, transportation, home care, check-ups, hospital visits, and even nursing home stays whenever necessary. If you have Medicare, Medicare pays for all Medicare-covered services. If you have Medicare and Medicaid, you will either have small monthly payments or pay nothing for the long-term care portion of the PACE benefit. If you have Medicare but not Medicaid, you will be charged a monthly premium to cover the long-term care portion of the PACE benefit and a premium for Medicare Part D drugs. However, in PACE there is never a deductible or copayment for any drug, service, or care approved by the PACE team of health care professionals.

PACE combines medical, social, and long-term care services for frail elderly people who live in and get health care in the community. PACE programs provide all medically-necessary services, including prescription drugs. PACE is a joint Medicare and Medicaid program that may be available in states that have chosen it as an optional Medicaid benefit. PACE might be a better choice instead of getting care through a nursing home. PACE is available only in states that have chosen to offer it under Medicaid. The qualifications for PACE vary from state to state. A call to a state Medical Assistance (Medicaid) office will inform one who is eligible and if a PACE site is nearby, or you can also visit http://www.cms.hhs. gov/pace/pacesite.asp on the web for PACE locations and telephone numbers.

Based on a model created by On Lok Senior Services in San Francisco, this program began as a Medicare and Medicaid demonstration project initially tested at ten (10) sites. The Balanced Budget Act of 1997 expanded PACE to become an option open to all states. PACE targets frail elderly persons living at home who are eligible for nursing home care. The program integrates health and long-term care services in an adult day care setting and uses a multidisciplinary case management team of providers, including physicians, nurses, social workers, nutritionists, occupational and speech therapists, and health and transportation personnel. PACE participants are required to attend an adult day care center regularly.

Unlike the Social Health Maintenance Organization project, PACE providers receive most of their funding from Medicaid. The funding is allocated according to a fixed monthly capitated fee for each participant based on the frailty of enrollees. The project serves to link acute care under Medicare and long-term care under Medicaid.

The Balanced Budget Act of 1997 established PACE as a state option to furnish comprehensive health care to persons who are enrolled with an organization that has contracted to operate the PACE program, who are eligible for Medicaid, and who receive Medicaid solely through the PACE program. The salient characteristics of PACE offered as a state option are set forth below.

I. PROVIDERS.

PACE providers may be public or private not-for-profit entities. During the three- (3) year period beginning in August 5, 1997, the Secretary of HHS was required to give priority to entities operating a PACE demonstration waiver program, and then to entities that have applied to operate a program as of May 1, 1997. The number of PACE program agreements that may be effective on August 5 of each year is limited.

II. ELIGIBILITY.

Persons eligible for PACE must be 55 years of age or older; require nursing facility level of care that would be covered under a state's Medicaid program; reside in the service area of the PACE program; and meet such other eligibility conditions as may be imposed under the PACE program agreement. Eligible individuals include both Medicare and Medicaid beneficiaries. Medicare participants not enrolled in the PACE program through Medicaid must pay premiums equal to Medicare capitation. PACE enrollees will be reevaluated annually to determine if they continue to need nursing facility level of care.

III. SERVICES.

Under a PACE agreement, a provider at a minimum must provide eligible persons all care and services covered under Medicare and Medicaid. The services must be provided without any limitation or condition as to amount, duration and scope and without application of deductibles, copayment, coinsurance or other cost sharing that would otherwise apply under Medicare or Medicaid. The services must be provided twenty-four (24) hours per day, every day of the year through a comprehensive multi-disciplinary health and social services delivery system which integrates acute and long-term services.

IV. PRIMARY CARE PHYSICIANS.

Primary medical care for a PACE enrollee must be furnished by a primary care physician who serves as a gatekeeper for access to treatment by specialists. CMS may grant waivers of this requirement. A primary care physician, registered nurse, medical director, program director, other health professionals and a governing body to guide the operation must be part of the multi-disciplinary team.

V.   CAPITATION.

States will make a prospective monthly capitation payment for each enrollee in an amount specified in the PACE agreement. PACE agreements are for one year, but may be extended for additional contract years at the discretion of the Secretary of HHS.

(continued on next page)

*Prostate Screening (PSA Test)/Medicare

Medicare covers a digital rectal exam and Prostate Specific Antigen (PSA) test once every 12 months for men over 50 (coverage for this test begins the day after your 50th birthday). You pay nothing for the PSA test. You pay the doctor 20% of the Medicare-approved amount, and the Part B deductible applies for the doctor's visit. In a hospital outpatient setting, you also pay the hospital a copayment.

Prostate Cancer Screening/Medicare

Commencing January 1, 2000, Medicare Part B began to cover annual prostate cancer screening tests for men age 50 or older, including a digital rectal exam and prostate-specific antigen (PSA) blood test. The annual Part B deductible and the twenty- (20%) percent coinsurance requirement do not apply to the PSA test, but do apply to the digital rectal exam.

Prosthetic Devices/Medicare

Medicare Part B helps to pay for prosthetic devices, other than dental, needed to substitute for all or part of an internal body organ when furnished incidental to a physician's services or on his/her orders. These devices include Medicare-approved corrective lenses needed after a cataract operation, ostomy bags and certain related supplies and breast prostheses (including surgical brassiere) after a mastectomy. Medicare also helps pay for artificial limbs and eyes, trusses and for arm, leg, back and neck braces. Medicare does not pay for orthopedic shoes unless they are an integral part of leg braces and the cost is included in the charge for the braces.

Protected Resource Amount/Medicaid
See *Community spouse's resource allowance (CSRA)/Medicaid.*

Protective Services

Almost every state has created a wide variety of programs to help individuals who because of seriously impaired physical or mental functions, or a combination of both, need assistance in managing their financial and personal business affairs. These services are commonly known as protective services. An individual can voluntarily and privately arrange for such services, or in some instances a court can order them, to prevent abuse and exploitation. Services may be limited to a specified period or may run indefinitely. Examples of types of protective services include: representative payees, living wills and health proxies, guardianship and court created trusts under the Uniform Custodial Trust Act.

Provider/Medicare

The doctor, hospital, home health agency, hospice, skilled nursing facility, or therapist that delivers medical services.

Provider Network/Medicare Advantage

This network includes the providers with which a Medicare Advantage organization contracts or makes arrangements to furnish health care services to Medicare enrollees under a Medicare Advantage coordinated care or network medical savings account plan.

Provider-Sponsored Organization/Managed Care

A provider-sponsored organization (PSO) is a public or private entity that is established or organized under state law and operated by a health care provider or a group of affiliated health care providers such as hospitals and physicians. The PSO provides a substantial proportion of the required services under a contract directly through the provider or group of providers. A PSO directly enrolls individuals. No insurance carrier participates in the arrangement. Providers in a PSO share substantial financial risk in providing health services and have at least a majority stake in the entity.

Provider-sponsored Organization (PSO)/Medicare Advantage
See *Medicare Advantage (MA)/Provider-sponsored Organization (PSO)*.

Provisional Income/Social Security
See also *Modified adjusted gross income/Social Security*.

Provisional income is the sum of a taxpayer's modified adjusted gross income plus one-half of "net Social Security benefits received" during the year; the quoted phrase means the Social Security benefit payments after statutory reductions and adjustments have been made (amounts withheld to pay Medicare Part B provisions count as benefits received).

*Proxy (Health Care)/Medicare

A health care proxy (sometimes called a "durable power of attorney for health care") is used to name the person you wish to make health care decisions for you if you aren't able to make them yourself. Having a health care proxy is important because if you suddenly aren't able to make your own health care decisions, someone you trust will be able to make these decisions for you.

Proxy
See also *Advance directive; Durable power of attorney for health care.*

A person, commonly referred to as an agent or attorney-in-fact, legally authorized by another person to make decisions on his/her behalf, for example the power to vote on shares of stock.

Psychiatric Care/Medicare

Medicare Part A will help to pay up to one-hundred ninety (190) days of inpatient care in a participating psychiatric hospital. This is a lifetime benefit period. Psychiatric care provided in a general hospital is not subject to the one-hundred ninety- (190) day limit. Inpatient care in a participating psychiatric hospital is subject to the same terms, conditions, deductibles and copayments as those for other Medicare inpatient hospital care.

Under certain conditions, Medicare Part B helps to pay for partial hospitalization for mental health services furnished by hospital outpatient units and by qualified community mental health centers. Partial hospitalization means an ambulatory program of active care that lasts less than twenty-four (24) hours a day.

In addition, Medicare helps pay for services received for non-hospital (outpatient) treatment of mental illness. This includes services from doctors, comprehensive outpatient rehabilitation facilities, physician assistants, psychologists and clinical social workers. Services for non-hospital treatment of a mental illness are subject to a special payment rule. Once the annual deductible is met, Medicare Part B pays only forty (40%) percent of approved charges for these services, not the eighty (80%) percent customary for other services. (This coinsurance amount for outpatient treatment of mental illnesses will decrease until it reaches twenty (20%) percent in 2014.) Partial hospitalization services for treatment of mental illness are not subject to this special payment rule.

*Pulmonary Rehabilitation/Medicare

Medicare covers a comprehensive pulmonary rehabilitation program if you have moderate to very severe chronic obstructive pulmonary disease (COPD) and have a referral from the doctor treating your chronic respiratory disease. You pay the doctor 20% of the Medicare-approved amount if you get the service in a doctor's office. You also pay the hospital a copayment per session if you get the service in a hospital outpatient setting.

(continued on next page)

Q

QTIP Trust
See *Terminable interest property*.

Qualified Disabled and Working Individual/Medicaid/Medicare

The term refers to individuals with incomes below two-hundred (200%) percent of the Federal poverty level who are entitled to Medicare on the basis of disability, who are in a trial work period and are entitled to continue Medicare coverage while they are in that work period, whose resources do not exceed twice SSI resource levels ($4,000 for individuals and $6,000 for couples) and who are not otherwise eligible for Medicaid. State Medicaid programs must pay Medicare Part A premiums for these individuals. They are not entitled to other Medicaid services.

Qualified Independent Contractors/Medicare

CMS has established new entities called qualified independent contractors (QICs) to conduct a second level of administrative reviews (called reconsideration) of Part A claim denials made by fiscal intermediaries, carriers and QIOs. The QIC's participation in the claims appeal process, commencing January 1, 2006, constitutes a replacement of the fair hearing level of appeals of Part B claims.

Qualified Long-Term Care Insurance Contract
See *Long-term care insurance, tax status; Qualified long-term care services*.

The Health Insurance Portability and Accountability Act of 1996 extends certain tax advantages to a qualified long-term care insurance contract, sometimes informally called a tax-qualified policy. The law defines such a contract as a guaranteed renewable life insurance contract or as a rider to a life insurance contract, under which the only insurance protection provided is coverage of qualified long-term care services. A qualified LTCI contract does not pay or reimburse expenses reimbursable by Medicare, except for coinsurance or

All entries preceded by an asterisk (*) are culled or copied from the official U.S. government **Medicare** handbook (*Medicare & You 2011*).

deductible amounts. Nor may a qualified LTCI contract provide for a cash surrender value or other money that can be paid, pledged or borrowed. Further, certain consumer protection provisions set forth in the Long-term Care Services Model Regulations and Model Act of the National Association of Insurance Commissioners must be part of the contract.

To be qualified, LTCI contracts sold after January 1, 1997 must meet Federal standards explained above. Policies issued prior to this date that have met existing standards are considered qualified policies though they may not meet the Federal requirements.

Qualified Long-Term Care Services

See *Long-term care insurance, tax status*.

The Health Insurance Portability and Accountability Act of 1996 defines qualified long-term services as necessary diagnostic, preventive, therapeutic, curing, treating, mitigating and rehabilitative services and maintenance or personal care services which are required by a chronically ill individual and provided pursuant to a plan of care prescribed by a licensed health care provider. The phrase "maintenance or personal care services" means any care, the primary purpose of which is the provision of needed assistance with any of the disabilities as a result of which the individual is chronically ill, including severe cognitive impairment. The cost of qualified long-term services can be counted as a medical expense deduction for income tax purposes.

Qualified Medicare Beneficiary (QMB)/Medicare/Medicaid

Federal law requires state Medicaid programs to "buy-in" Medicare coverage for low-income Medicare beneficiaries generally unable to afford the required payments to obtain Medicare benefits. Their buy-in consists of payment of deductibles and coinsurance costs under Medicare Part A and Part B, and payment of premiums under Medicare Part B, and where necessary, under Part A. These beneficiaries are known as qualified Medicare beneficiaries. QMBs who are not dual eligibles are entitled only to the buy-in of their Medicare coverage.

QMBs must meet the following requirements:

They must be entitled to Part A hospitalization. If they otherwise would be eligible for QMB benefits but are not automatically eligible for Medicare

Part A, the state must pay their Part A premium to make them eligible for Part A.

They must meet federally mandated income and resource standards. Individuals must have income below one-hundred (100%) percent of the Federal poverty level. The resources of QMBs cannot exceed twice the SSI resource standard ($4,000 for an individual and $6,000 for a family of two).

QMBs are a subset of a group known as dual eligibles who are individuals who have low assets and are eligible for full coverage under both Medicare and Medicaid. They are exempt from mandatory enrollment in Medicaid managed care. Virtually all individuals receiving Medicaid or age 65 and over are entitled to Medicare Part B at least. A state's Medicaid program pays the Medicare Part B premiums for dual eligibles and should also pay Medicare Part A premiums for those not entitled to Part A by virtue of receiving Social Security retirement benefits. All dual eligibles are qualified Medicare beneficiaries (QMBs), but not all QMBs are dual eligibles.

Qualified Personal Residence Trust (QPRT)
See *Grantor retained interest trust (GRIT)*.

Qualified Plan/Pension or Benefit Plan

A pension or benefit plan conforming to requirements of the Internal Revenue Code. An employer's contributions to a qualified plan are tax deductible by employers within permitted limits and non-taxable to an employee until received.

Qualified Prescription Drug Coverage Plan/Medicare Part D Drug Coverage

A qualified prescription drug coverage plan must be either: (a) standard prescription drug coverage with access to negotiated prices; or (b) alternative prescription drug coverage which is at least actuarially equivalent. Both of these coverages are considered basic coverage; there is no supplemental coverage. Supplemental prescription drug coverage may be offered by plans that offer basic prescription drug coverage. The supplemental coverage offers reductions in cost-sharing or coverage of optional drugs.

Qualified Terminable Interest Property (QTIP)
See *Terminable interest property*.

Qualifying Criteria/Medicare

See also *Reasonable and necessary/Medicare; Qualifying skilled services/Medicare.*

A person must meet the following qualifying criteria in order to be eligible for Medicare home health care benefits:

The person must be eligible for Medicare. (The largest group of eligible persons is those aged 65 and over and entitled to receive Social Security retirement benefits).

The person must be homebound, need qualifying skilled services (i.e., skilled intermittent nursing care or skilled therapy) and must obtain the services from a Medicare-certified home health care agency, pursuant to a physician's plan of care.

The service must be reasonable and necessary for the patient's illness or injury.

Qualifying Interest for Life

See *Terminable interest property.*

Qualifying Skilled Services/Medicare

For purposes of home health care, there are three (3) basic qualifying skilled services: skilled nursing care, physical therapy and speech-language pathology. In addition, occupational therapy is considered a qualifying skilled service under certain conditions mentioned below. To be covered by Medicare for home health care, a beneficiary must need one of these skilled services.

To be covered by Medicare, skilled nursing services must be reasonable and necessary. The determination must be based solely upon the beneficiary's unique condition and needs, without regard to whether the injury or illness is acute, chronic or terminal.

Therapy services, to be covered by Medicare, also must be reasonable and necessary. To be considered such, the services must be a specific, safe and effective treatment for the beneficiary's condition. The required services must be sufficiently complex or the condition of the beneficiary such that the services can be performed only by a qualified therapist. There also must be an expectation that the beneficiary's condition will improve materially in a reasonably predictable period of time or that such services are necessary to establish a safe maintenance program. The services must relate directly and specifically to a treatment regimen established by a physician, after any needed consultation with the qualified therapist, and designed to treat the beneficiary's illness or injury. The therapy services cannot merely relate to activities for the general physical welfare of the beneficiary.

Occupational therapy services, as distinct from other therapy services, are qualified for coverage as a qualifying skilled service only if they are part of a plan that also includes intermittent skilled nursing care, physical therapy or speech-language pathology services. Thus, a patient who initially needs just occupational therapy will not qualify for Medicare-covered home health services. However, if the patient's eligibility for occupational therapy was already established by a prior need for skilled nursing care or physical/speech therapy, the patient will qualify for continued occupational therapy.

*Quality Improvement Organization (QIO)/Medicare

A group of practicing doctors and other health care experts paid by the Federal Government to check and improve the care given to people with Medicare.

With a fast appeal, an independent reviewer, called a Quality Improvement Organization (QIO), will decide if your services should continue. You must call your local QIO to request a fast appeal no later than the time shown on the notice you get from your provider. Use the telephone number for your local QIO listed on your notice.

Quality Improvement Organization/Medicare

Medicare independent review entities, consisting of groups of practicing physicians and other health care experts, participate (as private contractors for HHS) in the administration of the Medicare program. These entities are called Quality Improvement Organizations (QIO) (formerly known as Peer Review Organizations (PRO)). The QIO's functions consist of the following: (i) responsibility for making determinations regarding the necessity and reasonableness of health care provided by Medicare; (ii) reviewing of non-coverage notices issued by hospitals to Medicare beneficiaries changing coverage of their continued stay; (iii) evaluating the efficiency and economy of the health care services provided; (iv) ensuring that such services meet professional and accepted medical quality of care standards; and (v) reviewing the professional activities of prescription drug sponsors pursuant to contracts under Medicare Part D. In addition, the QIOs review complaints by beneficiaries relating to the quality of care in settings such as inpatient hospitals, hospital outpatient departments, hospital emergency rooms, skilled nursing facilities, home health agencies, private fee-for-service plans, and ambulatory sites. QIOs make initial determination in hospital cases, but do not issue payments; they authorize the appropriate contractor to issue payment.

Quarters of Coverage/Social Security
See also *Work credits/Social Security.*

Quarters of coverage are now called Social Security work credits, but the old terminology is still frequently used. A quarter of coverage was earned by earning a minimum amount in covered employment in a calendar quarter (three (3) months). The maximum annual number of quarters of coverage therefore was four (4). A worker can now earn up to four (4) Social Security work credits annually, but the four (4) credits can be earned in one calendar quarter. For every $780 in earnings, a worker earns one work credit.

(continued on next page)

R

Radiation Therapy/Medicare

Medicare Part B helps pay for radiation therapy with x-rays, radium and radioisotopes given under the supervision of a doctor.

Reasonable and Necessary/Medicare
See also *Exclusions/Medicare; Qualifying skilled services/Medicare.*

In addition to specifically excluding coverage of a number of services in several broad categories such as routine or preventive care, Medicare applies a general exclusion for the coverage of any service that is not reasonable or necessary for the diagnosis, treatment of illness or injury to improve the function of a malformed body member.

There are no judicial decisions interpreting this term. However, the legislative history and Medicare manuals recognize that reasonable and necessary care needs to be practical and individualized. CMS in turn has established many policies applying the general exclusion provision, frequently referred to as the "medical necessity" exclusion. Further, Medicare coverage decisions relating to this exclusion frequently are made on a case-by-case basis by Medicare carriers and intermediaries and by providers of health services which often consult with utilization review committees and professional review organizations.

In respect to home care, the determination of whether skilled nursing care or skilled therapy is required entails the need to determine whether the services are reasonable and necessary. In practice, the following are among general principles applied to these skilled services:

> **Skilled Nursing.** To be considered reasonable and necessary, these services must be provided by a registered nurse or licensed (vocational) nurse under the supervision of a registered nurse to assure safety and effectiveness. The

All entries preceded by an asterisk (*) are culled or copied from the official U.S. government **Medicare** handbook (*Medicare & You 2011*).

determination is based upon the patient's unique condition and individual needs. While not binding on Medicare, the physician's plan of care is given great weight.

Therapy Services. These services, among other things, must be provided with the expectation, based upon a physician's assessment of the patient's potential, that his/her condition will improve materially in a reasonable and generally predictable length of time or that the services are necessary for the establishment of a safe maintenance program.

Reasonable Charge/Medicare

See also F*ee schedule charge/Medicare; Lesser of cost or charge principle/Medicare.*

This term, formerly used as part of the phrase "reasonable, prevailing and customary charge," has been replaced by Medicare's fee schedule charge. The term continues to be used by Medicare, however, when applying the lesser of cost or charge principle.

Reconsideration Determination/Medicare

See also *Appeals/Medicare; Appeals/Medicare Advantage.*

This is a part of the appeals process from a Medicare determination. The applicant seeks reconsideration by the carrier or fiscal intermediary of its denial of his/her claim.

Recovery Against Personal Injury Award/Medicaid

Should a Medicaid recipient have an action pending for personal injuries, Medicaid may impose a lien upon an award or judgment, or upon a settlement, in order to recover Medicaid payments covering the injury.

Recovery of Costs/Medicaid

In certain instances explained below, Medicaid may recover the cost of the Medicaid-paid expenses for nursing home and certain other long-term care services received by the recipient.

Medicaid Recovery from Community Spouse. When a community spouse has excess resources over and above the community spouse's resource allowance and the community spouse refuses (spousal refusal) to turn over his/her resources available to meet the Medicaid recipient's needs, states may and are likely to seek recovery of costs expended on the Medicaid recipient's care.

Medicaid Recovery from Estate of Deceased Recipient. Federal law mandates that each state place into effect an estate recovery program which provides for recovery from a Medicaid recipient of medical assistance for him/her. Estate recovery can occur: (i) only after the death of the Medicaid recipient who received Medicaid care when age 55 or older in a medical institution (e.g., nursing home or at home waivered home and community-based services); and (ii) only if there is no surviving spouse, disabled children or children under age 21. The estate of a Medicaid recipient is sheltered from recovery, in whole or in part, if the recipient purchased a long-term care insurance policy under the Robert Wood Johnson program, referenced below.

The term estate refers to all real and personal property and other assets included within an individual's estate under state probate law. In connection with its recovery program, Medicaid permits states to use a broader definition of the term to include whether or not the asset is the subject of probate, any real or personal property and other assets in which an individual had an interest at the time of death such as an interest in jointly owned property. The term estate does not include special powers of appointment under trusts which are expressly stated not to be an asset conveyed to a survivor.

The amount of an annuity will be subject to estate recovery upon the death of the Medicaid recipient unless (i) there is a surviving spouse or disabled or minor child or (ii) the annuity is sheltered because of his/her participation in the Robert Wood Johnson program (see *Robert* Wood *Johnson Long-term Care Insurance Program/LTCI*).

*Referral/Medicare

A written order from your primary care doctor for you to see a specialist or to get certain medical services. In many Health Maintenance Organizations (HMOs), you need to get a referral before you can get medical care from anyone except your primary care doctor. If you don't get a referral first, the plan may not pay for the services.

Referral/Medicare

A written order from a primary care doctor for an individual to see a specialist or to obtain certain medical services. Health Maintenance Organizations (HMOs) usually require that an individual obtain a referral before he/she can obtain medical care from anyone except his/her primary care doctor.

Regional Plan/Medicare Advantage (MA)

A coordinated care plan structured as a preferred provider organization (PPO) that serves one or more entire regions. An MA regional plan must have a network of contracting providers that have agreed to a specific reimbursement for the plan's covered services and must pay for all covered services whether provided in or out of the network.

Registered Nurse (RN)

A nurse who has passed a state registration examination and is licensed to practice nursing. Duties may include nursing care of patients, patient assessment and operating medical equipment.

Registry

A list of professionals and paraprofessionals in a professional field. A registry screens people listed and handles related personnel and bookkeeping tasks. In the hiring of home health workers for example, professional caregivers or elderly persons have the option of dealing directly with a registry rather than a home health agency.

Rehabilitation Services/Medicaid

These services are Medicaid long-term care services which the states at their option may provide to individuals eligible for Medicaid to treat mental, physical, occupational and speech disabilities. States must pay for skilled rehabilitation service in a nursing facility.

Rehabilitation Services/Medicare

See also Occupational therapy, physical therapy and speech-language pathology, home care/Medicare; Outpatient occupational therapy, physical therapy and speech-language pathology/Medicare.

These services consist of the restoration of the functioning of a body part after injury or disease. Rehabilitation therapy services include physical, occupational or speech therapy or any combination of such services and treatment of mental disorders. These services may be provided in such settings as acute care hospitals, outpatient rehabilitation facilities, inpatient rehabilitation hospitals, skilled nursing facilities or a patient's home.

Rehabilitation Facility
See also *Rehabilitation hospital coverage/Medicare*.

A hospital or facility that provides health-related, social, and/or vocational services to disabled persons to help them attain maximum functional capacity.

Rehabilitation Hospital Coverage/Medicare

Medicare will cover rehabilitation hospitalization in a freestanding rehabilitation hospital or in a rehabilitation unit of an acute care hospital. Coverage is dependent upon satisfying certain requirements:

> The care must be reasonable and necessary and not be available in a skilled nursing facility or on an outpatient basis.

> The hospital must be a certified Medicare facility.

> A physician must certify that the patient needs impatient hospital rehabilitation.

Relative Value Unit/Medicare
See *Physician fee schedule/Medicare; Resource-based relative value scale (RBRVS)/Medicare*.

*Religious Non-medical Health Care Institution/Medicare

Medicare will only cover the non-medical, non-religious health care items and services (like room and board) in this type of facility for people who qualify for hospital or skilled nursing facility care, but for whom medical care isn't in agreement with their religious beliefs. Non-medical items and services like wound dressings or use of a simple walker during your stay don't require a doctor's order or prescription. Medicare doesn't cover the religious aspects of care.

Religious Fraternal Benefits Plan (RFBP)/Medicare Advantage

See also *Medicare Advantage/Religious Fraternal Plans.*

A RFBP plan is an entirely new type of coordinated care plan that may be offered under the Medicare Advantage program. An organization offering a Medicare Advantage RFBP plan must do more than merely pay health care claims on behalf of its beneficiaries. The plan must meet the definition of a coordinated care plan. As such, it must have a network of health professionals and meet the applicable access, availability, and service area and quality assurance requirements of a coordinated care plan. Unlike other coordinated care plans, a RFBP plan may be offered only to the members of the church, convention or affiliated group and must permit all members to enroll without regard to health status.

The religious fraternal benefit society offering a RFPP plan must:

Be as described under Section 501(c)(8) of the Internal Revenue Code and be exempt from taxation under Section 501(a) of that legislation;

Be affiliated with, carry out the tenets of and share a religious bond with a church, convention, association or churches or an affiliated group of churches;

Offer, in addition to the RFBP plan, at least the same level of health coverage to individuals not entitled to Medicare benefits, who are members of the church, convention or group; and

Not limit membership in the society due to the prospective members' health status.

As with other types of coordinated care plans, an entity offering a RFBP plan must be organized and licensed under state law as a risk-bearing entity eligible to offer health insurance or health benefits coverage in each state in which it offers a Medicare Advantage plan. The RFBP plan must meet all other licensing requirements of the state.

Remainderman

This is a person or other entity designated in a trust as the beneficiary entitled to the principal or corpus of the trust after the income-paying stage comes to an end, that is, after the income beneficiary of the trust has been paid in full in accordance with the terms of the trust.

Rental Assistance (Federal)

See also *Federal housing program for the elderly*.

A rental assistance program, often called Section 8 (referring to a part of the Housing and Development Act) or housing vouchers. The program is designed to help those who, because of low income, have trouble paying rent. In most cases, rental assistance enables the program participant to pay approximately thirty (30%) percent of household income for rent. The subsidy pays the landlord the remaining portion of the fair market rent.

Eligible households usually must have an income no higher than fifty (50%) percent of the median in the geographic area, adjusted for family size. Preference is given to families who occupy substandard housing, or involuntarily displaced or are paying over fifty (50%) percent of their income for rent.

Replacement Rate/Social Security

See *Primary insurance amount (PIA)/Social Security*.

Representative Payee

Under Federal laws a representative payee may act as a surrogate on behalf of an individual who is not capable of making cognitive decisions, for the purpose of receiving and handling cash benefit checks of a Social Security or Supplemental Security Income recipient. The legal authority of the surrogate is usually limited to merely managing the benefits received for the well-being of the original beneficiary. A representative payee can be a public agency, non-profit organization, bank or an individual.

The designation of a representative payee generally is a protective arrangement for incapacitated persons. It is less restrictive, simpler and less expensive than alternative protective arrangements such as guardianship or conservatorship and does not require a judicial finding of incompetency or incapacity. The arrangement can be terminated if the recipient regains cognitive ability to handle the government benefits to which he/she is entitled.

623

Reserve Period/Medicare

A hospital inpatient is entitled under Medicare Part A to only ninety (90) days full coverage per spell of illness, with the exception that the patient must pay for the first day. In addition, a patient is entitled to a lifetime reserve of sixty (60) days of hospital care. Thus, after the ninety (90) days of coverage, a patient may utilize his/her lifetime reserve in part or whole, that is from the ninety-first (91st) through the one-hundred fiftieth (150th) day of a hospital stay. Before the ninetieth (90th) day of the hospital stay, the hospital must be notified of a beneficiary's intention to use the reserve days. Anytime lifetime reserve days are used, Medicare will pay all eligible charges, but the patient is required to pay the daily coinsurance equal to one half of the paid deductible.

Residential Apartment
See *Independent living retirement community.*

Residential Care Home
See also *Assisted living facility.*

Residents in this non-medical residential facility cannot function independently but are not sick enough to qualify for nursing homes. Resident care homes provide a supervised living mode. They offer residents meals, shelter and personal care.

The facility may be defined institutionally in terms of beds rather than in terms of independent living units. These facilities are also known as adult homes and homes for the aged.

Residential Village
See *Independent living retirement community.*

Resident's Bill of Rights
See *Nursing home reform law.*

Resource-based Relative Value Scale (RBRVS)/Medicare
See also *Fee schedule charge/Medicare; Physician fee schedule/Medicare.*

An index that assigns weights to each medical service provided by physicians. The weights represent the relative amount to be paid for each service. To fix the fee for a service, the relative value for that service is multiplied by a dollar amount, known as the conversion factor. The RBRVS used in the development of the

Medicare physician fee schedule consists of three (3) components: physician services (i.e., time, skill and intensity involved in the services), practice expenses (i.e., all direct and indirect costs relating to these services) and malpractice expenses. For each of the components of the fee schedule there is a geographic practice cost index. This index reflects the relative costs of the three (3) components in an area compared to the national average for each component.

Since 1992 Medicare has paid physician services according to a fee schedule. Physician practice expenses, however, were charge-based, not resource-based, between 1992 and 1998. The Balanced Budget Act of 1997 mandated that over a four- (4) year transition period beginning in 1999 the relative value units for physician practice expenses should be instituted so that by 2002 all these expenses would be fully resource-based. Beginning in 2000, physician malpractice expenses shifted to a resource-based methodology. Thus, since 2002, the physician fee schedule is entirely resource-based.

Resource Utilization Group (RUG)/Medicaid
See *Nursing facility/Medicaid.*

Resources/Medicaid

This term is defined, generally, by reference to the SSI program and is one of the elements taken into account in determining eligibility. That program considers resources to be assets that can be liquidated to provide food, clothing or shelter. Resources can be bank accounts, certificates of deposit, securities, life insurance, houses and other real estate, businesses, cars, household furnishings and personal possessions. Certain resources, such as a house under most circumstances, a car and household possessions of limited value, a burial plot, a burial fund, life insurance of limited value and $2,000 in cash are exempt from consideration in the eligibility determination. A state Medicaid program may be more generous in its resource exemptions than SSI, but it cannot be less generous, unless it is in a 209(b) state.

Respite Care

This is a service that provides temporary care by a surrogate caregiver for an older person to allow the primary caregiver some short-term relief from day-to-day responsibilities. Respite care may be rendered in home as a part of an in-home program provided by respite agencies or home care agencies that have such programs, or as home visits by volunteers affiliated with a community program.

Respite care can also be provided out of the home, at hospitals (in-hospital beds), freestanding respite facilities, some board-and-care homes and nursing homes on a private pay basis for a limited period of time. A majority of states have some sort of respite program, funded in part by Medicaid, grants and/or private funds.

Respite Care/Medicare

One of the hospice care benefits covered by Medicare is respite care. Patients can be charged a copayment of about $5 per day, depending on the area of the country where they live. Inpatient respite care at an institution that is a participating provider of hospice services is limited to no more than five days per stay.

Retirement Age
See also *Social Security Program (Title XVI), section VI.B.*

The age at which an employee stops working. Also, the age at which retirement benefits are payable. The Age Discrimination in Employment Act provides a minimum mandatory retirement age of 70 years.

*Retiree Health Insurance/Medicare
If you have retiree coverage, Medicare pays first.

Retirement Benefit Entitlement/Social Security
See also *Social Security Program.*

A worker must be fully insured and at least age 62 to be eligible for retirement benefits. A spouse is eligible for retirement benefits if married to a retired worker and is at least age 62.

Retirement Community
See also *Independent living retirement community.*

The residents of a retirement community, also known as a retirement village, engage in independent living and share services and common areas with other residents in a housing environment. Residents generally have an equity interest in their own apartments or town houses. Their functional abilities may be somewhat limited, but they are basically healthy. Retirement communities often provide social club houses, including golf and other social amenities. Some offer a level of care such as personal care services resembling somewhat those of a continuing care retirement community.

Retirement Equity Act

A 1984 Federal statute (P.L. 98-397) intended to make pension payments fairer to the non-employed spouses of married workers.

Retirement Village

See *Retirement community; Independent living retirement community.*

Retroactive Disability Benefits/Social Security

See also *Disability benefit entitlement/Social Security.*

Disability benefits may be paid for up to twelve (12) months prior to the date of application provided the five- (5) month waiting period requirement is satisfied.

Reverse Mortgage

See also *Home equity conversion plans.*

A reverse equity mortgage allows senior citizens who are house rich and cash poor to obtain a loan based on the equity in their home. They retain title to their home as long as they continue to live there. According to the terms of most mortgages currently available, the loan, interest and other costs such as origination fees do not have to be paid back until the owner vacates the property through a move or death. Almost all reverse mortgages now provide a guarantee of lifetime tenancy. Most reverse mortgages are non-recourse loans which means the lender can look only to the value of the home for repayment.

Payments to a homeowner from a reverse mortgage can be in the form of a single lump sum of cash, regular monthly advances or a line of credit. New mortgage plans allow a combination of payment methods. The amount of the loan is seldom for the full value of the property; most lenders place minimum and maximum limits on the size of mortgages they are willing to establish. Loan periods can vary.

Some mortgages combine a reverse mortgage with an annuity, thereby guaranteeing individuals monthly income for their lifetime regardless of whether they continue to live in their homes or not. The monthly payments are considered annuity advances and thus partially taxable. For purposes of Medicaid eligibility, these payments may be counted as income.

Reverse mortgages are currently available in all states, except Texas, and the District of Columbia. Several different plans are available, some more widely than others. Plan features offered by the same lender can vary from state to state. The Home Equity Conversion Mortgage is federally insured through the U.S. Department of Housing and Urban Development and is the most widely available plan. In 1995 the Federal National Mortgage Association began a program called Home Keeper. The three (3) main private for-profit plans are offered by Transamerica HomeFirst, Freedom House Equity Partners, and Household Senior Services.

Review Period/Medigap

A person has thirty (30) days from the date he/she receives a policy to review it. If the person returns the policy within this time period, the company must fully refund the premium paid.

Revocable Living Trust

See *Trust, Medicaid eligibility rules*.

Rider

A separate, supplemental contract of insurance that is attached to an insurance policy. Sometimes there is a separate premium for the rider; sometimes it is furnished without additional charge. In the context of long-term insurance, home health benefits are sometimes furnished as riders to LTCI policies. Benefits for institutional and/or home care may be available under accelerated benefits riders to life insurance policies.

Right to Die

See also *Advance directive; Living will*.

The legal right of an individual to refuse lifesaving or life-sustaining (or alternatively, death-prolonging) procedures.

Rights of Enrollees/Medicare Part D Drug Coverage

Generally, enrollees have the right to have a grievance heard, the right to timely coverage determinations, reconsiderations, and expedited determinations and reconsiderations, and appeal to an independent review entity contracted by Medicare.

Risk HMO

See *Medicare HMO Overview; Medicare Risk Contract/Managed Care.*

Risk-sharing Contractor/Managed Care

See also *Health Maintenance Organization.*

An HMO, health care service contractor, or competitive medical plan that has entered into a risk-sharing contract with HCFA.

Robert Wood Johnson/LTCI

A.   Original Program Limited to Certain States.

Several states following pilot projects funded by grants from the Robert Wood Johnson Foundation have enacted long-term care insurance (LTCI) programs integrating the purchase by an individual of a qualified state long-term care insurance policy with his/her eligibility for Medicaid.   California, Connecticut, Indiana, Iowa and New York approved such plans in 1993. Federal law (COBRA 1993) previously banned extension of this type of program to other states. The Deficit Reduction Act of 2005 (DRA) has authorized the other states to adopt the program.

According to this plan linking LTCI with Medicaid eligibility rules, if and when private insurance benefits are exhausted, the assets of policyholders are not counted in whole (New York) or in part (the other specified states) in determining their Medicaid eligibility.   However, all of their income will be counted. Under the New York plan, a person who purchases a LTCI policy may establish his/her eligibility for Medicaid when the insurance benefits run out and thereby shelter an unlimited amount of assets from recovery by Medicaid. In the four other states, a purchase of an LTCI policy will shelter assets on a dollar-for-dollar basis. The individual purchaser is able to retain an amount of assets free from Medicaid recovery equal to the amount of LTCI purchased.

B.   Programs Extended to All States.

The DRA provides that states now may amend their Medicaid plans to include qualified long-term care partnership programs that disregard assets or resources equal to the amount of insurance benefit payments made to or on behalf of a beneficiary under a LTCI policy if the statutorily specified requirements are met regarding the insured and the policy. Under DRA, the programs in California, Connecticut, Indiana and New York are "grandfathered" into the new provisions so long as the Secretary of HHS determines that each state's consumer protection standards are no less stringent than the standards applicable as of December 31, 2005. Other states that wish to offer the program may amend their Medicaid statutes to provide for the program.

C. Requirements of a Qualified State Long-term Care Insurance Policy.

In order to qualify as a qualified state long-term care insurance partnership policy, the policy must satisfy seven (7) requirements:

> The insured must be a resident of the state at the time coverage first becomes effective;

> The policy must be a qualified LTCI policy as defined in Internal Revenue Code Section 702B(b);

> The policy must meet nine (9) specified sections of the Long-term Care Insurance Model Act and nineteen (19) specified sections of the Model Regulations of the National Association of Insurance Commissioners;

> The policy must provide for compound annual inflation protection for persons under age 61 as of the purchase date and must also provide some level of inflation protection for persons between the ages of 61 and 75. From age 76 on, inflation protection is optional;

> The state Medicaid agency must provide information and technical assistance to the state insurance department to make sure that agents selling LTCI receive training and demonstrate understanding of the partnership LTCI policies and how they relate to other private and public coverage of long-term care;

> The insurer must provide regular reports to the Secretary of HHS regarding the performance of the program; and

> The state may not impose requirements on partnership policies that are not imposed on all LTCI policies.

Rollover

A technique of avoiding taxation on a payment from a qualified pension plan or IRA by placing (i.e., rolling over) the payment into another qualified plan or IRA.

Roth IRA

See *Individual retirement account (IRA)*.

The Roth IRA, named after Senator Roth who created it under the Taxpayer Relief Act of 1997, is a non-deductible individual retirement account. Several significant differences exist between a traditional or deductible IRA and a Roth IRA:

- Eligibility to contribute to a Roth IRA is subject to special adjusted gross income limits. An individual whose modified adjusted gross income (MAGI) is $125,000 (2012) or more cannot contribute to a Roth IRA; and for couples who filed joint tax returns, the amount is $183,000 (2012).

  The amounts set forth above are the maximum amounts (full contribution) that a single or joint filing taxpayer (both MAGI top levels stated above) may contribute. Otherwise, MAGI below the stated top level MAGI contributions (i.e., partial contributions) run proportionately throughout a MAGI range as follows:

  > Single filers: Up to $110,000 (2012) (to qualify for a full contribution); $110,000 - $125,000 (to be eligible for a partial contribution)

  > Joint filers: Up to $173,000 (to qualify for a full contribution); $173,000 - $183,000 (to be eligible for a partial contribution)

- Contributions to a Roth IRA are not deductible.

- A Roth IRA can continue for the life of a participant. Roth IRA contributions may be made after the owner has attained the age of 70½; and

- Qualified distributions from a Roth IRA are not included in gross income (are tax free) or subject to the minimum distribution rules if the following conditions are met: (i) a distribution may not be made within five (5) years of the taxpayer's initial contribution year (so-called seasoning period); (ii) a justification must exist, such as the taxpayer reaching the age of 59.5 years of age; (iii) disability; or (iv) being a first-time home buyer using the qualified distribution (not to exceed $10,000) to finance home buying expenses. Rephrased: Withdrawals from a Roth IRA are tax exempt only if: the account has been in existence for at least five (5) years and the taxpayer is at least 59½, has died, or is disabled; or a distribution of no more than $10,000 is made to finance the first-time home buying expenses of a taxpayer, his/her spouse or children, grandchildren, or ancestors of a taxpayer or spouse.

As with a traditional IRA, the income earned on the assets of a Roth IRA is tax free prior to distribution.

The total contributions allowed per year to all IRAs is the lesser of the taxpayer's taxable compensation (which is not the same as adjusted gross income) and the initial amounts as seen below (this total may be split up between any number of traditional and Roth IRAs. In the case of a married couple, each spouse may contribute the amount listed):

	Age 49 and Below	Age 50 and Above
2008 – 2012	$5,000	$6,000

An individual may make a regular contribution to both a traditional IRA and a Roth IRA for a taxable year. In such a case, a maximum contribution limit for a Roth IRA is the lesser of an amount determined under the dollar limitation reduced by the amount contributed to a traditional IRA for the taxable year, or, the amount determined under the adjusted gross income limitation. Eligible taxpayers may contribute to both the Roth IRA and a deductible IRA by dividing their contribution between the two.

Routine Physical Examination/Medicare
See *Physical examination/Medicare*.

Rule of Deeming
See *Deeming/Medicaid*.

(continued on next page)

S

1634 States/Medicaid

These are states that have entered into an agreement with the Federal government under which eligibility for Medicaid is determined using the same process that determines eligibility for SSI. They are called 1634 states after the section of the Social Security Act that authorizes the agreement. Since most states must cover SSI recipients in their Medicaid programs, the 1634 arrangement saves the individuals the added steps of pursuing a separate process in a separate agency and saves the states some of the cost of processing an additional application.

"Same as"/Medicare Part D Drug Coverage.

A term used to describe if another drug insurance program has the same as or better drug cost to the beneficiary than a Medicare prescription drug plan.

Sandwich Generation

A popular term to describe people, usually women, who have become primary caregivers for parents and/or other elderly relatives and are sandwiched between the caregiving responsibilities for the elderly and their own children.

Seat Lift Chair/Medicare
See also *Durable medical equipment/Medicare.*

This equipment is covered by Medicare.

*Second Surgical Opinions/Medicare

Covered in some cases for surgery that isn't an emergency. In some cases, Medicare covers third surgical opinions. You pay 20% of the Medicare approved amount, and the Part B deductible applies.

All entries preceded by an asterisk (*) are culled or copied from the official U.S. government **Medicare** handbook (*Medicare & You 2011*).

Second Opinion/Medicare

Before any surgery, Medicare recommends an opinion from a second doctor to help clarify the patient's decision. Medicare will help pay for both a second and, if necessary, a third opinion, if the first and second opinions contradict each other.

Secondary Payer/Medicare

When another health insurance plan covers a person, Medicare, both Part A and Part B, considers that plan to be the primary payer of a beneficiary's claim. Thus for example, Medicare pays only the remaining part of medical benefits after the benefits of Blue Cross/Blue Shield plans have been paid to persons who are eligible under these plans.

Secretary of the United States Department of Health and Human Services

The Secretary advises the President on health, welfare, and income security plans, policies, and programs (including Medicare and Medicaid) of the Federal government. The Secretary directs department staff in carrying out the approved programs and activities of the department and promotes general public understanding of the department's goals, programs, and objectives. The Secretary administers these functions through the Office of the Secretary and its four (4) operating divisions.

Section 8 Rental Subsidy Program
See *Federal housing programs for the elderly; Rental assistance.*

Section 1115 Demonstration Waivers/Medicaid
See also *Section 1915 program waivers/Medicaid.*

States may obtain from CMS either of two types of waivers of Medicaid requirements in order to design programs without being subject to certain Federal requirements such as a beneficiary's freedom to choose his/her provider. These waivers are program waivers under Section 1915 of the Social Security Act and demonstration waivers granted under Section 1115 of the Social Security Act.

Section 1115(a) of the Social Security Act allows the Secretary of HHS to approve demonstration projects to promote the objectives of the Medicaid program. The authorized demonstrations are for a limited time, usually three (3) to five (5) years.

Several states have implemented health reform projects under this Medicaid demonstration authority, while a few others have received approval for demonstrations.

According to the Balanced Budget Act of 1997, during the six- (6) month period ending one year before a demonstration waiver expires, a state may request that a demonstration project initially approved be extended up to three (3) years. If the Secretary of HHS fails to respond to the state's request within six (6) months of a waiver's expiration date, the request is automatically granted.

Section 1915 Program Waivers/Medicaid

See also *Section 1115 demonstration waivers/Medicaid; Medicaid mandatory managed care.*

Waivers under section 1915 of the Social Security Act permit states to mandate enrollment in managed care and develop home-based and community-based care programs.

Under Section 1915(b) of the Social Security Act, CMS can waive certain Federal requirements (e.g., freedom of choice, uniform statewide operation, and comparability of benefits) to allow states to implement alternative health delivery systems or provider payment arrangements. To receive approval, a state must demonstrate that the program will be cost effective and that access to quality care will not be impaired. These waivers are granted for two (2) years and can be renewed.

Most states have 1915(b) waivers for managed care programs. Michigan, for example, has waivers that allow it, in selected counties, to limit Medicaid beneficiaries' choice of providers to primary care case management and HMOs.

The Balanced Budget Act of 1997 authorizes states, without the necessity of a 1915(b) waiver, to require individuals eligible for Medicaid medical assistance to enroll with a Medicaid managed care entity.

Section 202 Housing Program

See *Federal housing programs for the elderly.*

Section 209(b) States/Medicaid
See also *Medicaid, section I.B.2.*

Section 209(b) states have chosen a Medicaid option (commonly referred to as 209(b) option and named for the section of Federal Public Law 92-603 which authorized the option) that allows them to use more restrictive income, resources or disability definition standards than those used by the SSI program for their Medicaid populations eligible on the basis of age, blindness or disability. The option was included in Medicaid at the time the SSI program changed from being a fully Federal program to being a Federal-state program. Had states been required to serve all SSI-eligible individuals under their Medicaid programs, they might have been overwhelmed by the increase in the rolls and opted out of the program altogether. To avoid this, Congress included the above provision, allowing them to use less generous standards if they used those standards as of January 1, 1972. Today, 13 states exercise the Section 209(b) option. They are Connecticut, Hawaii, Illinois, Indiana, Minnesota, Nebraska, Missouri, New Hampshire, North Carolina, North Dakota, Ohio, Oklahoma and Virginia. These states must offer all SSI-related individuals with incomes above each state's income cut-off the chance to spend down any excess income.

Section 221(d) Housing Program
See *Federal housing programs for the elderly.*

Section 236 Housing Program
See *Federal housing programs for the elderly.*

Self-directed Pension Plan

A pension plan that gives an employee some measure of control over the way his/her pension account is invested.

Semi-private Room/Medicare

A hospital room with two (2) to four (4) beds is covered by Medicare Part A.

Senior Center
See *Older Americans Act.*

*Service Area/Medicare

A geographic area where a health insurance plan accepts members if it limits membership based on where people live. For plans that limit which doctors and hospitals you may use, it's also generally the area where you can get routine (non-emergency) services. The plan may disenroll you if you move out of the plan's service area where the plan is available. You must live in a plan's service area to join. Companies decide the service area, and plans may not be available everywhere.

Service Area

A geographic area where a health insurance plan accepts Medicare members if it limits membership based on where people live. For plans that limit which doctors and hospitals one may use, it is also generally the area where an individual can get routine (non-emergency) services. A health plan may disenroll an enrollee if he/she moves out of the plan's service area.

Settlor
See *Grantor of a trust.*

Shared Housing
See also *Alternative housing facilities.*

This type of housing offers two or more unrelated persons who are basically independent but who cannot or choose not to live alone the opportunity to share living quarters. Often, public or private community agencies own or operate houses or large apartments that house persons who have their own sleeping quarters, but share the rest of the rooms in the house or apartment.

Private individuals may also make rooms in their own homes available to other persons in return for rent, services or a combination or both. A distinct advantage of this housing type is that it enables homeowners to remain in their neighborhoods and promotes community and neighborhood stability.

While shared housing residents do not require residential or in-home health care, they do benefit by sharing household finances, cooking, shopping, housekeeping and other minimal support services which help them continue living independently.

There are two (2) distinct models of shared housing:

> The match-up model pairs a homeowner or apartment dweller with a home-seeker.

> The group-shared residence, sometimes called a group home, houses three (3) or more persons living together as an unrelated family, sharing the responsibilities of making household decisions and pitching in on chores to the best of their abilities.

*Shingles Vaccine/Medicare

Medicare drug plans must cover all commercially available vaccines (like the shingles vaccine) when medically necessary to prevent illness except for vaccines covered under Part B.

Shoes/Medicare

Medicare generally does not cover the cost of shoes except that it will help pay for therapeutic shoes and shoe inserts for patients with severe diabetic foot disease, subject to two (2) limitations and requirements. One pair of therapeutic shoes and inserts is covered per calendar year. (Shoe modification may be substituted for inserts.) Shoes and inserts must be prescribed by a podiatrist and furnished by a podiatrist, orthotist or prosthetist.

Shopping/Medicare
See also *Homemaker services*.

Not covered by Medicare.

Single Life Annuity
See *Annuity*.

Skilled Nursing Care

The term refers to a level of care which must be furnished by or under direct supervision of licensed nursing personnel and under the general direction of a physician in order to assure the safety of the patient and achieve the medically desired result. The service involves observation and assessment of the total needs of the patient, planning and management of a treatment plan, and rendering direct services to the patient. As long as a patient needs skilled nursing care, it makes no difference whether his/her condition is acute, chronic or terminal.

Examples of skilled nursing care are:

>Management and evaluation of the patient's care plan, as established by the patient's doctor;

>Intravenous injections;

>Tube feeding;

>Kidney dialysis;

>Colostomy care;

>The use of medical gases;

>Catheter care;

>Wound care;

>Observation and monitoring of a patient's unstable condition;

>Changing sterile dressings;

>Supervision of non-skilled personnel; and

>Teaching or training family members to provide care that is needed and that can be performed by them.

Expressly excluded from the term is any service that could be safely and effectively performed (or self-administered) by the average non-medical personnel without the direct supervision of a licensed nurse.

*Skilled Nursing Facility (SNF) Care/Medicare

Skilled nursing care and rehabilitation services provided on a continuous, daily basis, in a skilled nursing facility. Examples of skilled nursing facility care include physical therapy or intravenous injections that can only be given by a registered nurse or doctor. Medicare only pays for medically necessary skilled nursing facility care or home health care if you meet certain conditions.

Skilled Nursing Facility/Medicaid
See also *Nursing facility/Medicaid.*

Formerly, Medicaid distinguished between a skilled nursing facility and an intermediate care facility, with the former providing care primarily by or under the direct supervision of licensed nursing personnel. Since October 1990, Medicaid subsumed these two facilities under the term nursing facility. However, Medicaid does continue a separate category of intermediate care facility for the mentally retarded.

Skilled Nursing Facility/Medicare

A skilled nursing facility is specially staffed and equipped to provide intensive nursing and rehabilitative care to patients. Care is provided by registered and other licensed nursing or licensed therapists under the supervision of a doctor.

Medicare's requirement for admission to a skilled nursing facility, the benefits covered and the period of coverage are set forth below.

Requirements for Admission. Subject to certain limits, Medicare Part A will help pay for a patient's care in a Medicare-participating skilled nursing facility if a patient meets all of the following six (6) requirements:

> The patient's condition must require daily skilled nursing or skilled rehabilitation services which, as a practical matter, can only be provided in a skilled nursing facility.

> The patient must have been in a hospital at least three (3) days in a row (not counting the day of discharge) before admission to a participating skilled nursing facility.

> The patient must be admitted to the facility within a short time (generally thirty (30) days) after leaving the hospital.

> The patient's care in the skilled nursing facility must be for a condition that was treated in the hospital or for a condition that arose while receiving care in the skilled nursing facility for a condition which was treated in the hospital.

> A physician must certify that the patient needs and receives daily skilled nursing or skilled rehabilitation services.

The Medicare intermediary must not disapprove the patient's stay.

Covered Benefits. The covered Medicare services provided to a patient in a skilled nursing facility include: blood transfusions furnished by the facility; diagnostic or therapeutic services; drugs, biologicals, supplies (e.g., splints and casts), appliances (e.g., wheelchair) and equipment; meals; medical services provided by a resident or intern in training; medical social services; nursing care provided by or under the supervision of a registered nurse; physical, occupational or speech-language therapy; and a semi-private room with two to four beds.

Medicare will not provide a private nurse or attendant. Nor will Medicare provide personal care services or custodial care. The Medicare blood deductible (i.e., beneficiary must pay for the first three (3) pints) applies to skilled nursing facility care if it was not paid during the patient's prior hospital stay.

Period of Coverage. Inpatient skilled nursing care, known as "extended care services," is furnished to a patient in a skilled nursing facility up to one-hundred (100) days of each spell of illness, depending on the patient's condition. Medicare Part A will pay one-hundred (100%) percent of covered services for the first twenty (20) days. For each day from the 21st to the 100th day, the patient must pay a coinsurance amount of \$144.50 (2012) per day, with Medicare paying the balance.

Skilled Nursing Requirements/Medicare
See also *Intermittent care/Medicare; Part-time care/Medicare; Part-time or intermittent care/Medicare.*

For Medicare to cover skilled nursing services as a home health care service, such services must be: reasonable and necessary; provided and performed by a registered nurse or practical (vocational) nurse obtained through a certified home health agency; and, provided on an intermittent or part-time basis to a homebound patient under a doctor's plan of care.

Skilled Services/Medicare
See *Qualifying skilled services/Medicare.*

Snapshot Day/Medicaid
See *Snapshot rule/Medicaid.*

Snapshot Rule/Medicaid

See also *Community spouse's resource allowance (CSRA)/Medicaid.*

This colloquial term refers to the act of assessing, for purposes of Medicaid eligibility, the value of a couple's resources at the beginning of a period of institutionalization of one member of the couple. Because Medicaid allows the at-home spouse to keep a certain amount of resources, it is necessary to identify a point in time, the so-called "snapshot day," to measure the couple's resources so that the protected amount is not spent on nursing home care. Thus, a "snapshot" of the couple's resources is taken when one begins a nursing home stay expected to last thirty (30) days or more, regardless of whether an application for Medicaid is made at that time.

Social Health Maintenance Organization (SHMO)/Managed Care

These organizations are a variant of classic HMOs and very limited in number (see below). They supplement Medicare benefits available through a traditional HMO and in addition provide services which include care coordination, prescription drug benefits, chronic care benefits including short-term nursing home care, a full range of home and community based services such as homemaker, personal care services, adult day care, respite care, and medical transportation. Other services that may be provided include eyeglasses, hearing aids, and dental benefits. SHMO enrollees are locked in and may receive Medicare coverage only from that organization. Financing is through prepaid capitation funded jointly by Medicare and Medicaid (for Medicaid-eligible enrollees) and through member premiums and copayments. Capitation payments and premium amounts differ from SHMO to SHMO.

There are currently four SHMOs participating in Medicare, and each SHMO has eligibility criteria. These SHMO plans (their sponsor's name in parentheses) are located in Portland, Oregon (Kaiser Permanente); Long Beach, California (*SCAN*); Brooklyn, New York (Elderplan); and Las Vegas, Nevada (Health Plan of Nevada). The criteria for Elderplan in Brooklyn, New York are described as follows:

> The enrollee must be 65 years of age or older, must have Medicare Part A and Part B, must continue to pay the Part B premium and must live in Elderplan's service area. The enrollee cannot have end-stage renal disease. In order to receive chronic care benefits, the enrollee must meet state nursing home certifiable criteria.

Social Security Act

This Federal legislation was passed in 1935 and created the Old Age and Survivors Insurance program, commonly referred to as Social Security. Disability insurance was added in 1956. The Social Security Act and various amendments are responsible for a substantial part of the Federal safety net, including Aid to Families with Dependent Children, Medicare, Medicaid, SSI, unemployment insurance, public health services, maternal and child health services and social services block grants.

Social Security Administration
See also *Administration of Social Security program/Social Security*.

The Federal agency responsible for administering the Old Age, Survivors and Disability Insurance program and the Supplemental Security Income program.

Social Security Benefits
See *Social Security Program (Title II)*.

Social Security Eligibility
See also *Social Security Program (Title II); Insured status/Social Security*.

Social Security benefits are payable based on an individual's work record. An entire family may receive benefits (see *Dependent Benefits/Social Security*).

However, the benefits are based on the earnings record of one worker. That individual must have worked in employment that is covered by the Social Security system and must have worked long enough to have acquired insured status.

(continued on next page)

SOCIAL SECURITY PROGRAM (TITLE II)

INTRODUCTION

The several sections of the Social Security Act (Act) relevant to the elderly are:

> Title II Federal Old Age, Survivors, and Disability Insurance (OASDI) programs. This is the retirement and disability section of the Act.

> Title XVI Supplemental Security Income for the Aged, Blind and Disabled (SSI).

> Title XVIII Health Insurance for the Aged and Disabled (Medicare).

> Title XIX Medical Assistance Program (Medicaid).

> Title XX Block Grants to States for Social Services.

Social Security is the popular name for the Old Age, Survivors and Disability Insurance program authorized under Title II of the Social Security Act. Administered by the Social Security Administration (SSA), it is a social insurance program funded through employee and employer payroll taxes called Federal Insurance Contributions Act (FICA) taxes.

Social Security taxes are based on the amount of wages paid by the employer to the employee. The term wages generally refers to salary payments of cash. There is an annual wage limit on the amount of wages subject to a Social Security tax. The maximum limitation is $110,000 (2012); wages in excess of that amount are exempt from Social Security taxes. There is no hospital insurance (Medicare Part A) tax ceiling.

The taxes levied by the Act consist of both Old Age and Disability insurance taxes (called Social Security taxes), and the Hospital Insurance (Medicare Part A) taxes. Taxes imposed by the Act are paid at the same annual rate as percentage of wages by both the employer and the employee. The 2010 Social Security tax rate on wages was 7.65 percent (6.2 percent plus 1.45 percent for Medicare Part A hospital insurance) each for employer and employee, for a total rate of 15.3 percent.

Note: The Tax Relief, Unemployment Insurance Reauthorization, and Job Creation Act of 2010, reduced the Social Security payroll tax by 2% on the portion of the tax paid by the worked in 2011. This reduction was extended through the end of February 2012 by the Temporary Payroll Tax Cut Continuation Act of 2011 and under the Middle Class Tax Relief and Job Creation Act of 2012, the reduction was extended through December 2012.

Salient features of the Social Security program are set forth below.

I. SOCIAL SECURITY NUMBERS.

Every employee and every self-employed worker covered by the Act must have a Social Security number from the SSA, which is used to maintain the individual's earnings record. Earnings credited to an individual are one of the factors used to determine whether the worker is insured under the Social Security system. Earnings are also a factor in determining the amount of benefits payable to the worker and/or his or her dependents or survivors based on the worker's retirement, disability, or death.

Applications for a Social Security number must be submitted on Form SS-5, which may be obtained at the Social Security Administration's website, www.ssa.gov/online/ss-5.pdf., at any local Social Security office, U.S. Postal Service offices (except the main office in cities served by a Social Security office), offices of the district director of the Internal Revenue Service, any U.S. Foreign Service post, or U.S. military posts outside the United States. Parents may apply for a Social Security number for their baby when they apply for the baby's birth certificate. Parents may apply for a Social Security number for their baby when they apply for a birth certificate. The state that issues birth certificates will share the information with SSA.

II.   CRITERIA TO OBTAIN BENEFITS.

An individual must fulfill the following requirements during his or her working life to receive benefits:

the individual must have been an employee or have been self-employed;

the individual's job must be "covered employment;"

the individual must pay Social Security taxes on wages received or net earnings from self-employment;

the individual must accumulate sufficient work credits (sometimes called quarters of coverage), based on earned income, to meet the requirements for insured status necessary for a particular benefit; and,

the individual must attain a prescribed age.

- Workers, spouses, and divorced spouses can receive early retirement benefits beginning at age 62. Surviving spouses and divorced spouses are eligible to receive benefits beginning at age 60, or age 50 if disabled. Benefits for early retirees, including disabled widows or widowers, are subject to early retirement reductions.

- Retirement benefits are reduced a fraction of a percent for each month that benefits are paid prior to the month in which the retiree reaches full retirement age. Because full retirement age is increasing, these reductions increase along with the increase in full retirement age. Early retirement reductions vary for workers, spouses, widows and widowers.

- The normal retirement age is 65 years of age for workers and spouses born in 1938 or before. Since December 31, 1999, the normal retirement age has been gradually increasing until it reaches age 67 years of age for those born in 1960 or later.

III.   TYPES OF BENEFITS.

As discussed below (see section VII), there are three types of Social Security benefits under Title II of the Act: (i) retirement benefits and disability benefits paid to insured workers; (ii) dependents' benefits paid to qualified family members of retired or disabled workers; and (iii) survivor benefits paid to qualified surviving family members of a deceased worker, in a single lump-sum death benefit payable to the deceased worker's qualified spouse or child.

IV. CONSUMER PRICE INDEX ADJUSTMENT OF BENEFITS.

Monthly benefits increase automatically each January, based on increases, if any, in the Consumer Price Index from the previous year. (They are 3rd quarter to 3rd quarter calculations.)

V. PRIMARY INSURANCE AMOUNT (PIA).

The PIA is the figure from which plans of all Social Security basic benefits are derived. The PIA figure is based upon a formula consisting of statutorily prescribed percentages (see below), at successive earnings levels (see below), of a worker's average wage-indexed monthly earnings (AIME, see below), from covered employment averaged over a working lifetime (defined as thirty-five (35) years). The worker's monthly earnings are determined by (a) averaging the worker's thirty-five (35) highest earning years that have been indexed to wage growth and (b) dividing by the number of months in those years. Earning years are indexed by wage growth not inflation. (Only benefits are indexed to inflation.) The AIME of workers born before 1925, disabled workers, and workers who die before retirement is based on record (i.e., actual) years.

The successive earnings levels to which the statutory percentages apply, are referred to as bend points. Up to the first bend point, Social Security replaces ninety (90%) percent of AIME. Between the first and second bend points, Social Security replaces thirty-two (32%) percent of the worker's average indexed monthly earnings. Above the second bend point, Social Security replaces fifteen (15%) percent of AIME.

The term replacement rate describes the amount of Social Security benefits received in the first year of retirement as a percentage of the amount of earnings in the last year of employment. It is not used to calculate how much a Social Security check will be.

VI.   ELIGIBILITY.

A.   Insured Status.

Eligibility for all benefits, whether paid directly to a retired worker (age 62 or older), disabled worker, a worker's dependent or a worker's survivor, depends on whether the worker has earned the required number of work credits calendar (quarters of coverage) in covered employment, thereby entitling the worker to insured status. The amount of earnings that is required to earn a work credit or quarter of coverage is $1,180 (2012).

Covered employment generally consists of any type of work, including self-employment, part-time work and employment as a domestic worker, provided the employer has complied with reporting requirements. It includes the services of United States citizens whether rendered in or outside of the United States. It includes the services of aliens provided the services are performed in the United States, and provided the aliens are lawfully in the United States and legally permitted to perform such services in the United States.

There are three (3) basic types of insured status: fully insured, currently insured and disability insured. The requirements for insured status are defined below:

Fully Insured. A fully insured person generally is one who has worked ten (10) years or has forty (40) credits. This applies to persons born on January 2, 1929 or later; variations are prescribed for persons born on an earlier date.

Currently Insured. A currently insured person is a worker who has at least six (6) quarters of coverage during the thirteen (13) quarters ending with the quarter the worker died, became disabled or became entitled to Social Security retirement benefits.

Disability Insured. A worker has disability insured status if he/she has worked twenty (20) credits during a forty- (40) quarter period (five (5) of the last ten (10) years) in covered employment.) This general rule varies in the case of younger workers.

B.   Retirement Age.

Historically. Age 65 was the age entitling the worker to full retirement and benefits. However, since January 1, 2000, full retirement age has been gradually increasing toward age 67. Early retirement remains at age 62.

Increased Retirement Age. Under the 1983 amendments to the Social Security Act, the age at which a worker may receive his/her full benefit amount is gradually increasing to 67: (i) the retirement age was first increased by two (2) months per year for six (6) years, effective beginning with workers who reached age 62 in 2000, so that the full retirement age is set at age 66 for workers reaching age 62 in 2005; (ii) ten (10) years later, the retirement age is further raised, in two- (2) month increments over a six- (6) year period, so that the full retirement age is set at 67 for workers reaching age 62 in 2022 and beyond.

The following table shows how the full retirement age will gradually increase.

Years of attainment at age 62	Full Retirement Age
Years through 1999	65
2000	65+2 months
2001	65+4 months
2002	65+6 months
2003	65+8 months
2004	65+10 months
2005 through 2016..................	66
2017	66+2 months
2018	66+4 months
2019	66+6 months
2020	66+8 months
2021	66+10 months
2022 and beyond....................	67

Note: Individuals born on January 1 of any given year are deemed to have attained age 62 on the last day of the preceding year. Thus, while the 62nd birthday of an individual born January 1, 1955, will occur on January 1, 2017, because this person will have attained age 62 on December 31, 2016, the individual will reach full retirement at age 66.

Reduction and Increase of Worker's Retirement Benefits Based on Age. The Social Security benefits are available as follows:

When a fully insured worker attains full retirement age, he/she qualifies for full benefits, which is one-hundred (100%) percent of an amount referred to as the primary insurance amount (PIA).

An insured worker's Social Security benefits will be reduced by a prescribed percentage of the PIA for each month he/she retires before full retirement age. Payment to the worker is reduced 5/9 of one percent for each month of early retirement up to thirty-six (36) months and 5/12 of one percent for each additional period.

If the worker defers receiving benefits until after full retirement age, then his/her benefits are increased by prescribed percentages from full retirement age to age 70.

A fully insured individual between the ages of 62 and full retirement age is eligible for Social Security benefits even if he/she continues to work as long as his/her annual earnings do not exceed a prescribed maximum allowable amount, commonly referred to as the earnings limit. The earnings limit, is $14,640 ($1,220 per month) in 2012, and increases annually based on wage growth. Should such individuals continue to work, their Social Security benefits are reduced $1 for every $2 above the earnings limit, until full retirement age.

Individuals who reach full retirement age and who continue to work can earn any amount without a reduction in their Social Security benefits. However, in the year such beneficiary reaches full retirement age, there is an earnings limit for those months occurring within the calendar year in which full retirement age is attained; earnings above $38,880 (2012) that are earned in the month(s) before the full retirement age is attained will reduce Social Security benefits by $1 for every $3 earned.

VII.   BENEFITS OF BENEFICIARIES.

A.   Workers' Retirement and Disability Benefits.

Retirement Benefits. To receive retirement benefits, a worker must be age 62 or over and fully insured.

Disability Benefits. To qualify for disability benefits, the worker must be under full retirement age, disability insured and must meet the definition of disability. Disability is defined as the inability to do substantial gainful activity (i.e., earn more than $1,010 per month in 2012) as a result of any medically determined physical or mental impairment that has lasted or can be expected to last for a continuous period of not less than twelve (12) months or result in death.

The amount of the disability insurance benefit is equal to the insured individual's primary insurance amount, except in the relatively uncommon case where an actuarial reduction applies. The benefit is payable beginning with the first month after the waiting period in which he or she becomes entitled to benefits and ending with the month preceding whichever of the following months is the earliest: the month in which the individual dies, the month in which he or she attains full retirement age, or the third month following the month in which disability ceases. The term waiting period means the earliest period of five (5) consecutive calendar months throughout which the individual has been given disability status; however, the waiting period cannot begin more than seventeen (17) months before the month in which an application for disability insurance benefits is filed.

Note: Disability benefits convert to retirement benefits at full retirement age.

B.   Dependents' Benefits – Spouses, Divorced Spouses and Children of Retired and Disabled Workers.

Spousal benefits and children's benefits are available only if the worker upon whom those benefits depend has met the requirements specified in Section A above and is receiving those benefits.

Spousal benefits are available if the spouse is age 62, or is younger and caring for a child age 16 years or younger who is entitled to benefits.

The spousal benefits are reduced if old age benefits commence in a month prior to the month the beneficiary attains full retirement age. Payment is reduced by 25/36 of 1% times the number of months of early application up to thirty-six (36) months – a reduction of twenty-five (25%) percent – with an additional deduction of 5/12 of 1% for each additional month up to a total of forty-seven (47) months.

If a spouse is taking care of a child who is either under age 16 or disabled and receiving Social Security benefits, such spouse gets fifty (50%) percent of the worker's PIA benefits, regardless of the spouse's age.

Children's benefits are available if the child is under age 18 and unmarried, or over age 18, but disabled before he/she became 22 years old.

The amount of dependent's benefits is statutorily fixed as a percentage of the worker's primary insurance amount for each category of dependent. Subject to the family maximum, and to early retirement reductions, dependents are eligible to receive the percentages, of the worker's primary insurance amount, set forth below:

Spouse and/or divorced spouse 50%

Child (unmarried and under age of 18) of retired
or disabled worker 50%

Child (unmarried and under age of 18) of
deceased worker* 75%

Mother/father with child-in-care 75%

Widow, widower, surviving divorced spouse* 100%

Dependent parent of deceased worker* 82.5%

Two dependent parents of deceased
worker (each) 75%

*For more details, see section C below.

The family maximum varies according to a statutory formula which is based upon statutorily fixed percentages of a worker's primary insurance amount. The worker always receives the full benefit payable. If the family maximum is reached, each dependent receives a prorated share of the remainder. Benefits to a divorced spouse or to the surviving divorced spouse of a deceased worker are payable without regard to the family maximum and do not affect benefits to other eligible dependents.

C. Dependent(s) Benefits of Widow or Widower, Divorced Widow/er, Parent, Child of a Deceased Worker.

If a worker was fully insured at the time of death, survivor benefits are available to the following individuals:

Surviving spouse or surviving divorced spouse benefits. Benefits are available if the recipient is age 60 or over or age 50-59 and disabled. The test for disabled widow is more restrictive than that for a disabled worker.

Parent benefits. Benefits are available if the parent is a dependent of the deceased worker and is over age 62.

If a worker was currently or fully insured at the time of death, survivorship benefits are available to the following individuals:

Surviving spouse or surviving divorced spouse. If caring for a worker's child under age 16 or disabled prior to age 22, a surviving spouse or surviving divorced spouse, regardless of age, may receive benefits.

Child. A child under age 18 and unmarried or over 18 but disabled before the child became age 22.

Note: When benefits are available to the survivors of a deceased worker, the dependents are respectively entitled to the percentage of the workers PIA set forth in the table in section III.B above.

D. Lump-Sum Death Benefit for Surviving Spouse, Child.

When a deceased worker was fully or currently insured, the following survivors are entitled to a single lump-sum death payment (LSDP) of $255 in the following order:

Surviving spouse. The spouse must either be living with the worker at the time of his/her death or, if not living with the worker, be eligible to receive dependent benefits on the worker's account.

Child. If there is no spouse to whom the LSDP can be paid, a child of the deceased worker may claim the LSDP, but only if eligible for benefits on the worker's earnings record in the month of death.

VIII. APPLICATION FOR BENEFITS.

A. Retirement Benefit.

An application can be completed online at *www.SSA.gov* or filed at the claimant's local Social Security office. The application can be requested by phone, but is not considered filed until the SSA receives a completed and signed form.

An application may be filed before the claimant is actually eligible for payment of the benefit. Many claimants will file several months before they reach early retirement age (age 62) so that by the time they reach retirement age (i.e., 62 or older) the application will have been approved.

Claimants who attain full retirement age and older and who delay filing an application may be eligible for up to six (6) months of benefits prior to the date the application is filed, provided they meet all eligibility requirements prior to filing an application.

Claimants who reach full retirement age and delay filing for benefits will receive a percentage increase, called delayed retirement credit, added automatically from full retirement age until the person takes benefits or reaches age 70.

The full retirement age is 65 years of age for workers and spouses born in 1938 or before. The full retirement age gradually increases until it is 67 years of age for those born in 1960 or later.

B. Disability Benefits.

Disability applications can be done online by going to *http://www.socialsecurity.gov/applyfordisability* or can be made at one of SSA's local offices, or depending on the disability, a claims representative may be sent to the applicant's home. The application is more complicated than an application for retirement benefits. The applicant is required to submit essentially the same documents as Social Security requires in support of applications for benefits, plus medical and employment-related information. Eligibility depends on the inability of the worker to work due to a medical condition. This disability must last or be expected to last at least one year or result in death.

C. Lump-Sum Death Benefit.

Applications for the lump-sum death benefit generally must be filed within two (2) years after a worker's death unless an extension is granted for good cause or because the deceased was a service man who died overseas.

IX.   TAXATION OF BENEFITS.

Taxpayers must report all of their gross income, excepting certain express statutory exclusions. Prior to 1984, benefits paid under the Social Security program were excluded from gross income. Since 1984, a portion of these benefits has been included in gross income and therefore taxable every month. Social Security retirement benefits are taxed in part, any amounts withheld to pay Medicare Part B premiums are included in the amount received, plus any foreign earned income, exclusions for certain U.S. possession sources and tax-exempt interest (cumulatively the foregoing are called modified adjusted gross income or MAGI). The Social Security retirement benefits are included in MAGI only if the beneficiary's modified adjusted income plus one-half of the Social Security benefit received in a year exceeds the statutory base thresholds: $32,600 for married couples or $24,000 for single persons – the foregoing is called the base amount or first threshold; and $44,000 for married couples or $34,000 for single persons – the foregoing is called the adjusted base amount or a second threshold.

For taxpayers whose provisional income is within the first threshold, he/she is required to pay taxes up to fifty (50%) percent of Social Security benefits. For taxpayers whose provisional income is above the first threshold (i.e., within the second threshold), he/she is required to pay taxes up to eighty-five (85%) percent of the Social Security benefits.

A beneficiary is required to pay Federal income tax on up to fifty (50%) percent of Social Security benefits when his/her modified adjusted gross income plus one-half Social Security benefits (provisional income) received is within a first threshold of $32,000 for married couples or $25,000 for single persons. Taxpayers whose modified adjusted gross income plus one-half Social Security benefits received (provisional income) exceeds a second threshold of $44,000 for married couples or $34,000 for single persons may be taxed on up to eighty-five (85%) percent of benefits.

X.   APPEALS.

All claims and all questions relating to benefits are initially acted upon by the Social Security Administration, which makes an initial determination. (In the case of a disability claim, the initial determination is made after a determination as to disability by the State Disability Determinations Service Agency in accordance with rules and regulations of the SSA.) In each case the persons concerned are notified in writing of the decision. If they are dissatisfied with the SSA's findings, they may pursue the following process: (1) reconsideration by the SSA; (2) hearing before an administrative law judge (ALJ) or hearing examiner; (3) review by an appeals council; and then (4) a civil suit in the Federal courts. Requests for reconsideration must be filed within sixty (60) days after notice of the decision is received.

The SSA will provide video teleconferencing in the case of hearings before ALJs for claimants in remote locations.

Note: New Approach to Improve the Disability Determination Process

The Centers for Medicare and Medicaid Services (CMS) has presented a new approach to improve the disability determination process.

This new approach, set forth below, as proposed by CMS in its rules on July 21, 2005 and September 25, 2005, maintains some of the significant features of the existing disability determination process.

> The appropriate state agency (Agency) will continue to adjudicate claims for benefits.

> Administrative law judges will continue to conduct *de novo* hearings and issue decisions.

> Claimants will still be able to appeal the Agency's final decision to the Federal courts.

> A quick disability determination process will be established at the outset of the claims process to identity people who are clearly disabled.

> Medical and vocational expertise within a new Federal expert unit will be available to disability decision makers at all levels of the process, including the Agencies, reviewing officials, and administrative law judges.

Following the initial Agency determination, a Federal reviewing official will review the claim upon the claimant's request. The reviewing official is authorized to issue an allowance or to deny the claim. If the reviewing official does not allow the claim, he or she will be required to explain why the disability claim should be denied.

If requested by a claimant who is dissatisfied with the reviewing official's decision, an ALJ will conduct an administrative hearing. If the ALJ determines that a favorable decision should be made, the ALJ will explain the basis for disagreeing with the reviewing official's decision. (The appeals council stage of the current process will be eliminated.) A portion of ALJ decisions will be reviewed by a centralized quality control staff. If the administrative law judge's decision is not chosen to be reviewed by the centralized quality control staff, the decision of the administrative law judge would become the final Agency decision.

If the centralized quality control staff disagrees with an ALJ's decision, the disability claim will be referred to an oversight panel known as the decision review board consisting of two (2) ALJs and one administrative appeals judge. The oversight panel can affirm, modify, or reverse the ALJ's decision, making the panel's decision the final Agency decision.

The decision review board is an administrative review body comprising experienced adjudicators who can advance the objective of ensuring fair, consistent, and efficient decision making.

Cases will continue to be received by the appeals council while CMS implements the proposed rules. Once the proposed rules are fully implemented nationwide, this review function will be transferred to the decision review board.

CMS will not use these rules until it evaluates the public comments it receives on them, determines whether to issue them as final rules and issues final rules to the Federal Register. Until the effective date of any final rules, CMS will continue to use its current rules.

SOCIAL SERVICES BLOCK GRANTS

INTRODUCTION

Social services block grants from the Federal government primarily enable states to either directly provide, or contract with public and non-profit agencies to provide, social services to eligible individuals and families.

The most frequently provided services to older persons are home and community-based care such as adult day care, preparation and delivery of meals, protective services and access to service. Eligibility standards vary from state to state.

Block grants are also made under the Community Service Block Grant program, Community Mental Health Service Act, the rural Transit Assistance Act and the Mass Transportation Assistance Act.

The block grants are made by the Federal government to states under Title XX of the Social Security Act (42 U.S.C. Section 1397(a)). These grants are directed at a number of general goals including "preventing or reducing inappropriate institutional care by providing for community-based care, home-based care or other forms of less intensive care...." The grants enable states to provide these services and achieve the objectives of the grants either directly or by contract with public and non-profit agencies.

The social services block grants program is managed at the Federal level by the Secretary of HHS. The administration of the grants at the state level varies from state to state.

(continued on next page)

I.   ELIGIBILITY.

Basically, the statue and regulations leave eligibility and coverage standards to the state. The eligibility standards vary from state to state. One advantage of the block grant home care programs is that the caregivers can be family members. Other advantages are that the beneficiaries need not be homebound, nor meet Medicaid financial eligibility requirements, although priority will be given to needy applicants.

II.   SERVICES.

Services made possible by the social services block grants include: homemaker and chore services; adult day care; transportation services; family planning services; training and related services; employment services; information referral and counseling services; home-delivered meals; health support services; and protective and legal services.

Social welfare agencies and community organizations perform the services set forth below.

Homemaker services to assist in light house-cleaning or personal assistance, as well as services to assist with heavier chores in the house.

Community pharmacies and grocery stores may provide delivery, often free within the service area.

Community volunteers are often available to serve as home companions to run local errands, help with small household tasks, accompany the elderly person to a physician's office, etc.

Most communities offer transportation services at a reduced cost. In some communities door-to-door transportation services are provided such as vans or minibuses which accommodate wheelchairs, walkers and other devices.

Most communities have an emergency number to dial in time of crisis.

Some communities may offer volunteer or for-pay respite services which provide short-term, temporary care for an impaired person so as to relieve family members who provide daily care to their relative.

To reassure older persons living alone, many communities provide daily telephone contact, friendly visiting, the U.S. Postal Service's carrier alert program and emergency assistance program.

Some communities may have a telephone reassurance program. Calls are made to homebound people on a regular basis to check their safety and provide them with a personal contact. Usually this is a free service provided by religious or civic organizations or by hospitals and, sometimes, home health agency volunteers.

(continued on next page)

Social Worker/Home Care

A trained professional employed by a home health agency, hospital or a social service department who is available to help a person adjust to confinement at home. The social worker also counsels family members in caring for the patient. If community services or financial assistance are needed, the social worker can recommend sources for help.

Sonogram
See also *Ultrasonic diagnostic services*.

An image produced by ultrasonography; for example, a sonogram of a kidney.

*Special Enrollment Period/Medicare

If you didn't sign up for Part A and/or Part B (for which you pay monthly premiums) when you were first eligible because you're covered under a group health plan based on current employment, you can sign up for Part A and/or Part B as follows:

Any time that you or your spouse (or family member if you're disabled) are working, and you're covered by a group health plan through the employer or union based on that work.

During the 8-month period that begins the month after the employment ends or the group health plan coverage ends, whichever happens first.

Usually, you don't pay a late enrollment penalty if you sign up during a Special Enrollment Period. This Special Enrollment Period doesn't apply to people with End-Stage Renal Disease (ESRD). You may also qualify for a Special Enrollment Period if you're a volunteer serving in a foreign country.

If you have COBRA coverage or a retiree health plan, you don't have coverage based on current employment. You're not eligible for a special enrollment period when that coverage ends.

Special Enrollment Period/Medicare
See *Eligibility and Enrollment/Medicare, section II.2.*

Special Needs Individual/Medicare Advantage (MA)

See also *Institutionalized special needs individual/Medicare Advantage.*

A special needs individual is an MA-eligible individual who is institutionalized, is entitled to medical assistance under a state plan under Title XIX of the Social Security Act, or has a severe or disabling chronic condition and would benefit from enrollment in a special needs MA plan. Institutionalized means continuously residing or being expected to continuously reside for ninety (90) days or longer in a long-term care facility that is a skilled nursing facility (SNF), an intermediate care facility for the mentally retarded, or an inpatient psychiatric facility. CMS may also consider as institutionalized those individuals living in the community but requiring a level of care equivalent to that of those individuals living in these long-term facilities.

*Special Needs Plan (SNP)/Medicare

You generally must get your care and services from doctors or hospitals in the plan's network (except emergency care, out-of-area urgent care, or out-of-area dialysis). All SNPs must provide Medicare prescription drug coverage (Part D). You must choose a primary care doctor. In most cases a referral is necessary. However, certain services like yearly screening mammograms don't require a referral.

A plan must limit membership to the following groups: (1) people who live in certain institutions (like a nursing home) or who require nursing care at home, or (2) people who are eligible for both Medicare and Medicaid, or (3) people who have specific chronic or disabling conditions (like diabetes, ESRD, or HIV/AIDS). Plans may further limit membership.

Special Needs Trust

See *Supplemental needs trust.*

Specified Low-income Medicare Beneficiary (SLMB)/Medicare, Medicaid

An individual entitled to Medicare Part A benefits whose income is between one-hundred (100%) percent and one-hundred twenty (120%) percent of Federal poverty guidelines and whose non-exempt resources are $4,000 or less ($6,000 in the case of a couple) is eligible to have Medicaid pay his/her Medicare Part B premium.

This individual is referred to as a SLMB under the Qualified Medicare Beneficiary program. The program is managed by the state agency that provides medical assistance under Medicaid.

*Speech-language Pathology/Medicare

Evaluation and treatment given to regain and strengthen speech and language skills including cognitive and swallowing skills when your doctor certifies you need it. There may be limits on these services and exceptions to these limits. You pay 20% of the Medicare-approved amount, and the Part B deductible applies.

Speech-language Pathologist
See also *Occupational therapy, physical therapy and speech-language pathology, home care/Medicare.*

A speech-language pathologist assesses a patient's problem, designs a treatment program and provides therapy to help the patient regain or maintain speech or language skills. This professional holds a graduate degree and is certified by the American Speech-Language-Hearing Association.

Speech Therapist
See also *Speech-language pathologist.*

A person trained in the application and use of the techniques aimed at improving language and speech disorders.

Speech Therapy

See also Occupational therapy, physical therapy and speech-language pathology, home care/Medicare; Outpatient occupational therapy, physical therapy and speech-language pathology/Medicare.

The study, examination and treatment of defects and diseases of the voice, speech, and spoken and written language, as well as the use of appropriate substitution devices and treatment.

Spell of Illness/Medicare

Under Medicare Part A, a spell of illness begins on the first day a patient is admitted as an inpatient to a hospital or skilled nursing facility and extends until he/she has been out of the hospital or skilled nursing facility for sixty (60) consecutive days. For each spell of illness, Medicare Part A covers up to ninety (90) days of hospital care and up to one-hundred (100) days of care in a skilled nursing facility. Medicare deductibles are applicable to each new spell of illness so that, for example, two (2) spells of illness require payment of two (2) Medicare deductibles.

Spend Down/Medicaid

Spend down refers to the process of applying, when applicable, incurred medical expenses to reduce an individual's income to a state-prescribed level for purposes of becoming eligible for Medicaid. Some states also utilize a resource spend down, applying the same principle.

Spend down occurs in two (2) particular areas of Medicaid eligibility. First, individuals in 209(b) states whose income is higher than the state's prescribed financial levels have the right of spend down so as to become Medicaid-eligible. Second, persons eligible under a state's optional medically needy program can spend down to the state's prescribed levels of financial eligibility and thereby become Medicaid-eligible.

The process works roughly as follows:

> An individual not receiving cash assistance applies for Medicaid. If he/she does not fit into one of the groups designated as optional categorically needy, and if the state has a medically needy program or is a 209(b) state, the state must apply all incurred medical expenses to reduce the applicant's income when determining eligibility.
>
> If he/she still does not meet the medically needy income level (MNIL) – or in a 209(b) state, the income standard that the state uses – Medicaid will advise the individual of the amount he/she is over income, or, in some cases, over resource. This amount is called the spend down.
>
> The incurred medical expenses that the state must consider in determining both eligibility and subsequently the point when the spend down is met must include health insurance premiums and other cost-sharing, as well as other medical and remedial expenses recognized under state law, whether or not they are covered by the state's Medicaid plan.

The prospective period during which an applicant must spend down his/her income or resource is called the budget period. Once the individual has incurred medical expenses that reduce his/her income to the MNIL or the 209(b) standard, he/she is entitled to have Medicaid pay for covered care and services for the duration of the budget period.

The categorically needy and optional categorically groups have no right of spend down. In addition, some states restrict spend down, even though they have a medically needy program, have imposed income caps for qualification for Medicaid nursing coverage, and do not permit nursing home expenses to be calculated in determining spend down expenses. These states – Arizona, Arkansas, Florida, Iowa, Kansas, Louisiana (subject to the availability of state funds for individuals above the income cap), Oklahoma and Oregon plus Texas which does not cover the elderly – do not permit nursing home expenses to be counted in calculating spend down expenses.

Splint/Medicare

See *Medical supplies/Medicare*.

Split Dollar Life Insurance

An arrangement whereby the cost of paying for life insurance premiums for a shareholder or corporate employee is split between the company and the employee/shareholder. The shareholder/employee generally pays for the current insurance value. The corporation receives back its cost on payment or surrender of the policy. This form of arrangement eases the after-tax costs of the insurance to the employee/shareholder.

Sponsor/Medicare Part D Drug Coverage

A non-governmental entity approved by Medicare to offer a Part D prescription drug plan.

Sponsoring Agency/Home Care

A home health agency providing home health care services which are customarily under a physician's orders. The services include nursing care, physical therapy, speech and hearing therapy, occupational therapy, homemaker/home health aide services, nutrition counseling, social services, laboratory services, dental care, transportation services and medical equipment and supplies.

Spousal Impoverishment/Medicaid

See also *Minimum monthly maintenance needs allowance/Medicaid; Community spouse's resource allowance (CSRA)/Medicaid.*

This term is used somewhat colloquially to refer to the body of Medicaid law that is designed to prevent the impoverishment of at-home spouses (community spouses) of institutionalized Medicaid recipients needing long-term care. Its basic components are income and resource allowances set aside for the at-home spouse that can be paid out of the income and resources belonging to the Medicaid recipient before determining what he/she must pay to the nursing home or other long-term care provider.

Spousal Refusal/Medicaid

Spousal refusal occurs when the community spouse of a Medicaid applicant receiving long-term care refuses to turn over resources considered by the Medicaid agency as available to the Medicaid recipient to pay for his/her needs. As long as the state Medicaid agency has legal authority, either granted by the Medicaid applicant explicitly or inherent in state law, to seek repayment from the community spouse for the resources withheld, the Medicaid applicant cannot be denied eligibility.

However, when a community spouse has excess resources over and above the community spouse's resource allowance, states may and are likely to seek recovery of costs expended on the Medicaid recipient's care. In cases where Medicaid does pursue the community spouse for reimbursement of the institutionalized spouse's expenses, the Medicaid claim may be based upon a variety of theories including an implied contract running from the community spouse to Medicaid or an assignment of the spouse's statutory obligation to the state to support his/her spouse.

Spouse Benefits/Social Security

See *Social Security program; Dependent benefits/Social Security.*

Spray Trust

See also *Sprinkler trust.*

A trust in which the trustee has the discretion to distribute principal among several beneficiaries.

Springing Power of Attorney

A durable power of attorney that does not become effective until the person creating the power becomes incapacitated.

Sprinkler Trust

A trust in which the trustee has the discretion to distribute income among several beneficiaries.

SSI State/Medicaid

An SSI state is one that determines eligibility for Medicaid by using Supplemental Security Income (SSI) financial and citizenship criteria. In SSI states, persons who receive SSI benefits due to age, blindness or disability are automatically eligible for Medicaid and are mandatorily considered categorically eligible. This essentially entitles them to the best benefit package the state offers.

Staff Model/Managed Care
See *Health Maintenance Organization, section I.*

Standard Coverage/Medicare Part D Drug Coverage
See also *Alternative prescription drug coverage plan/Medicare Part D Drug Coverage.*

All Medicare beneficiaries have access to the basic standard drug benefit. The drug plans are allowed to provide limitations and restrictions on available drugs and other specifications, but the benefit offered must be at least equal to the standard benefit.

For the standard benefit in 2012, the individual must pay the following amounts in addition to a monthly premium (which varies depending on the plan chosen):

A yearly deductible of $320 (2012);

Twenty-five- (25%) percent co-pay of the yearly drug costs of $2,610 (2012), representing the costs between $320 and $2,930 (initial coverage limit) which amounts to $652.50. The plan pays the other seventy-five (75%) percent (plan cost share) which represents $1,957.50 (2012); and

Additional out-of-pocket expenses (called doughnut hole) of $3,727.50 (2012).

The aggregate of the foregoing deductible, co-pay, and additional out-of-pocket expenses totals $4,700 (2012).

Part D drug plans are not required to offer the standard drug benefit, but instead may offer alternative prescription drug coverage.

Start Date/Annuity

The first date on which a payment is received under an annuity.

State Pharmaceutical Assistance Program (SPAP)/Medicare Part D Drug Coverage

A state-operated program (other than Medicaid) that provides Medicare beneficiaries with financial assistance to purchase prescription drugs in selected states. SPAPs can provide assistance to enrollees with their premiums, deductibles, and coinsurance, under a Part D plan.

State Prescription Drug Plans/Medicare Part D Drug Coverage

States may offer prescription drug plans. The plans must coordinate benefits between Part D plans and state plans for premiums, coverage and payment for supplemental prescription drug benefits.

State Unit on Aging (SUA)
See also *Older Americans Act*.

Each state is mandated to have a state unit on aging which is part of state government. Together with the U.S. Administration on Aging, SUAs are part of the national aging network created by the Older Americans Act to plan and coordinate the work of local area agencies on aging and to help provide a wide range of home and community-based services.

State-wideness/Medicaid

This term reflects a Federal Medicaid requirement that any benefits offered by a state under the Medicaid program must be offered throughout the state. The state-wideness requirement can be explicitly waived under the programs that allow states to experiment with or otherwise permit different ways of providing services with advance approval of the Federal government.

Status Test/Medicaid
See *Medicaid, section II.A.*

Step-down Requirement
See also *Prior hospitalization/LTCI.*

Some insurance policies impose a step-down requirement denying benefit payments for a particular level of care unless care has already been received at a higher level – for example, no custodial care benefits are allowed unless skilled care has already been received, and no home care benefits are allowed unless institutional care has been received. Step-downs are banned by some states because they are contrary to the normal pattern of long-term care use. People usually get sicker and more dependent, not less. Step-downs also make it very difficult for policyholders to collect benefits.

Stop-loss Protection/Managed Care
See *Health Maintenance Organization.*

Subacute

Somewhat or moderately acute; between acute and chronic.

Subacute Care

This high level of skilled care consists of medical and skilled nursing services, such as I.V. therapy, wound care, intensive rehabilitation and enteral/parenteral feeding, and is provided to patients who are not in an acute phase of illness. It is generally short term – fifteen (15) to one-hundred (100) days and is covered by Medicare.

Subacute care is, generally speaking, a term defined by the industry rather than by governmental payers. Its usual definition, however, is very similar to that for skilled nursing services under Medicare.

To achieve greater profitability, skilled nursing facilities are increasingly converting parts of their facilities to what they term subacute care, and upgrading medical staff and equipment to support this higher level of care. Governmental payers do not, at this time, recognize subacute as a separate level of care.

Subsidized Apartments for the Elderly

See also *Federal housing programs for the elderly*.

Rental units, generally in the form of garden apartments or apartments in high-rise or mid-rise buildings. The units have been specially designed for, and are limited to, older persons who are at least 62 years old or to non-elderly handicapped individuals. Construction or rental costs are generally financed by the state or Federal government. Sponsors of this housing include non-profit or limited profit organizations or public housing authorities. There are income limitations for eligibility for this type of housing, and the rents are usually subsidized, with the amount of rent based upon the income of the household.

Summary Notice/Medicare

After the provider of Medicare-covered services such as a hospital, skilled nursing home or home health agency sends a claim to a fiscal intermediary or carrier, Medicare will forward to the Medicare beneficiary a Medicare Summary Notice (MSN) for Part A and/or Part B services. The MSN lists all the services or supplies that were billed to Medicare for a thirty- (30) day period – the amount the provider billed, and the amount paid by Medicare to the provider for unassigned claims. In addition, the MSN, among other things lists the Medicare-approved charges for the listed services and supplies; the amount that the beneficiary may be billed by the provider for deductibles and coinsurance; appeals information and a notice that the beneficiary may request an itemized statement. The MSN may or may not state the reasons to explain a denial; it may merely state that the care provided was not reasonable and necessary.

Supplemental Benefits/Medicare Advantage

These refer to health benefits normally not covered by Medicare, purchased at the option of the Medicare Advantage enrollee and paid for by him/her in the form of a premium or cost-sharing.

Supplemental Benefits/Medicare Part D Drug Coverage

Benefits which are additional to the basic, standard Part D prescription drug coverage including a reduced or eliminated deductible, reduced co-sharing percentage or co-pay, coverage for some or all of the doughnut hole, or a different formulary.

Supplemental Needs Trust

See also *Trust, Medicaid eligibility rules*.

This type of trust, also known as a special needs trust, is an irrevocable trust, sometimes funded by assets of a third party, created for a disabled beneficiary, and intended to supplement government benefits. The trust prohibits the trustee from spending trust assets in diminution of government benefits. The beneficiary has no power to control distributions.

For SSI and generally for Medicaid, disbursements from the trust are governed by SSI income principles. If payments are made for food, clothing or shelter, or if payments are made directly to the beneficiary, the amounts are counted as income for purposes of eligibility and will disqualify the beneficiary's Medicaid eligibility status. The more common arrangement with such trusts is for the trustee to make direct payments to vendors of services or goods that are not food, clothing or shelter; such payments are not considered income to the beneficiary.

In addition to these general rules, Medicaid has special rules governing the treatment of a trust established by and for a Medicaid recipient or his/her spouse during their lifetime. These rules are discussed under the entry *Trust, Medicaid eligibility rules*.

*Supplemental Policy (Medigap)/Medicare

Original Medicare pays for many, but not all, health care services and supplies. A Medigap policy, sold by private insurance companies, can help pay some of the health care costs ("gaps") that Original Medicare doesn't cover, like copayments, coinsurance, and deductibles. Some Medigap policies also offer coverage for services that Original Medicare doesn't cover, like medical care when you travel outside the U.S. If you have Original Medicare and you buy a Medigap policy, Medicare will pay its share of the Medicare-approved amount for covered health care costs. Then your Medigap policy pays its share. Medicare doesn't pay any of the premiums for a Medigap policy.

Every Medigap policy must follow federal and state laws designed to protect you, and it must be clearly identified as "Medicare Supplement Insurance." Medigap insurance companies can sell you only a "standardized" Medigap policy identified in most states by letters. All plans offer the same basic benefits but some offer additional benefits, so you can choose which one meets your needs. In Massachusetts, Minnesota and Wisconsin, Medigap policies are standardized in a different way.

Commencing June 1, 2010, the types of Medigap Plans that you can buy have changed:

There are two new Medigap Plans – Plans M and N.

Plans E, H, I, and J are no longer available to buy. If you bought Plan E, H, I, or J before June 1, 2010, you can keep that plan.

In some states, you may be able to buy another type of Medigap policy called Medicare SELECT (a Medigap policy that requires you to use specific hospitals and, in some cases, specific doctors to get full coverage). If you buy a Medicare SELECT policy, you also have rights to change your mind within 12 months and switch to a standard Medigap policy.

You must have Part A and Part B

You pay a monthly premium for your Medigap policy in addition to your monthly Part B premium.

If you're under 65, you won't have this open enrollment period until you turn 65, but state law might give you a right to buy a policy before then.

*If you have a Medigap policy and join a Medicare Advantage Plan (like an HMO or PPO), you may want to drop your Medigap policy. Your Medigap policy **can't** be used to pay your Medicare Advantage plan copayments, deductibles, and premiums. If you want to cancel your Medigap policy, contact your insurance company. If you drop your policy to join a Medicare Advantage plan, in most cases you won't be able to get it back.*

If you have a Medicare Advantage plan, it's illegal for anyone to sell you a Medigap policy unless you're switching back to Original Medicare. Contact your State Insurance Department if this happens to you.

If you join a Medicare Health Plan for the first time, and you aren't happy with the plan, you will have special rights to buy a Medigap policy if you return to Original Medicare within 12 months of joining.

If you had a Medigap policy before you joined, you may be able to get the same policy back if the company still sells it. If it isn't available, you can buy another Medigap policy.

The Medigap policy can no longer have prescription drug coverage even if you had it before, but you may be able to join a Medicare Prescription Drug Plan.

You can't have prescription drug coverage in both your Medigap policy and a Medicare drug plan.

If you have a Medigap policy and join a Medicare Advantage plan (like an HMO or PPO), you will probably want to drop your Medigap policy. You can't use it to pay for any expenses (copayments, deductibles and premiums) you have under a Medicare Advantage plan. If you drop your Medigap policy, you may not be able to get it back.

*Supplemental Security Income (SSI)

If you have limited income and resources, you might qualify for help to pay for some health care and prescription drug costs.

SSI is a cash benefit paid by Social Security to people with limited income and resources who are disabled, blind, or 65 or older. SSI benefits help people meet basic needs for food, clothing, and shelter.

People who live in Puerto Rico, the Virgin Islands, Guam or American Samoa can't get SSI.

(continued on next page)

SUPPLEMENTAL SECURITY INCOME

INTRODUCTION

The Supplemental Security Income (SSI) program (Title XVI of the Social Security Act) was enacted in 1972 by Congress and commenced in 1974. Like the Social Security program, the SSI program is administered by the Social Security Administration. Unlike Social Security, SSI is a means-tested program, and eligibility is (among other criteria) conditioned on a person's limited income and resources, each of which may not exceed prescribed limits. Certain items, though considered income and resources by definition, are statutorily excluded, and do not constitute countable income and resources. One of the requirements to receive SSI is that the individual's income must be below certain limits. These limits may vary based on the state the individual lives in, the number of people living in the residence, and the type of income. The resource limit is $2,000 for an individual with no spouse, and $3,000 for a married couple. The purpose of the program is to provide benefits based upon need to individuals who are aged, blind or disabled. The program replaced previously existing federally supported welfare programs for individuals who were aged, blind, or disabled.

SSI benefits (Federal basic benefit) come from the U.S. Treasury and the state. In many states the two (2) amounts are combined into a single monthly check. The Federal basic benefit is paid, based on certain factors such as: whether the SSI claimant is single, or has an eligible spouse (i.e., who is also eligible for SSI benefits). The benefits vary with the claimant's living arrangements (e.g., living alone, living in the household of another). The claimant's monthly benefit is determined by deducting the claimant's countable income (i.e., income counted, after exclusions from income, in determining SSI eligibility), from the monthly Federal basic benefit.

(continued on next page)

I.   ELIGIBILITY – APPLICATION FOR SSI BENEFITS.

A.   Eligibility.

To be eligible for SSI, a person:

> must be age 65 or over, blind or disabled;
>
> must be a U.S. resident for thirty (30) consecutive days, and a citizen or alien (lawfully admitted to the United States for permanent residence) in a qualified alien category who meets certain exception standards (see Note below).
>
> must not have income or resources that exceed certain levels for individuals and couples. It is not necessary for a person to have no income to qualify for SSI, but such other income as the person has must be less than the SSI benefit income level.
>
> must not be a resident in a non-medical public institution (e.g., prison).
>
> must not be a fleeing felon, escaped prisoner or person in violation of probation or parole.

Note: There are seven (7) categories of qualified aliens based on Department of Homeland Security (DHS) immigration statuses:

> those lawfully admitted for permanent residence (LAPR);
>
> those granted conditional entry pursuant to Section (a)(7) of the Immigration and Nationality Act (INA);
>
> those paroled into the U.S. under Section 212(d)(5) of the INA for a period of at least one (1) year;
>
> those who are refugees admitted to the U.S. under Section 207 of the INA;
>
> those granted asylum under Section 208 of the INA;
>
> those whose deportation is being withheld under Sections 243(h) or 241(b)(3) of the INA; and,
>
> Cuban/Haitian entrants under Section 501(e) of the Refugee Education Assistance Act of 1980.

There are five (5) exception standards:

having already been receiving SSI on 8/22/1996;

having forty (40) qualifying credits (using SSI as a supplement to retirement or disability insurance benefits) when in LAPR status;

being a veteran, active duty member of the U.S. military service, or being the spouse or dependent child of an individual who is;

having been lawfully residing in the U.S. on 8/22/1996 and being blind and disabled (excluding aged individuals); and,

being deemed an alien of one of five immigration statuses within seven (7) years of being eligible for SSI.

B.   Application for Benefits.

An application for SSI benefits is made on a form prescribed by the Social Security Administration and filed at a Social Security office or other office designated to receive SSI applications. It is signed by the claimant or by a person authorized to sign for the claimant.

C.   Benefits.

The SSI program provides monthly Federal cash assistance of up to $698 (as of 2012) for an individual to help meet the costs of basic needs of food, shelter and clothing.

Payments for SSI are made on the first day of the month, unless the first of the month is on a weekend or a legal holiday, in which case the payment is made on the first day prior that is not a weekend or a legal holiday.

II.   INCOME AND RESOURCES.

A.   Income.

The term income generally consists of the receipt by a person of cash and/or something of in-kind value that is expended to meet personal needs of food or shelter. Income consists of four (4) categories: earned income; unearned income; in-kind income; and deemed income. There is a basic income exemption of $20 per month, which is not counted in determining eligibility applicable to any income source, without regard to any other income exclusions.

Certain items, though considered income by definition, are statutorily excluded (exclusions) from earned income and unearned income, and therefore are not countable income in determining SSI eligibility. The different types of income the income excluded under each type are defined below:

Earned Income. Some types of earned income are: wages, self-employment income, and payment of goods sold or services rendered.

Exclusions from earned income are as follows:

> The first $65 per month of earned income plus one-half of remaining earned income;
>
> Special provisions for blind and disabled persons; and,
>
> $10 per monthly of infrequent or irregular income that is received only once in a calendar quarter from a single source not reasonably eligible.

Unearned Income. Some types of unearned income are: Social Security, pensions, annuities, worker compensation awards (excluding portions intended to pay medical expenses), alimony or support payments, dividends, interest, royalties, rents, proceeds from life insurance policies and public assistance benefits (except food stamps).

Exclusions from unearned income are as follows:

> The first $20 of unearned income each month;
>
> A grant, scholarship of fellowship used for educational expenses, except for any portion used for room and board; and,
>
> Up to $20 of unearned income in a month if received on an irregular or infrequent basis.

In-Kind Income. This is a non-cash benefit, such as receipt of a payment of rent and/or utilities; payment of bills directly to the supplier of food which is provided to a SSI recipient; and the provision of meals to a SSI recipient.

Gifts of or the provision of clothing are not considered in-kind income of an SSI recipient.

In-kind income for room and board can result in a one-third reduction of the SSI grant. (This reduction can be partially offset if the SSI recipient pays something towards room and board or if he/she provides his/her own meals.)

Deemed Income. The term deemed income is used to describe the process of attributing the income of another person to the SSI claimant, thereby reducing the claimant's SSI benefits. For example, if a SSI recipient should lose a spouse, or a child of the age 18 or less, or loses a parent, then the income of the non-applying spouse or parent is deemed available to the SSI claimant.

B.   Resources.

Resources consist of cash, financial instruments convertible to cash (liquid resources); and real and personal property (non-liquid resources) that a person may readily liquidate, provided such property is readily convertible into cash and usable for food or shelter (countable resources). Not all resources are counted in determining SSI eligibility. Resources of a third person (deemed resources) may be treated as assets of a claimant in certain cases.

Deemed resources consist of certain resources of another person which are attributed to a SSI-eligible person, though not owned by the eligible person.

> An eligible spouse with a spouse not eligible for SSI benefits will have the ineligible spouse's resources deemed to the eligible spouse.

> A child seeking SSI benefits living in the same house as the parents will have the parents' resources deemed to the child in excess of $2,000 for one parent, $3,000 for two (2) parents or a parent and his/her spouse.

Resource exclusions are non-countable resources and consist of:

A person's home. (Rent received is countable and will affect eligibility. However, household and personal effects are not countable resources.)

The value of an automobile necessary for a job, appointments with a doctor, or for a handicapped person.

The value of an automobile used for transport of the person by members of his/her family.

Life insurance up to a face value of $1,500.

$1,500 of burial expenses for the individual or immediate family (burial space, including a cemetery plot, mausoleum, a headstone or any other depository).

Property of a trade/business essential for self-support of a claimant. This exclusion does not exempt property (e.g., a certificate of deposit) not used in a trade/business, where the monthly interest payments contribute to an applicant's self-support.

Non-business property essential for the claimant's self-support (e.g., tools, equipment or uniforms required by an employer, or an additional or specially modified car or truck needed for transportation because of climate, terrain, or distances.

Resources of a blind or disabled person needed to fulfill an approved plan for achieving self-support.

Payments from another Federal benefit program which requires exclusion of that payment (e.g., food stamps, children's school lunches, grants and loans to college students, work incentive allowances, housing assistance).

Cash or in-kind replacement received from any source (e.g., an insurance company) to repair or replace a lost, damaged, or stolen resource, as long as the cash is spent for that purpose within nine (9) months, which can be extended for another nine (9) months with good cause.

Certain stock held by Alaskan Natives and restricted allotted land owned by an enrolled member of an Indian tribe.

III.   RESOURCE TRANSFER PENALTIES.

The resource transfer penalties are substantially the same as the Medicaid transfer penalty rules. Two differences are:

The period (months) of ineligibility in the case of SSI by reason of a resource transfer for less than fair market value (uncompensated value), is calculated as follows: dividing

the uncompensated value of the resource transfer by the amount of the SSI benefit equals the number of months of ineligibility.

The cap on the period of ineligibility is thirty-six (36) months.

(continued on next page)

Supplier/Medicare

A provider of health care services, other than a practitioner, that is permitted to bill under Medicare Part B. Suppliers include independent laboratories, durable medical equipment providers, ambulance services, orthotists, prosthetists and portable x-ray providers.

*Surgical Dressing Services/Medicare

For treatment of a surgical or surgically treated wound. You pay 20% of the Medicare-approved amount for the doctor's services. You pay a fixed copayment for these services when you get them in a hospital outpatient setting. You pay nothing for the supplies. The Part B deductible applies.

Swing-bed Hospital/Medicare

See also *Administratively necessary days of care.*

A hospital participating in the Medicare swing-bed program. This program allows rural hospitals with fewer than one-hundred (100) beds to provide either acute care or skilled post-acute care services in acute care beds, depending on demand.

Syringe/Medicare

See also *Medicare supplies/Medicare.*

This medical supply item is covered by Medicare.

_____

(continued on next page)

T

209(b) State/Medicaid
See *Medicaid, section II.B.2.*

2176 Waivers/Medicaid
See also *Medicaid waivers; Waivered services/Medicaid.*

Medicaid 2176 waivers are authorized by the 1981 Medicaid amendments which permit states to apply to the Federal government for waiver of certain Medicaid program requirements in order to provide home care to persons who would otherwise be likely to be institutionalized. The term "2176" refers to a specific section of the amendments and is distinguished from other waivers in the Medicaid statute.

300% Program/Medicaid
See *Optional categorically needy/Medicaid; Income cap states/Medicaid.*

Taxes on Benefits/Social Security
See *Social Security, section IX.*

Taxes on Wages/Social Security
See also *Social Security Introduction; Earnings limit/Social Security.*

The maximum amount of wages subject to Social Security taxes is $110,000 (2012).

*Telehealth/Medicare

Includes a limited number of medical or other health services, like office visits and consultations provided using an interactive two-way telecommunications system (like real-time audio and video) by an eligible provider who isn't at your location. Available in some rural areas, under certain conditions, and only if you're located

---

All entries preceded by an asterisk (*) are culled or copied from the official U.S. government **Medicare** handbook (*Medicare & You 2011*).

at one of the following places: a doctor's office, hospital, rural health clinic, federally-qualified health center, health-based dialysis facility, skilled nursing facility, or community mental health center. You pay 20% of the Medicare-approved amount, and the Part B deductible applies.

Tenancy by the Entirety

In some states the combined ownership of property, usually real estate, by a married couple creates a tenancy by the entirety. Each of the spouses has to agree upon all matters while both are living and married to each other. There is no right of partition or other means for one spouse to sever his/her interest from the other's nor to encumber, sell or mortgage the property without the other's consent. Upon the death of one spouse, his/her interest automatically passes to the survivor.

Term Life Insurance

A life insurance policy that provides coverage for a specified period at a level premium. The policy may be renewed for another period at a higher premium based on the older age of the insured. The policy does not create any cash reserve.

Terminable Interest Property

This is an interest in property that will terminate after a lapse of time (e.g., a term of years, a lifetime, an annuity), on the occurrence of a contingency (e.g., should the surviving spouse remarry) or on the failure of an occurrence of a contingency (e.g., should the surviving spouse not live for five (5) years).

A terminable interest property is not deductible from a decedent's gross estate for estate and gift tax purposes, when it passes for less than fair market value from the decedent. Hence, the transfer to a spouse of non-deductible terminable interest property will not qualify for the marital deduction. A notable exception is a transfer of qualified terminable interest property (QTIP).

A qualified terminable interest property is a transfer by a decedent to a surviving spouse of a qualifying interest for life in the decedent's property. In connection with this transfer, the estate executor irrevocably elects to take the marital deduction on the decedent's estate tax return. The transfer may be in the form of a life estate to the surviving spouse or in the form of a trust, commonly known as a QTIP trust, coupled in each instance with an election of the executor to take the marital deduction.

A surviving spouse has a qualifying income interest for life in the QTIP trust if he/she is entitled to all of the income from the trust, payable at least annually, and if no person has the power to appoint any part of the property to any person other than the surviving spouse.

Terminally Ill
See also *Hospice care/Medicare; Accelerated benefits, tax status.*

An illness, disease or injury where recovery can no longer be reasonably expected. For purposes of Medicare-covered hospice care, a person with a terminal illness has a life expectancy of six (6) months or less, as certified by a physician, if the illness runs a normal course. In the context of tax regulations governing accelerated benefits, a terminally ill person has a reasonable life expectancy of twenty-four (24) months or less.

*Tests/Medicare

Includes x-rays, MRIs, CT scans, EKGs, and some other diagnostic tests. You pay 20% of the Medicare-approved amount, and the Part B deductible applies. If you get the test at a hospital as an outpatient, you also pay the hospital a copayment that may be more than 20% of the Medicare-approved amount, but it can't be more than the Part A hospital-stay deductible.

Testamentary Trust
See *Trust, Medicaid eligibility rules.*

Testator

The person who creates a will.

Therapeutic Substitution/Medicare Part D Drug Coverage.

Refers to a request by a Part D-eligible individual that his/her physician prescribe an alternate, preferred drug in the same category or class.

Therapy Services/Medicare
See *Qualifying skilled service/Medicare.*

Third Party Payer

This insurance term relates to any organization that pays for medical expenses on behalf of a beneficiary such as non-profit insurers, commercial insurance companies, Medicaid and Medicare. The payer making the payment in place of the beneficiary is a third party payer.

Threshold Override Application/Medicaid
See *Utilization threshold program/Medicaid.*

Time Limit, Part B Claims/Medicare

For Medicare to make payments on Part B claims, they must be submitted within fifteen (15) months of the date of a procedure or service.

*Tiers (drug formulary)/Medicare Part D Drug Coverage

Many Medicare drug plans place drugs into different "tiers" on their formularies. Drugs in each tier have a different cost. For example, a drug in a lower tier will generally cost you less than a drug in a higher tier. In some cases, if your drug is on a higher tier and your prescriber thinks you need that drug instead of a similar drug on a lower tier, you can file an exception to ask your plan for a lower copayment.

Tiered Cost-sharing/Medicare Part D Drug Coverage

A formulary that has different levels of cost-sharing or co-pay for different drugs that could be used to treat the same disease or condition.

Transfer of Assets/Medicaid
See also *Transfer penalty (civil)/Medicaid; Transfer penalty (criminal)/Medicaid; Exempt transfers/Medicaid.*

Used almost exclusively in the Medicaid context, this term refers generally to the act of transferring assets without receiving fair value for them. Under certain circumstances, individuals are denied Medicaid eligibility for nursing facility services and certain other long-term care services because of such transfers.

Transfer Penalty (Civil)/Medicaid
See also *Medicaid; Period of ineligibility/Medicaid; Trust , Medicaid eligibility rules; Trust, Medicaid transfer penalty rules.*

The civil transfer penalty is a period of ineligibility for Medicaid imposed under certain circumstances on people seeking Medicaid to pay for long-term care. Generally, when a person transfers any asset for less than fair market value, called uncompensated value of transferred assets, and applies for Medicaid assistance to pay for certain long-term care services within a prescribed period after the transfer, called the look-back period, then the Medicaid agency must determine if the individual must be penalized (i.e., rendered ineligible) for a period of time.

The term look-back period refers to a number of months prior to the Medicaid application for which the Medicaid agency will ask the applicant to account for any transfers of assets for less than fair market value. Historically, the look-back period was thirty-six (36) months for all transfers, except that transfers into a trust were subject to a sixty- (60) month look-back period. The thirty-six- (36) month period has been extended to sixty (60) months. Hence the look-back period currently is sixty (60) months for all transfers.

The commencement date of the look-back period in the case of an institutionalized person is the date the individual is deemed both an institutionalized person and an applicant for state Medicaid assistance. In the case of a non-institutionalized person, the commencement date is the date the individual applies for state Medicaid aid, or, if later, the date the individual disposes of assets for less than fair market value.

The transfer penalty must be applied in cases of individuals seeking nursing home care, or its equivalent, and waivered home care services. It affects Medicaid non-waivered (i.e., other than waivered) home care services, only if a state so elects.

A number of transfers are exempt from the civil penalty rule. These are enumerated under the entry *Exempt transfers/Medicaid.* States must waive transfer penalties if their application would cause undue hardship.

Transfer Penalty (Criminal)/Medicaid
See also *Transfer penalty (civil)/Medicaid.*

The Balanced Budget Act of 1997 (Act) makes it a Federal crime for an individual for a fee to knowingly and willfully counsel or assist another individual to dispose of the latter's assets so that such individual can become eligible for Medicaid. More specifically, the Act provides: "whoever ...for a fee knowingly and willfully counsels or assists an individual to dispose of assets (including by any transfer in trust) in order for an individual to become eligible for medical assistance under a state plan under Title XIX . . . if disposing of the assets results in the imposition of a period of ineligibility for such assistance . . . shall . . . be guilty of a misdemeanor and upon conviction thereof fined not more than $10,000 or in prison for not more than one year or both." This provision is directed solely to the individual who counsels and advises, and not to the person who is so advised. The constitutionality of the above provisions of the Act has been successfully challenged in lower Federal courts. The U.S. Attorney General has publicly stated that the Department of Justice will not take any steps to enforce the Act's provision.

Only transfers that result in the imposition of a period of ineligibility for Medicaid assistance are made criminal; those specifically protected by existing law from penalty are not. The transfers that remain legally permissible are enumerated in the entry *Exempt transfers/Medicaid.*

It appears likely that certain other transfers will not be considered by the Act to be criminal transfers:

> Transfers made outside the statutory look-back period, that is more than sixty (60) months prior to application for Medicaid. Since such transfers are made outside the statutory look-back period, they do not result in any imposition of a period of ineligibility.

> Transfers for which a period of ineligibility, less than the look-back period, has run out by the time of application for Medicaid assistance. The new law is less clear about these transfers. The only assured protection from criminal prosecution is to avoid applying for benefits during the look-back period.

> Transfers by homebound individuals applying for or receiving non-waivered Medicaid services in states which have opted not to apply Medicaid transfer penalties to non-waivered services. A transfer will not make such individuals ineligible for receipt of the non-waivered services. That is, such a transfer will not result, under civil transfer penalty rules, in a denial of reimbursement from Medicaid for non-waivered services. The absence of the imposition of a period of ineligibility suggests such transfer should not be subject to criminal penalties.

As mentioned, the penalty provisions of the Act state that the crime covered by it is a misdemeanor punishable by a fine up to $10,000 or one year in prison, or both. According to the felony portion of the Act, "any persons . . . furnishing . . . items or services . . . under the program [is] guilty of a felony and upon conviction thereof are fined not more than $25,000 or imprisoned for not more than five years, and/or both." This appears to apply only to the providers of services for Medicare or Medicaid recipients and not to the recipients or persons advising them.

*Transplant Services/Medicare

Includes doctor services for heart, lung, kidney, pancreas, intestine, and liver transplants under certain conditions and only in a Medicare-certified facility. Medicare covers bone marrow and cornea transplants under certain conditions.

Transportation
See also *Ambulance/Medicare.*

Transportation for medical appointments, shopping and other purposes is a frequent and often unmet need of many older persons. The Older Americans Act and social services block grants help support some transportation services, and some community programs also provide limited assistance. The support can take the form of money given to underwrite van or bus service or to provide vouchers for taxi or bus rides. Senior centers may finance a van and a driver to help seniors get around town and/or to the center.

Medicare does not cover transportation other than for an ambulance. Medicaid, however, gives states the option to cover transportation as a long-term care service for Medicaid-eligible persons.

*Travel/Medicare, Medigap

Some Medigap policies offer coverage for services that Original Medicare doesn't cover, like medical care when you travel outside the United States.

Trigger/LTCI

An LTCI policy's trigger is the event or events making benefits payable. For example, the trigger may be a medical necessity, cognitive impairment, ADL limitations or some combination of these. Combined triggers make payment for benefits more difficult to access.

Trigger Trust
See also *Trust, Medicaid eligibility rules.*

Also referred to as a convertible trust, a trigger trust automatically becomes irrevocable, and the grantor's interest terminates, in the event that grantor applies for Medicaid or enters a nursing home. Since OBRA '93, the law treats the trust assets as if they were transferred for less than fair market value. This causes a period of ineligibility for Medicaid based on the value of the trust interest deemed transferred.

Trust

A trust is a legal entity created by an owner (grantor, settlor or creator) of property, who places the property into trust by signing a legal document transferring title to the property to a trustee for the benefit of designed beneficiaries. The trustee has a fiduciary responsibility to manage the property for the benefit of the beneficiaries.

Trust/Medicaid
See also *Trust, Medicaid eligibility rules.*

The term trust is defined in the Federal Medicaid statute to include any legal instrument or device that is similar to a trust. It may also include an annuity, but only to the extent and in the manner specified by the Secretary of Health and Human Services.

The Medicaid law applies to any trust established, other than by will, by an individual, including the individual's spouse, a guardian, attorney-in-fact, a court, or administrative body acting with legal authority in place of or on behalf of the individual or the spouse, or acting at the direction or upon the request of either spouse, who subsequently applies for Medicaid.

Trust for Disabled Persons Under Age 65/Medicaid
See also *Trust, Medicaid eligibility rules.*

This is one of the three (3) categories of the types of trusts expressly exempted (exempt trust) from Medicaid's special rules for treatment of trusts. The assets of this trust are not considered available to the Medicaid applicant in determining his/her Medicaid eligibility. Payments from the trust are governed by general eligibility principles concerning the counting of income and resources.

Trusts, Medicaid Eligibility Rules

Medicaid trust rules govern the treatment of the income and principal of a trust for purposes of determining eligibility and of penalizing illegal transfers of assets.

The application of rules differs depending upon the type of the trust as set forth below:

Revocable Living Trust. A revocable living (*inter vivos*) trust is a trust created by a grantor during his/her lifetime and may be amended or revoked by the grantor at any time or at the end of a designated period. The trust may be funded at the time of the trust's creation by the transfer of assets to it, or unfunded until the occurrence of some event.

In the case of a revocable living trust, the entire principal is considered to be an available countable resource. All of the payments from the trust to or for the benefit of the grantor are considered available, countable income. Since the principal and the income are considered to be countable, they affect Medicaid eligibility.

Irrevocable Living Trust. An irrevocable living trust is created by a grantor during his/her lifetime for the purpose of irrevocably transferring assets to another beneficiary. The grantor loses all control over the trust's assets (principal) and may not amend or revoke the trust.

Only if and to the extent payments from the trust can be made to or for the benefit of the grantor, the portion of the principal (or the income on the principal) from which payment to the grantor can be made is considered an available resource of the grantor. All of the payments from any portion of the principal or income of the irrevocable trust, which are made to or for the benefit of the grantor, are considered available income of such individual, and therefore affect Medicaid eligibility.

Testamentary Trust. A testamentary trust is created by the last will and testament of the grantor (the testator) and becomes effective after the testator's death.

If the trust is a testamentary trust, generally neither the principal nor the income is considered to be countable and thus does not affect the applicant's Medicaid eligibility.

If the testamentary trust is created by a community spouse for the benefit of his/her surviving spouse who is institutionalized, to avoid the principal or income from being countable and available to the institutionalized spouse (and thereby affecting his/her Medicaid eligibility), the trust must contain provisions which prevent, under any circumstances, the distribution of the trust principal to the institutionalized spouse, and may permit the payment of the trust income for the comfort and happiness of the institutionalized spouse, but not for food, clothing or shelter.

Supplemental Needs Trust. This type of trust, also known as a special needs trust, is an irrevocable trust, funded by assets of a third party, created for a disabled beneficiary, and intended to supplement government benefits. The trust prohibits the trustee from spending trust assets in diminution of government benefits. The beneficiary has no power to control distributions.

Generally, for Medicaid eligibility purposes, payments from a supplemental needs trust are governed by SSI income principles. If payments are made for food, clothing or shelter, or if payments are made directly to the beneficiary, the amounts are counted as income to the beneficiary for purposes of eligibility and may disqualify the beneficiary's Medicaid eligibility status. The more common arrangement with supplemental needs trusts, which will not disqualify the beneficiary's Medicaid eligibility, is for the trustee to make direct payments to vendors of services or goods that are not food, clothing or shelter; such payments are not considered countable income to the beneficiary.

Trigger Trusts. These are trusts designed to divert from a Medicaid applicant income (or principal) that would otherwise be paid to such Medicaid applicant upon entry into a hospital or nursing home, and thereby excludes the income (or principal) as a countable resource in determining his/her Medicaid eligibility. Standards may vary from state to state as to the validity of these trusts for such purpose. The state of New York has, by statutory enactment, declared void any *inter vivos* trust which suspends, or diverts the payment of income (or principal) in the event of the creator's spouse applying for Medicaid assistance, hospital, nursing or long-term care.

Medicaid Qualifying Trust. The Medicaid qualifying trust, contrary to its name, actually disqualifies an individual for Medicaid eligibility. Under this trust an individual or his/her spouse may be the beneficiary of all or part of the payments of principal and/or income from the trust; the trustee has discretion as to the amounts to be distributed.

Note: The state Medicaid agency must establish procedures, in accordance with standards specified by the Secretary of HHS, whereby the state waives the application of the trust eligibility rules in cases where the individual establishes that these rules will cause undue hardship if applied to him or her.

Exempt Trusts. Certain categories of trusts (A – C below) are by statute expressly exempt from Medicaid income and resource eligibility rules. One trust (income-only, see D below), by virtue of an administrative ruling, is exempt, and the assets of such trusts are not considered available.

A. Trust for Disabled Person under Age 65.
This trust contains that person's assets and is established for his/her benefit by his/her parent, grandparent, legal guardian or a court. This trust is exempt from the Medicaid eligibility rules if it provides that the state will receive all amounts remaining in the trust upon the death of the disabled person up to the amount of Medicaid assistance provided to this person by the state.

B. Miller Trust.
Composed of an individual's pension and/or Social Security income, this trust is exempt from Medicaid eligibility rules if the following conditions are met:

> The trust is composed only of the individual's pension, Social Security or other income payable to the individual, including accumulated trust income. Neither the income transferred to this type of trust nor the right to recover the income is counted in determining the individual's eligibility for Medicaid.

> The state will receive all amounts remaining the trust upon the person's death up to the amount of Medicaid assistance provided to this person by the state.

> The individual resides in a state that does not have a medically needy program for nursing facility services and that uses a special income limit for eligibility for certain

long-term care services. Such a state is called an income cap state or three-hundred- (300%) percent state (see *Income cap states/Medicaid*).

Should any principal be transferred to a Miller trust, this will disqualify the trust from its exempt status. A transfer to the trust of the ownership rights to a stream of income (e.g., Social Security benefits) constitutes a transfer of a resource and will also cause the trust to lose its exempt status.

C. Pooled Trust.

Established for a disabled individual, regardless of age, this trust contains the assets of that individual. If it meets the following conditions, a pooled trust is exempt from Medicaid eligibility rules.

> The trust is established and managed by a non-profit association;
>
> Each trust beneficiary has a separate account, but the trust pools these accounts for investment and management of the funds;
>
> The accounts are established solely for the disabled individual's benefit by the individual, the individual's parent, grandparent, legal guardian or a court; and
>
> Any amounts remaining in the trust after the beneficiary's death and not retained by it are paid over to the state up to an amount equal to the total amount of Medicaid services provided to the beneficiary.

D. Income-only trust.

This is an irrevocable trust established by an individual which provides that income only from the trust shall be paid to the grantor for life, but excludes distribution of the trust principal to the grantor.

CMS has interpreted the trust Medicaid eligibility rules to preclude the counting of such trust's principal as available to the grantor since it cannot under any circumstances be distributed to, or for the benefit of, the grantor or his/her spouse.

Trust, Medicaid Transfer Penalty Rules
See *Transfer penalty (civil)/Medicaid.*

The Medicaid transfer penalty rules impose a penalty (a period of Medicaid Ineligibility) upon certain transfers of assets into and from certain kinds of trusts.

Revocable trust. A transferred principal to this trust is not subject to the transfer of assets rules. A payment from the trust is subject to the transfer rules and penalties only to the extent payment is made to or for the benefit of someone other than the individual applying for or receiving Medicaid.

Irrevocable trust. Transfers of assets into an irrevocable trust are penalized if the assets cannot be paid under any circumstances to the individual Medicaid applicant. Any portion of the assets which could be paid to or used for the benefit of the individual creating the trust is outside the purview of the penalty rules. Payments from this trust are penalized (i.e., such payment triggers the sixty- (60) month look-back period) if they are not actually paid to or for the benefit of the individual whose assets established the trust but are paid to or for the benefit of other individuals.

Trusts for the disabled. Transfer rules expressly exempt from coverage transfers to trusts established for a disabled child and to a trust established for disabled individuals under age 65. In addition, it would appear that, as in the case of transfers that are made outright, no penalty would be incurred if assets transferred to the trust are returned to the individual.

Irrevocable Miller Trust. The transfer of income into this trust will not be penalized if and to the extent that the trust instrument provides that such income will be used to pay for medical care provided to the individual. The transfer of any income not used (e.g., income which exceeds the amount paid for these medical services) will be penalized.

Pooled Trust. This trust is not exempt from the transfer of assets rules. However, a transfer to a pooled trust is exempt if the transfer is made by a disabled person under age 65 at the time the trust is established.

Income-only trust. The value of the trust principal will be treated, for transfer penalty purposes, as a transfer of assets for less than fair market value, and therefore is subject to transfer penalty.

Trustee

The trustee is the person or institution who holds legal title to trust property for the benefit of another individual or entity.

*TTY/Medicare

A teletypewriter (TTY) is a communication device used by people who are deaf, hard-of-hearing, or have a severe speech impairment. People who don't have a TTY can communicate with a TTY user through a message relay center (MRC). An MRC has TTY operators available to send and interpret TTY messages. TTY Users 1-877-486-2048.

(continued on next page)

U

Ultrasonic Diagnostic Service
See also *Sonogram*.

A unit of a hospital or other health care organization providing ultrasound imaging services. This service includes the use by a diagnostic medical sonographer of an ultrasonic graph – an apparatus that produces images obtained by ultrasonic waves.

Uncompensated Value of Transferred Assets/Medicaid
See also *Transfer penalty (civil)/Medicaid*.

This represents the value of a transferred asset less payment, if any, for the asset.

Unearned Income/Medicaid
See *Income, unearned/Medicaid*.

Unified Credit

Each person has a lifetime unified tax credit, which he/she may use to offset gift taxes, estate taxes or both (however, the maximum offset for lifetime transfer is $5,000,000). The unified tax credit (for 2012) is $1,772,800. The maximum exclusion amount for the estate of an individual (for 2012) is $5,120,000; thus, if a person dies without having drawn on the unified credit, it is sufficient to offset the estate tax liability on the first $5,120,000 (in 2012) of his estate.

Unitrust
See *Charitable remainder trust*.

All entries preceded by an asterisk (*) are culled or copied from the official U.S. government **Medicare** handbook (*Medicare & You 2011*).

Unused Capitation/Managed Care

When a physician or physician group participating in a prepaid health care organization successfully holds costs per patient below the capitation amount paid by an enrollee to an HMO, the difference is known as unused capitation.

*Urgently-Needed Care/Medicare, Medicare Advantage Plans

In all types of Medicare Advantage Plans, you're always covered for emergency and urgent care. You can't be asked to sign a private contract for emergency or urgent care.

Utilization Review Committee (URC)/Medicare
See also *Appeals/Medicare*.

The URC is responsible for making decisions as to the medical necessity and reasonableness of care for extended stays in hospitals and skilled nursing facilities. An adverse finding by a URC will likely lead to a denial of Medicare coverage. A URC decision is not an initial determination subject to appeal.

Utilization Threshold Program/Medicaid

This program relates to Medicaid outpatients only. Generally, a Medicaid outpatient is subject to specific utilization thresholds which are limitations on the number of services, such as laboratory, dental, and pharmacy, and the number of physician and clinic visits to which a Medicaid recipient is entitled. The limitations do not apply to elderly, blind or disabled individuals who utilize managed care programs or to emergency medical services.

When a patient approaches his/her threshold limit(s), the patient may apply to Medicaid to obtain an increase in a particular threshold limit or, in some instances, may obtain a complete exemption from the threshold limits. The application, known as the threshold override application, must be accompanied by a doctor's specific request for the increase or exemption.

(continued on next page)

V

*Vaccinations (shots)/Medicare, Medicare Advantage Plans

Medicare drug plans must cover all commercially-available vaccines (like the shingles vaccine) when medically necessary to prevent illness except for vaccines covered under Part B.

Vaccinations/Medicare

Medicare Part B covers flu vaccinations each fall, hepatitis B vaccinations for beneficiaries considered to be at high or intermediate risk of contracting the disease, and pneumococcal pneumonia vaccinations once in a beneficiary's lifetime.

Variable Annuity
See *Annuity*.

Vendorization/Medicaid

The process of qualifying a privately hired home care worker as a Medicaid vendor.

Venipuncture/Medicare

Venipuncture is drawing of blood from a patient to obtain a sample for diagnosis. It does not qualify for Medicare home health benefits based on needing intermittent skilled nursing care solely for venipuncture. It is treated as a laboratory benefit covered by Medicare Part B.

Vertical Comparability/Medicaid
See *Comparability/Medicaid*.

All entries preceded by an asterisk (*) are culled or copied from the official U.S. government **Medicare** handbook (*Medicare & You 2011*).

Vesting

See *Private pension.*

Viatical Settlement

See also *Accelerated benefits; Viatical settlement provider.*

This term denotes a transaction whereby an individual who is terminally or chronically ill and is insured under a life insurance contract on his/her life sells the contract or assigns the death benefits under such contract to a viatical settlement provider.

The insured, if chronically or terminally ill, may receive the proceeds of such a sale or assignment tax free. The proceeds received are excluded from gross income as if paid by reason of the death of the insured. This exclusion applies, as in the case of accelerated benefits paid to a chronically ill individual under a life insurance contract, only if:

> The payment received by the insured is for costs incurred for qualified long-term services rendered to the insured;

> Payment or reimbursement of such costs are not made by Medicare; and ,

> The life insurance contract complies with the consumer protection provisions of the Health Insurance Portability and Accountability Act applicable to long-term care insurance contracts.

Viatical Settlement Provider

Any person regularly engaged in the trade or business of purchasing or taking assignment of the death benefit of a life insurance contract of an insured who is terminally ill or chronically ill. Such person must be licensed for such purposes in the state in which the insured resides. Or in the case of an insured who resides in a state which does not require the licensing of such person, he/she must meet the requirements of the Viatical Settlement Model Act and Long-Term Care Insurance Model Act of the National Association of Insurance Commissioners.

*Vision/Medicare (Medicare Advantage Plans)

Medicare Advantage plans may offer extra coverage, such as vision, hearing, dental, and/or health and wellness programs.

700

Visit/Home Care

The unit of reimbursement for a home health aide visit. The normal visit is two and a half (2½) hours long.

Visiting Nurse Service/Home Care

Visiting nurses are major providers of skilled home health services. The Visiting Nurse Association has approximately four-hundred fifty (450) independently operated groups nationwide which can provide these services.

Volume Performance Standard/Medicare

A mechanism to record and adjust Medicare physician fee schedules based on how annual actual increases in Part B expenditures compare to previously determined rates of increase. By this method Medicare seeks to restrict physicians from rendering unnecessary services and thereby compensate for restraints in Medicare-allowed fees.

Voluntary Enrollee/Medicare
See also *Eligibility and enrollment/Medicare, section I.*

A voluntary enrollee is a person who: (a) has attained age 65; (b) is not eligible for either Social Security or Railroad Retirement benefits; (c) is a resident of the United States; and (d) is either a citizen of the U.S. or an alien lawfully admitted for permanent residence (who has continuously resided in the U.S. for not less than five (5) years immediately before the month in which application for Medicare enrollment is made). These individuals may purchase Medicare coverage by payment of a monthly premium that CMS determines annually. In order for a voluntary enrollee to receive coverage in Medicare Part A, he/she must enroll in Medicare Part B.

(continued on next page)

W

Waiting Period/Medigap

See also *Open enrollment period/Medigap.*

Medigap insurers may impose a waiting period, also known as an exclusion period, of up to six (6) months before a preexisting condition is covered except for individuals who have had a least six (6) months of creditable coverage before applying for Medigap insurance. See *Preexisting condition, waiting period/ Medigap.*

Waiver of Liability/Medicare

See also *Claims for service/Medicare.*

There is a presumption that claims are submitted by the patient and the provider of services in good faith and therefore are required to be paid by Medicare. Hence, when claims are submitted by patients and providers under circumstances where they did not know that coverage for services would be denied under the medical necessity exclusion, liability to Medicare for reimbursement will be waived. The presumption of good faith is lost when a provider errs in more than 2.5% of its decisions. When the presumption is lost, the loss is referred to as a loss of waiver status, the penalties for which include loss of a periodic advance on anticipated Medicare payments (prospective interim payments).

Waiver of Premiums/LTCI

Some long-term care insurance policies allow the insured, usually in connection with nursing home stays, to cease payment of premiums after receiving benefits for a certain number of days. Once the insured is well or discharged from a nursing home, the payment of premiums must resume. The policyholder pays nothing back, and nothing is deducted from his/her benefits.

All entries preceded by an asterisk (*) are culled or copied from the official U.S. government **Medicare** handbook (*Medicare & You 2011*).

Waiver Programs/Medicaid
See *Medicaid waivers; Waivered services/Medicaid.*

Waivered Services/Medicaid
See also *Medicaid waivers; 2176 waivers/Medicaid; Personal care/Medicaid.*

Through the process of obtaining a waiver from CMS of requirements that would otherwise be imposed by Federal law, states may provide Medicaid services beyond those required by Federal Medicaid regulations. The waiver programs most relevant to older and disabled individuals are those that:

Provide services to individuals at risk of institutionalization in a nursing home or intermediate care facility for the mentally regarded; and

Provide services to individuals age 65 or older at risk of institutionalization.

Waivers for home and community-based long-term care services have proven to be particularly helpful to older and disabled individuals. CMS periodically publishes a Medicaid waiver fact sheet that summarizes the waivers for home and community-based services for each state. Some of the waivered services relevant to long-term care (e.g., 2176 waivers for home care) include:

Adult Day Care	Medical Social Services
Case Management	Moving Assistance
Emergency Response Systems	Nutritional/educational services
Foster Care	Respite Care
Home-delivered Meals	Respiratory Therapy
Home Maintenance Tasks	Shift Nursing
House Improvement	Social Transportation

Walker/Medicare
See also *Durable medical equipment/Medicare.*

This item is covered by Medicare.

*Welcome to Medicare Physical Exam/Medicare

A one-time review of your health, education, and counseling about preventative services, and referrals for other care if needed. Medicare will cover this exam if you get it within the first 12 months you have Part B. Starting January 1, 2011, you pay nothing for the exam if the doctor accepts assignment. When you make your appointment, let your doctor's office know that you would like to schedule your "Welcome to Medicare" physical exam.

*Wellness Exam/Medicare

If you've had Part B for longer than 12 months, starting January 1, 2011, you can get a yearly wellness visit to develop or update a personalized prevention plan based on your current health and risk factors. You pay nothing for this exam if the doctor accepts assignment. This exam is covered once every 12 months.

Your first yearly "wellness" exam can't take place within 12 months of your "Welcome to Medicare" physical exam.

Wheelchair/Medicare
See also *Durable medical equipment/Medicare.*

This item is covered by Medicare.

Whole Life Insurance

A life insurance policy covering the entire life of an insured person at a level premium that is paid throughout the life of the insured. A reserve customarily accumulates for the insured's benefit. It may be converted to cash value upon surrender of the policy or borrowed against at low interest while the policy continues in effect.

Widow's (Widower's) Benefits/Social Security
See *Social Security Program.*

Withholds/Managed Care
See also *Health Maintenance Organization.*

To encourage physicians to refer patients to a specialist or to hospitalize them only when medically necessary, a prepaid health care organization may withhold from a physician's or a physician group's payment (i.e., salary, fees, or capitation) a percentage or fixed dollar amount. The amount withheld is set aside in pools to pay for any costs exceeding the amount budgeted for specialty referral services and inpatient hospital care. Should these costs exceed budget, part or all of the withhold may be forfeited. If the costs are below budget, part or all of the withhold may be returned to a physician or physician group.

Work Credit/Social Security
See also *Social Security Program (Title II), section VI.A.*

The term work credit was formerly known as quarter of coverage, which is still frequently used. A worker accumulates Social Security work credits by working in covered employment. For every $780 in earnings, a worker can earn one work credit up to an annual maximum of four. After a worker earns a minimum number of work credits and thereby gains insured status, he/she qualifies for various Social Security benefits.

Worker's Compensation/Medicaid

Worker's compensation, like private medical insurance, is considered a third-party payer by Medicaid. Generally speaking, Medicaid requires that worker's compensation payments for medical expenses be made before Medicaid will pay any difference. Medicaid is generally the payer of last resort. It will pay for injury-related medical costs only if and when there is a pending dispute between the worker-claimant and insurer and the worker's claim is not yet settled.

Following a settlement between the worker-claimant and the insurer, Medicaid has the right of reimbursement, against the amount settled, from the worker-claimant and the insurer. In arriving at a settlement, if the settlement makes no provision for future medical expenses, Medicaid will refuse coverage of these expenses.

If the settlement provides for further medical expenses, Medicaid will pay for them, only when the claimant has first incurred bills up to the aggregate sums allocated in the settlement amount. Hence, when the injury requires it, a settlement must provide for future expenses, and Medicaid coverage will be provided only when settlement allocation has been used up.

Wrap-around Coverage
See *Coordination of coverage/Medicare.*

(continued on next page)

X

X-rays/Medicare
See *Diagnostic tests/Medicare; Radiation therapy/Medicare.*

All entries preceded by an asterisk (*) are culled or copied from the official U.S. government **Medicare** handbook (*Medicare & You 2011*).

www.ingramcontent.com/pod-product-compliance
Lightning Source LLC
Chambersburg PA
CBHW080221270326
41926CB00020B/4109